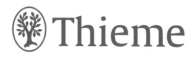

Medical Neuroscience Q&A

Manas Das, MD, MS
Associate Professor
Director of Clinical Anatomy (MS-3 & MS-4)
Director of Medical Embryology (MS-1 & MS-2)
Director of Medical Histology (MS-1 & MS-2)
Division of Translational Anatomy
Department of Radiology
University of Massachusetts Medical School
Worcester, Massachusetts

Lee A. Baugh, PhD
Associate Professor of Neuroscience
Division of Basic Biomedical Sciences
Director of Human Functional Imaging Core
Center for Genetics and Behavioral Health
Director, MS-1 Nervous Systems
Associate Director of Center for Brain and Behavior Research
Sanford School of Medicine
University of South Dakota
Vermillion, South Dakota

168 illustrations

Thieme
New York • Stuttgart • Delhi • Rio de Janeiro

Acquisitions Editor: Delia DeTurris
Managing Editor: Gaurav Prabhu
Director, Editorial Services: Mary Jo Casey
Production Editor: Shivika
International Production Director: Andreas Schabert
Editorial Director: Sue Hodgson
International Marketing Director: Fiona Henderson
International Sales Director: Louisa Turrell
Senior Vice President and Chief Operating Officer: Sarah Vanderbilt
President: Brian D. Scanlan

Library of Congress Cataloging-in-Publication Data
Names: Das, Manas, author. | Baugh, Lee A., author.
Title: Medical neuroscience Q&A / Manas Das, Lee A. Baugh.
Description: New York : Thieme, [2019] | Series: Thieme test prep
    for the USMLE |
Identifiers: LCCN 2018045373 (print) | LCCN 2018045693 (ebook) |
    ISBN 9781626235380 | ISBN 9781626235373 (paperback : alk.
    paper) | ISBN 9781626235380 (eISBN)
Subjects: | MESH: Nervous System Diseases | Diagnostic Techniques,
    Neurological | Examination Questions
Classification: LCC RC343.5 (ebook) | LCC RC343.5 (print) | NLM
    WL 18.2 | DDC 616.80076--dc23
LC record available at https://lccn.loc.gov/2018045373

© 2019 Thieme Medical Publishers, Inc.
Thieme Publishers New York
333 Seventh Avenue, New York, NY 10001 USA
+1 800 782 3488, customerservice@thieme.com

Thieme Publishers Stuttgart
Rüdigerstrasse 14, 70469 Stuttgart, Germany
+49 [0]711 8931 421, customerservice@thieme.de

Thieme Publishers Delhi
A-12, Second Floor, Sector-2, Noida-201301
Uttar Pradesh, India
+91 120 45 566 00, customerservice@thieme.in

Thieme Publishers Rio de Janeiro, Thieme Publicações Ltda.
Edifício Rodolpho de Paoli, 25º andar
Av. Nilo Peçanha, 50 – Sala 2508
Rio de Janeiro 20020-906, Brasil
+55 21 3172 2297

Cover design: Thieme Publishing Group
Typesetting by Thomson Digital

Printed in USA by King Printing Company, Inc.   5 4 3 2 1

ISBN 978-1-62623-537-3

Also available as an e-book:
eISBN 978-1-62623-538-0

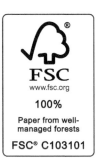

FSC
www.fsc.org
100%
Paper from well-managed forests
FSC® C103101

To Swapna, Parimal, Seema, Tutun, Mimi, and Ryan
for being family

To all my students, past and present
for being the inspiration

—Manas

Contents

Contents

Preface

Neuroscience stands out for its rationality in medicine. It has fascinated the medical fraternity for ages, and it is one of the most important (and challenging) topics tested in competitive and standardized medical exams. This book presents a collection of multiple-choice questions that test neuroscientific competencies of an aspiring physician, consistent with the testing standards of USMLE Step 1.

Most of these clinically-oriented questions are presented in a patient-centered vignette style that is used by the National Board of Medical Examiners (NBME). These questions link various basic science concepts and should be helpful for the student to synthesize information that might be obtained from a wide range of disciplines.

All questions belong to type A, i.e., there is one best answer for each. Each question is provided with a difficulty level of easy, moderate, or hard. While "easy" questions require, for the most part, simple recall of information, harder questions will require analysis and application of information. A brief explanation follows each of these questions, indicating why the author-indicated correct answer outmatches the distractors.

Each question is tagged with a learning objective. It is a direct measure of the learning outcome for the concept that is necessary to achieve the desired level of LCME-outlined competencies.

The book comprises 24 chapters. These are organized primarily according to neuroanatomical structures.

High-quality images have been incorporated throughout the text. These should add to integration, challenge the ability to analyze and interpret, and meet appropriate standards.

The book is also available on Thieme's online platform. Searchable tags (symptoms, organs, structures, etc.) have been provided with each question for ease of navigation.

Finally, this book is not a substitute for textbooks. Nor is it intended to be used as the primary resource for neuroscience. As with any other question bank, the use of this book should follow an initial understanding of the concepts gained from reading textbooks and lecture notes. The information used in this book has been drawn from a pool of standard textbooks used in medical schools. It is highly advisable to return to the pool for concept clarification.

Manas Das, MD, MS
Lee A. Baugh, PhD

Acknowledgements

We would like to express our gratitude to everyone who saw us through this book.

First, we would like to extend special thanks to the faculty and the student reviewers of the book for their valuable suggestions.

I (Manas) would like to thank Max Rosen, the Chair, Department of Radiology, at the University of Massachusetts Medical School, for his constant support and encouragement.

I (Manas) would also like to thank my colleagues at the University of Massachusetts Medical School for their support. Special thanks to Lela Giannaris, Julie Jonassen, Cristopher Cerniglia and Susan Gagliardi for their endorsement and well wishes.

Finally, we would like to acknowledge the role of Delia DeTurris (Associate Acquisitions Editor, Thieme Publishers) toward this publication. We thank her for the constant support, flexibility, willingness to accommodate, and for keeping us on track. I also sincerely thank her for lending us permission to use the image database of Thieme Publishers, which accounts for a large proportion of images used in the book.

How to Use This Series

Chapter Head

Section Header

Question Stem

Answer Options

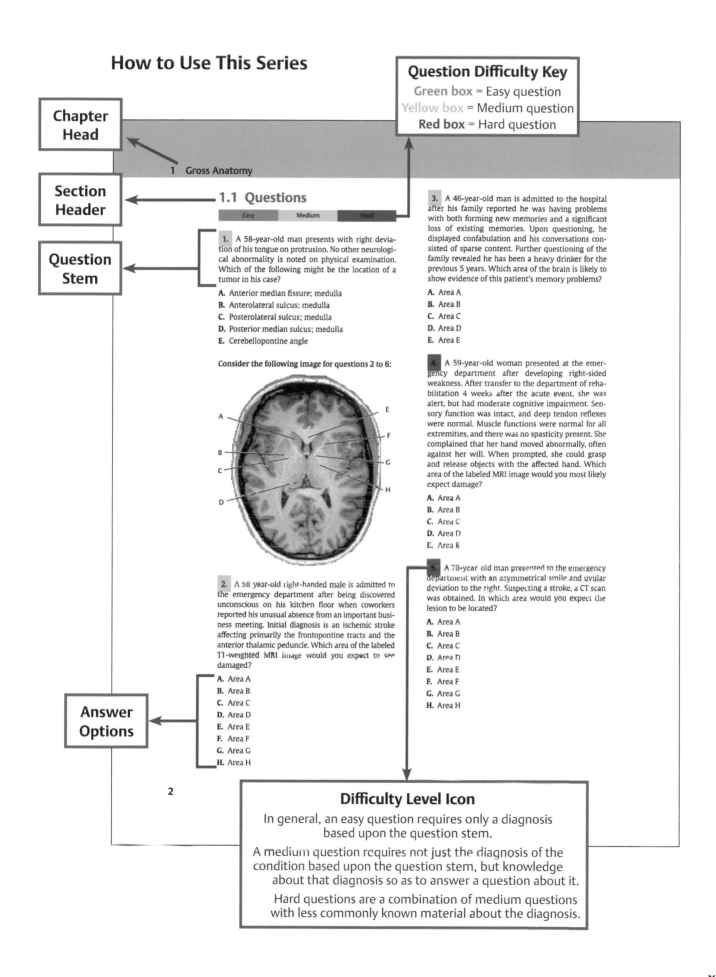

1 Gross Anatomy

1.1 Questions

| Easy | Medium | Hard |

1. A 58-year-old man presents with right deviation of his tongue on protrusion. No other neurological abnormality is noted on physical examination. Which of the following might be the location of a tumor in his case?

A. Anterior median fissure; medulla
B. Anterolateral sulcus; medulla
C. Posterolateral sulcus; medulla
D. Posterior median sulcus; medulla
E. Cerebellopontine angle

Consider the following image for questions 2 to 6:

2. A 58-year-old right-handed male is admitted to the emergency department after being discovered unconscious on his kitchen floor when coworkers reported his unusual absence from an important business meeting. Initial diagnosis is an ischemic stroke affecting primarily the frontopontine tracts and the anterior thalamic peduncle. Which area of the labeled T1-weighted MRI image would you expect to see damaged?

A. Area A
B. Area B
C. Area C
D. Area D
E. Area E
F. Area F
G. Area G
H. Area H

3. A 46-year-old man is admitted to the hospital after his family reported he was having problems with both forming new memories and a significant loss of existing memories. Upon questioning, he displayed confabulation and his conversations consisted of sparse content. Further questioning of the family revealed he has been a heavy drinker for the previous 5 years. Which area of the brain is likely to show evidence of this patient's memory problems?

A. Area A
B. Area B
C. Area C
D. Area D
E. Area E

4. A 59-year-old woman presented at the emergency department after developing right-sided weakness. After transfer to the department of rehabilitation 4 weeks after the acute event, she was alert, but had moderate cognitive impairment. Sensory function was intact, and deep tendon reflexes were normal. Muscle functions were normal for all extremities, and there was no spasticity present. She complained that her hand moved abnormally, often against her will. When prompted, she could grasp and release objects with the affected hand. Which area of the labeled MRI image would you most likely expect damage?

A. Area A
B. Area B
C. Area C
D. Area D
E. Area E

5. A 78-year-old man presented to the emergency department with an asymmetrical smile and uvular deviation to the right. Suspecting a stroke, a CT scan was obtained. In which area would you expect the lesion to be located?

A. Area A
B. Area B
C. Area C
D. Area D
E. Area E
F. Area F
G. Area G
H. Area H

2

Chapter Head

20. A 22-year-old right-handed male suffered head trauma following a fight in a bar. Upon admission to the emergency department, it was discovered that he had an acute deficit in the programming of saccadic eye movements into the right visual field. Tests of visual acuity revealed no deficits, suggesting the programming of eye movements to be the only deficit. In which area would you expect the damage to have occurred?

A. Area A

B. Area B

C. Area C

D. Area D

E. Area E

1.2 Answers and Explanations

| Easy | Medium | Hard |

1. Correct: Anterolateral sulcus; medulla (B)

The patient seems to be suffering from hypoglossal nerve palsy. Rootlets of the nerve emerge from the brainstem (medulla) at the anterolateral sulcus between the pyramid and the olive.

The anterior median fissure (**A**) and posterior median sulcus (**D**) of medulla do not give attachment to any cranial nerves.

Glossopharyngeal, vagus, and accessory nerves emerge from the medulla at the posterolateral sulcus (**C**).

The cerebellopontine angle (**E**) is closely related to the attachments of the facial and vestibulocochlear nerves.

Refer to the following image key for answers 2 to 6:

A, head of caudate nucleus; B, putamen; C, globus pallidus; D, thalamus; E, corpus callosum; F, anterior limb of internal capsule; G, genu of internal capsule; H, posterior limb of internal capsule.

2. Correct: Area F (F)

The frontopontine tract and the anterior thalamic peduncle are contained within the anterior limb of the internal capsule, between the caudate nucleus and the lentiform nucleus. In addition, the anterior limb contains fibers from the anterior and the medial nuclear groups of the thalamus to the cingulate gyrus and the prefrontal cortex, respectively.

3. Correct: Area D (D)

History and clinical features for this man are typical for Korsakoff's psychosis. Although Korsakoff's syndrome can cause general cerebral atrophy, the memory problems are most likely to represent damage to the thalamus and to the mammillary bodies of the hypothalamus.

4. Correct: Area E (E)

The patient is presenting with classical symptoms of alien hand syndrome, a relatively rare condition that includes autonomous activity of the affected limb, which is perceived by the patient as being outside of voluntary control. In this particular case, the patient is displaying an agnostic dyspraxia, in which the affected hand competitively interacts with the non-affected hand when attempting to perform motor commands. Damage to the anterior corpus callosum, and consequent lack of interhemispheric connection, is the most common underlying cause for these cases.

5. Correct: Area G (G)

Facial paralysis (cranial nerve VII involvement) accompanying with uvular deviation (cranial nerve X involvement) indicates damage of corticobulbar fibers. The genu of the internal capsule contains such fibers and is likely to be the site of lesion in his case.

6. Correct: Areas A and B (D)

The neostriatum comprises the caudate nucleus and the putamen. The globus pallidus (**C**) forms the paleostriatum.

7. Correct: C6–C7 disc herniation (D)

Clinical features for the woman are typical for C7 radiculopathy. This is commonly caused by C6–C7 disc herniation.

Cervical nerve roots exit above the correspondingly numbered vertebra (except C8, since there is no corresponding vertebra). These have a fairly horizontal course as they emerge from the dural sac near the intervertebral disc and exit through the intervertebral foramen. Cervical discs are usually constrained by the posterior longitudinal ligament to herniate laterally toward the nerve root, rather than centrally toward the spinal cord. In cervical cord, therefore, the nerve root involved usually corresponds to the lower vertebral bone of the disc space.

C3–C4 disc herniation (**A**) would cause C4 radiculopathy, which might present as sensorimotor deficits in the neck region.

C4–C5 disc herniation (**B**) would cause C5 radiculopathy. Motor weakness of deltoid, sensory loss over shoulder and upper lateral arm, and compromised biceps reflex would be characteristic.

C5–C6 disc herniation (**C**) would cause C6 radiculopathy. This would present with motor weakness of biceps brachii and wrist extensors, sensory loss over first and second digits and lateral forearm, and compromised biceps and brachioradialis (more specific) reflex.

Indicates Question Difficulty

Correct Answer

Correct Answer Explanation

Incorrect Answer Explanation

5

Abbreviations

ACA, anterior cerebral artery

ACommA, anterior communicating artery

ADC, apparent diffusion coefficient

ADH, antidiuretic hormone

AICA, anterior inferior cerebellar artery

ANT, anterior nucleus of thalamus

ATM, AT mutant

BAER, brainstem auditory evoked response

BPPV, benign positional paroxysmal vertigo

CBF, cerebral blood flow

CHARGE, coloboma, congenital *h*eart disease, choanal *a*tresia, growth *r*etardation, *g*enital abnormalities, and *e*ar abnormalities

CN, cranial nerve

CNS, central nervous system

CSF, cerebrospinal fluid

CT, computed tomography

DM, dorsomedial

DRG, dorsal root ganglion

DTR, deep tendon reflex

DVN, dorsal vagal nucleus

DWI, diffusion weighted imaging

ER, emergency room

18F-FDG, fluorodeoxyglucose

FEF, frontal eye field

FLAIR, fluid-attenuated inversion recovery

FSH, follicle-stimulating hormone

GBS, Guillain–Barré syndrome

GFAP, glial fibrillary acidic protein

GI, gastrointestinal

GnRH, gonadotropin-releasing hormone

H&E, hematoxylin and eosin

HMSN, hereditary motor and sensory neuropathies

ICP, intracranial pressure

INO, internuclear ophthalmoplegia

IV, intravenous

LGB, lateral geniculate body

LH, luteinizing hormone

LMN, lower motor neuron

MALT, mucosa-associated lymphoid tissue

MCA, middle cerebral artery

MCP, middle cerebellar peduncle

MGB, medial geniculate body

MLF, medial longitudinal fasciculus

MRI, magnetic resonance imaging

MS, multiple sclerosis

MSO, medial superior olive

NTD, neural tube defect

OCD, obsessive compulsive disorder

oVEMP, ocular vestibular-evoked myogenic potential

PAG, periaqueductal gray

PCA, posterior cerebral artery

PCommA, posterior communicating artery

PET, positron emission tomography

PICA, posterior inferior cerebellar artery

PMP22, peripheral myelin protein-22

PNS, peripheral nervous system

PPRF, paramedian pontine reticular formation

PTSD, posttraumatic stress disorder

riMLF, rostral interstitial nucleus of medial longitudinal fasciculus

SCA, superior cerebellar artery

SCDS, superior canal dehiscence syndrome

SCP, superior cerebellar peduncle

SIADH, syndrome of inappropriate antidiuretic hormone

SSRI, selective serotonin reuptake inhibitor

STN, subthalamic nucleus

SVA, special visceral afferent

TRN, thalamic reticular nucleus

UMN, upper motor neuron

VA, ventral anterior

VAmc, ventral anterior nucleus, magnocellular part

VApc, ventral anterior nucleus, parvocellular part

VL, ventral lateral

VLc, ventral lateral nucleus pars caudalis

VLo, ventral lateral nucleus pars oralis

VLPO, ventral lateral preoptic nucleus

VP, ventral posterior

VPL, ventral posterolateral

VPM, ventral posteromedial

WBC, while blood cell

Chapter 1

Gross Anatomy of the Nervous System

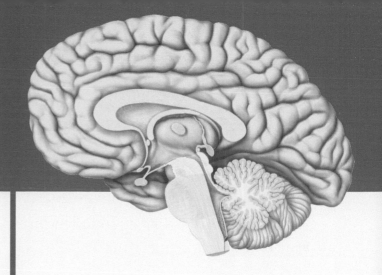

LEARNING OBJECTIVES

▶ Identify external features of brainstem through which cranial nerves emerge.

▶ Identify the location of the anterior limb of the internal capsule on a T1-weighted anatomical axial slice MRI. Describe the contents of the parts of the internal capsule.

▶ Recognize the role of the thalamus in the formation and recall of memory. Locate the thalamus on a T1 anatomical axial MRI image. Analyze the clinical features of Korsakoff's psychosis.

▶ Analyze the role of the corpus callosum in interhemispheric communication. Locate the corpus callosum on a T1-weighted anatomical MRI axial slice.

▶ Locate the genu of the internal capsule on a T1 anatomical MRI axial slice. Describe the contents of the parts of the internal capsule.

▶ Classify nuclei within the basal ganglia. Locate the neostriatum on at T1-anatomical MRI axial slice.

▶ Describe the supply for spinal nerve roots. Describe spinal nerve root involvement with disc herniation.

▶ Describe the origin, course, distribution, function, and effects of lesion for the abducens nerve.

▶ Describe the pathways for the corneal reflex. Identify external features of brainstem through which cranial nerves emerge.

▶ Trace visceromotor and viscerosensory sympathetic fibers for thoracic and abdominal organs.

▶ Trace the secretomotor pathway for lacrimation.

▶ Describe the innervation of the muscles of mastication. Identify the location of the pons on a T1-weighted anatomical MRI sagittal slice.

▶ Define the role of the cingulate gyrus within the limbic system. Locate the cingulate gyrus on a T1-weighted anatomical MRI sagittal slice.

▶ Analyze the inverted unilateral relationship between visual fields and primary visual cortex. Identify the location of the inferior bank of the calcarine sulcus on a T1-weighted anatomical MRI sagittal slice.

▶ Define the role of posterior paracentral lobule as the sensory area for the lower limbs and genitals.

▶ Define the boundaries of the fourth ventricle.

▶ Define the role of the posterior parietal cortex in attentional mechanisms. Identify the posterior parietal cortex on a T1-weighted anatomical MRI sagittal slice.

▶ Define the role of orbitofrontal cortex in emotion and executive functions. Identify orbitofrontal cortex on a T1-weighted anatomical MRI sagittal slice.

▶ Define the role of the frontal eye fields in the programming of horizontal saccades. Identify the location of the frontal eye fields on a T1-weighted anatomical MRI sagittal slice.

1.1 Questions

Easy	Medium	Hard

1. A 58-year-old man presents with right deviation of his tongue on protrusion. No other neurological abnormality is noted on physical examination. Which of the following might be the location of a tumor in his case?

A. Anterior median fissure; medulla

B. Anterolateral sulcus; medulla

C. Posterolateral sulcus; medulla

D. Posterior median sulcus; medulla

E. Cerebellopontine angle

Consider the following image for questions 2 to 6:

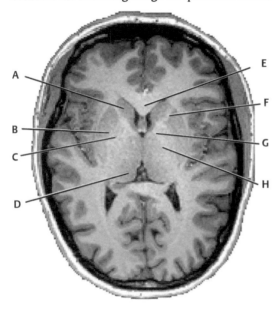

2. A 58-year-old right-handed male is admitted to the emergency department after being discovered unconscious on his kitchen floor when coworkers reported his unusual absence from an important business meeting. Initial diagnosis is an ischemic stroke affecting primarily the frontopontine tracts and the anterior thalamic peduncle. Which area of the labeled T1-weighted MRI image would you expect to see damaged?

A. Area A

B. Area B

C. Area C

D. Area D

E. Area E

F. Area F

G. Area G

H. Area H

3. A 46-year-old man is admitted to the hospital after his family reported he was having problems with both forming new memories and a significant loss of existing memories. Upon questioning, he displayed confabulation and his conversations consisted of sparse content. Further questioning of the family revealed he has been a heavy drinker for the previous 5 years. Which area of the brain is likely to show evidence of this patient's memory problems?

A. Area A

B. Area B

C. Area C

D. Area D

E. Area E

4. A 59-year-old woman presented at the emergency department after developing right-sided weakness. After transfer to the department of rehabilitation 4 weeks after the acute event, she was alert, but had moderate cognitive impairment. Sensory function was intact, and deep tendon reflexes were normal. Muscle functions were normal for all extremities, and there was no spasticity present. She complained that her hand moved abnormally, often against her will. When prompted, she could grasp and release objects with the affected hand. Which area of the labeled MRI image would you most likely expect damage?

A. Area A

B. Area B

C. Area C

D. Area D

E. Area E

5. A 78-year-old man presented to the emergency department with an asymmetrical smile and uvular deviation to the right. Suspecting a stroke, a CT scan was obtained. In which area would you expect the lesion to be located?

A. Area A

B. Area B

C. Area C

D. Area D

E. Area E

F. Area F

G. Area G

H. Area H

6. A 62-year-old woman presents with abrupt and jerky movements of her limbs. Neuroimaging reveals extensive degeneration of her neostriatum. Which of the area(s) is/are affected in her case?

A. Area A
B. Area B
C. Area C
D. Areas A and B
E. Areas B and C
F. Areas A and C

7. A 21-year-old woman presents with sensory loss affecting the left middle finger. There was considerable weakness noted for her left triceps muscle, and her triceps jerk was severely diminished. Which of the following might be the cause for her symptoms?

A. C3–C4 disc herniation
B. C4–C5 disc herniation
C. C5–C6 disc herniation
D. C6–C7 disc herniation
E. C7–C8 disc herniation

8. A 38-year-old man presents with medial deviation of his right eyeball. He walks forward with his head rotated toward his right shoulder. No other neurological abnormality is noted on physical examination. Which of the following locations might be spared during a radiological search for localizing a tumor in his case?

A. Midline pons, just beneath the fourth ventricle
B. Horizontal sulcus, medial pontomedullary junction
C. Horizontal sulcus, lateral pontomedullary junction
D. Cavernous sinus
E. Superior orbital fissure

9. A 28-year-old woman presents with an abnormal blink reflex during routine neurological testing. When her right cornea was touched with a wisp of cotton, her left but not the right eye blinked. Which of the following is true for the affected nerve in her case?

A. The nucleus is located in the midbrain at the level of superior colliculus.
B. The nucleus is located in the midbrain at the level of inferior colliculus.
C. The nerve emerges from the brainstem at the level of mid pons.
D. The nerve emerges from the brainstem via the horizontal sulcus at the medial aspect of the pontomedullary junction.
E. The nerve emerges from the brainstem via the horizontal sulcus at the lateral aspect of the pontomedullary junction.

10. A 21-year-old man presents with tachycardia. A senior resident explains to her intern the pathway for the sympathetic fibers to reach the pacemaker cells of the heart. Which of the following structures should be brought up in their discussion?

A. Dorsal root of T1 spinal nerve
B. Dorsal rami of T1 spinal nerve
C. Gray rami communicantes
D. White rami communicantes
E. Greater splanchnic nerve

11. A 12-year-old girl presents with dry eyes consequent to lack of lacrimation. Which of the following structures might be the site of lesion in her case?

A. Ciliary ganglion
B. Pterygopalatine ganglion
C. Otic ganglion
D. Superior cervical ganglion
E. Gasserian ganglion

Consider the following image for questions 12 to 14:

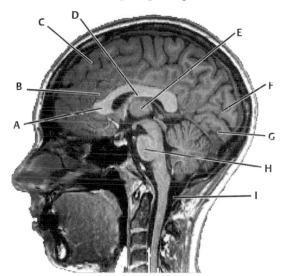

12. A 54-year-old man was admitted to the emergency department with deviated jaw. Physical examination revealed a lower motor neuron type of paralysis of the right lateral pterygoid muscle. Which of the following areas might be damaged in this patient?

A. Area A
B. Area B
C. Area C
D. Area E
E. Area H

13. You are referred a patient from a local psychiatrist for a neurological consult. The patient was described as having undergone an extreme change in mood. The 17-year-old boy was described as having been a happy, responsible, and quiet teenager. However, in recent months, he has been impulsive, prone to anger, and has been getting into fights at school. The psychiatrist believes these changes in behavior are not a result of "teenage angst." You order an MRI and a cortical tumor was found. What is the most likely location for this tumor?

A. Area A

B. Area B

C. Area C

D. Area D

E. Area E

14. A 77-year-old woman presents to the ophthalmologist with an upper quadrantanopia. A subsequent MRI revealed she had suffered from a cerebrovascular event. In which area would you expect the lesion to be?

A. Area C

B. Area D

C. Area E

D. Area F

E. Area G

15. A 48-year-old man presents with a 2-year history of severe, transient, and stabbing pain that initiates in the right side of throat. It gradually radiates to the base of tongue, right ear, and occasionally beneath the angle of right jaw. The paroxysmal attacks are frequently precipitated by swallowing of cold drinks. Which of the following might be the location of nerve irritation in his case?

A. Anterior median fissure; medulla

B. Anterolateral sulcus; medulla

C. Posterolateral sulcus; medulla

D. Posterior median sulcus; medulla

E. Cerebellopontine angle

16. A 56-year-old man presents with anesthesia of his leg, foot, and genitals. Which of the following might be the location of a cortical tumor in him?

A. Precentral gyrus, lateral hemisphere

B. Postcentral gyrus, lateral hemisphere

C. Anterior paracentral lobule

D. Posterior paracentral lobule

E. Superior parietal lobule

17. A 52-year-old man presents with a tumor affecting the roof of the fourth ventricle. Which of the following structures will be directly related to the tumor?

A. Medulla oblongata

B. Pons

C. Cerebellum

D. Thalamus

E. Hypothalamus

Consider the following image for questions 18 to 20:

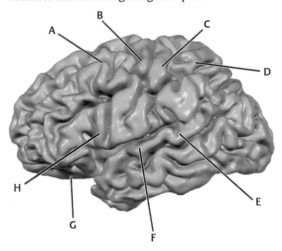

18. A 77-year-old left-handed woman is brought to the emergency department displaying severe right-sided hemispatial neglect. Which of the following area is most likely to be damaged resulting in this condition?

A. Area A

B. Area B

C. Area D

D. Area G

E. Area H

19. Following a motorcycle accident, a 17-year-old male is suspected of having undergone a traumatic brain injury. During psychological testing, he displays poor performance on the Wisconsin Card Sorting Task, and is prone to anger. Additionally, he scores poorly on general intellectual skills assessments. Which area best accounts for these symptoms, and therefore, was likely damaged in the motorcycle crash?

A. Area A

B. Area C

C. Area D

D. Area E

E. Area G

20. A 22-year-old right-handed male suffered head trauma following a fight in a bar. Upon admission to the emergency department, it was discovered that he had an acute deficit in the programming of saccadic eye movements into the right visual field. Tests of visual acuity revealed no deficits, suggesting the programming of eye movements to be the only deficit. In which area would you expect the damage to have occurred?

A. Area A

B. Area B

C. Area C

D. Area D

E. Area E

1.2 Answers and Explanations

Easy	Medium	Hard

1. Correct: Anterolateral sulcus; medulla (B)

The patient seems to be suffering from hypoglossal nerve palsy. Rootlets of the nerve emerge from the brainstem (medulla) at the anterolateral sulcus between the pyramid and the olive.

The anterior median fissure (**A**) and posterior median sulcus (**D**) of medulla do not give attachment to any cranial nerves.

Glossopharyngeal, vagus, and accessory nerves emerge from the medulla at the posterolateral sulcus (**C**).

The cerebellopontine angle (**E**) is closely related to the attachments of the facial and vestibulocochlear nerves.

Refer to the following image key for answers 2 to 6:

A, head of caudate nucleus; B, putamen; C, globus pallidus; D, thalamus; E, corpus callosum; F, anterior limb of internal capsule; G, genu of internal capsule; H, posterior limb of internal capsule.

2. Correct: Area F (F)

The frontopontine tract and the anterior thalamic peduncle are contained within the anterior limb of the internal capsule, between the caudate nucleus and the lentiform nucleus. In addition, the anterior limb contains fibers from the anterior and the medial nuclear groups of the thalamus to the cingulate gyrus and the prefrontal cortex, respectively.

3. Correct: Area D (D)

History and clinical features for this man are typical for Korsakoff's psychosis. Although Korsakoff's syndrome can cause general cerebral atrophy, the memory problems are most likely to represent damage to the thalamus and to the mammillary bodies of the hypothalamus.

4. Correct: Area E (E)

The patient is presenting with classical symptoms of alien hand syndrome, a relatively rare condition that includes autonomous activity of the affected limb, which is perceived by the patient as being outside of voluntary control. In this particular case, the patient is displaying an agnostic dyspraxia, in which the affected hand competitively interacts with the non-affected hand when attempting to perform motor commands. Damage to the anterior corpus callosum, and consequent lack of interhemispheric connection, is the most common underlying cause for these cases.

5. Correct: Area G (G)

Facial paralysis (cranial nerve VII involvement) accompanying with uvular deviation (cranial nerve X involvement) indicates damage of corticobulbar fibers. The genu of the internal capsule contains such fibers and is likely to be the site of lesion in his case.

6. Correct: Areas A and B (D)

The neostriatum comprises the caudate nucleus and the putamen. The globus pallidus (**C**) forms the paleostriatum.

7. Correct: C6–C7 disc herniation (D)

Clinical features for the woman are typical for C7 radiculopathy. This is commonly caused by C6–C7 disc herniation.

Cervical nerve roots exit above the correspondingly numbered vertebra (except C8, since there is no corresponding vertebra). These have a fairly horizontal course as they emerge from the dural sac near the intervertebral disc and exit through the intervertebral foramen. Cervical discs are usually constrained by the posterior longitudinal ligament to herniate laterally toward the nerve root, rather than centrally toward the spinal cord. In cervical cord, therefore, the nerve root involved usually corresponds to the lower vertebral bone of the disc space.

C3–C4 disc herniation (**A**) would cause C4 radiculopathy, which might present as sensorimotor deficits in the neck region.

C4–C5 disc herniation (**B**) would cause C5 radiculopathy. Motor weakness of deltoid, sensory loss over shoulder and upper lateral arm, and compromised biceps reflex would be characteristic.

C5–C6 disc herniation (**C**) would cause C6 radiculopathy. This would present with motor weakness of biceps brachii and wrist extensors, sensory loss over first and second digits and lateral forearm, and compromised biceps and brachioradialis (more specific) reflex.

C7–C8 disc herniation (**E**) would cause C8 radiculopathy. This will result in weakness of digit flexors and sensory loss affecting the ring and little fingers for the digits.

8. Correct: Horizontal sulcus, lateral pontomedullary junction (C)

The patient is suffering from abducens nerve palsy. This can be inferred from a paralyzed lateral rectus muscle (causing medial deviation of the eyeball). These patients turn the head horizontally toward the ipsilateral shoulder for forward vision. The abducens nerve is not related to the lateral part of the horizontal sulcus at the pontomedullary junction and therefore will be spared in the case of a tumor affecting this location.

The abducens nucleus is located in the pons just beneath the fourth ventricle (**A**). The nerve emerges from the pontomedullary junction near the midline at the horizontal sulcus (**B**). It then courses through the cavernous sinus (**D**) to enter the orbit through the superior orbital fissure (**E**). Tumors located in each of these locations therefore could affect the nerve.

9. Correct: The nerve emerges from the brainstem via the horizontal sulcus at the lateral aspect of the pontomedullary junction. (E)

Corneal (blink) reflex consists of bilateral eye closure in response to stimulation of either cornea. The afferent limb of this reflex is formed by the ophthalmic division of the trigeminal nerve. The efferent limb comprises motor fibers that begin in the sensory nucleus of trigeminal, project bilaterally on facial motor nuclei, and supply orbicularis oculi muscles. A lesion of trigeminal nerve abolishes both ipsilateral and contralateral eye closure. A lesion of the facial nerve, as in this case, abolishes only ipsilateral eye closure. Facial nerve emerges from the brainstem via the horizontal sulcus at the lateral aspect of the lateral pontomedullary junction.

Oculomotor and trochlear nerve nuclei are located in the midbrain at the levels of superior (**A**) and inferior (**B**) colliculi, respectively. The trigeminal nerve emerges from the brainstem at the level of mid pons (**C**). The abducens nerve (**D**) emerges from the brainstem via the horizontal sulcus at the medial aspect of the pontomedullary junction.

10. Correct: White rami communicantes (D)

Preganglionic sympathetic fibers arise from the lateral horn cells of T1–T5 spinal segments, travel via the ventral roots and the ventral rami of the spinal nerves, and reach the corresponding thoracic sympathetic ganglia via white rami communicantes. Some of these fibers reach the cervical sympathetic ganglia by running up the sympathetic trunk. Postganglionic fibers from the cervical and the thoracic ganglia reach the heart via cardiac splanchnic nerves.

Dorsal roots (**A**) contain central processes of afferent fibers from skin and viscera; dorsal rami (**B**) contain motor fibers to skeletal muscles and sensory fibers for skin of the back; gray rami communicantes (**C**) contain postganglionic sympathetic fibers for blood vessels, sweat glands, and arrector pili muscles; and greater splanchnic nerves (**E**) contain preganglionic visceromotor and peripheral processes of viscerosensory sympathetic fibers for abdominal organs.

11. Correct: Pterygopalatine ganglion (B)

The pterygopalatine ganglion contains cell bodies for the postganglionic neurons that supply secretomotor fibers to the lacrimal, nasal, and palatine glands.

The ciliary ganglion (**A**) is involved in pupillary constriction, and contains cell bodies for the postganglionic neurons that supply the sphincter pupillae and ciliary muscles.

The otic ganglion (**C**) is involved in salivation, and contains cell bodies for the postganglionic neurons that supply secretomotor fibers for the parotid gland.

The superior cervical ganglion (**D**, a sympathetic ganglion formed by fusion of the upper four cervical paravertebral sympathetic ganglia) and gasserian ganglion (**E**, a sensory ganglion of the trigeminal nerve) are not involved in lacrimation.

12. Correct: Area H (E)

The basilar portion of the pons (H in the image) contains the motor trigeminal nucleus, which contains the cell bodies for the lower motor neurons that supply the muscles of mastication (including the lateral pterygoid muscle). Damage to this area would result in jaw deviation.

Area A (**A**) in the sagittal slice corresponds to the anterior corpus callosum. It provides the major pathways for interhemispheric communication, with damage possibly resulting in alien hand syndrome, alexia without agraphia, and other clinical manifestations of split-brain.

Area B (**B**) represents the anterior cingulate gyrus. Damage to the area is associated with problems in error detection, task switching, attention deficits, appreciation of reward, emotional instability, and social anxiety.

Area C (**C**) in the labeled sagittal slice corresponds to the medial frontal gyrus. Damage to this region typically results in dysfunctions of working memory and decision-making.

Area E (**D**) in the sagittal slice corresponds to the thalamus. Thalamic damage often results in Dejerine–Roussy syndrome, which involves unilateral, contralesional, dysesthesia, and allodynia.

13. Correct: Area B (B)

The cingulate gyrus is part of the limbic system, which is heavily involved in the regulation of emotional behavior. Tumors within this region can result in drastic changes in personality.

Area A (**A**) in the sagittal slice corresponds to the anterior corpus callosum. It provides the major pathways for interhemispheric communication, with damage possibly resulting in alien hand syndrome, alexia without agraphia, and other clinical manifestations of split-brain.

Area C (**C**) in the labeled sagittal slice corresponds to the medial frontal gyrus. While damage to this region could result in personality changes, it is more commonly linked to dysfunctions of working memory and decision-making.

Area D (**D**) in the sagittal slice indicates the fornix, the major output formation of the hippocampal system. As part of the limbic system, disruption of these fibers is most often associated with memory loss, in particular recalling long-term episodic memory.

Area E (**E**) in the sagittal slice corresponds to the thalamus. Thalamic damage often results in Dejerine–Roussy syndrome, which involves unilateral, contralesional, dysesthesia, and allodynia.

14. Correct: Area G (E)

Primary visual cortex is located on the superior and inferior banks of the calcarine sulcus and receives information from the lateral geniculate nucleus pertaining to the contralateral visual field. The inferior bank represents the superior visual field. Therefore, an upper quadrantanopia would be associated with a unilateral lesion of the inferior bank of the calcarine sulcus (area G [**E**]).

Area C (**A**) in the labeled sagittal slice corresponds to the medial frontal gyrus. While damage to this region could result in personality changes, it is more commonly linked to dysfunctions of working memory and decision-making.

Area D (**B**) in the sagittal slice indicates the fornix, the major output formation of the hippocampal system. As part of the limbic system, disruption of these fibers is most often associated with memory loss, in particular recalling long-term episodic memory.

Area E (**C**) in the sagittal slice corresponds to the thalamus. Thalamic damage often results in Dejerine–Roussy syndrome, which involves unilateral, contralesional, dysesthesia, and allodynia.

Damage to area F (**D**) in the labeled image (the superior bank of the calcarine sulcus) would result in a visual deficit of the inferior visual field.

15. Correct: Posterolateral sulcus; medulla (C)

The clinical features of the patient are typical of glossopharyngeal neuralgia. The glossopharyngeal nerve emerges from the medulla at the posterolateral sulcus.

Rootlets of the hypoglossal nerve emerge from the brainstem (medulla) at the anterolateral sulcus (**B**) between the pyramid and the olive.

The anterior median fissure (**A**) and posterior median sulcus (**D**) of medulla do not give attachment to any cranial nerves.

The cerebellopontine angle (**E**) is closely related to the attachments of the facial and vestibulocochlear nerves.

16. Correct: Posterior paracentral lobule (D)

The posterior paracentral lobule (postcentral gyrus on the medial hemisphere) represents the cortical area for sensation of the lower limbs and genitals.

The precentral gyri on the lateral (**A**) and the medial (**C**, anterior paracentral lobule) hemispheres are related to motor areas for the upper and lower body, respectively.

The postcentral gyrus on the lateral hemisphere (**B**) represents the cortical area for sensation of the upper limbs and trunk.

The superior parietal lobule (**E**) lies posterior to the postcentral gyrus and is a complex sensory association area. A lesion to this region might produce astereognosis and other forms of agnosia but anesthesia would be uncommon.

17. Correct: Cerebellum (C)

The fourth ventricle is formed as a cavity within the hindbrain or rhombencephalon. The cerebellum can be conceptualized as the roof of the fourth ventricle, while both the pons (**B**) and medulla oblongata (**A**) lie on its floor. The thalamus (**D**) and hypothalamus (**E**) derive from diencephalon and are not related to the fourth ventricle.

18. Correct: Area D (C)

The posterior parietal cortex (area D [**C**]) plays a large role in the modulation of visual attention. Therefore, damage to the area may result in failures to orient attention toward the contralesional hemifield.

Area A (**A**) in the labeled image corresponds to the lateral aspect of the superior frontal gyrus. Damage to this region is most likely to result in a loss of horizontal eye movements (due to the superior frontal gyrus' role in producing conjugate deviation of the eyes, ultimately through innervation of the superior colliculus).

The primary motor cortex responsible for control of the arm (area B [**B**]) projects axons to the spinal cord and activity within this region directly correlates with volitional movement. Damage to this region would result in an upper motor neuron lesion of the contralateral arm.

Area G (**D**) in the labeled image corresponds to the orbitofrontal cortex, which plays a prominent role in higher order intellectual functions and some aspects of emotional behavior.

Broca's area (area H, inferior frontal gyrus [**E**]) has a prominent role in speech production.

19. Correct: Area G (E)

The orbitofrontal cortex (area G [**E**]) is involved in higher order intellectual functions and some emotional behavior. Following damage to this region, changes in personality and emotions are possible.

Area A (**A**) corresponds to the lateral aspect of the superior frontal gyrus. Damage to this region is most likely to result in a loss of horizontal eye movements (due to the superior frontal gyrus' role in producing conjugate deviation of the eyes, ultimately through innervation of the superior colliculus).

The primary somatosensory cortex is immediately adjacent to the central sulcus (area C [**B**]). Damage to this region would result in a loss of sensation (vibration, tactile, and pressure) of the contralateral body part. The precise location of the deficit would depend on the portion of sensory homunculus affected.

Area D (**C**), the superior parietal lobule, is involved in the attention. Damage to this region can cause a hemispatial neglect for contralesional visual space and other disorders of attention, such as tactile agnosia.

Area E (**D**) marks the dorsal border of the superior temporal gyrus, and in combination with adjacent portions of parietal cortex makes up Wernicke's area. This region is critical for the understanding of both written and spoken words.

20. Correct: Area A (A)

The frontal eye fields, located on the superior and middle frontal gyri (area A [**A**]), send signals to the superior colliculus to initiate eye movements. Damage to this region usually results in an inability to produce saccades into the contralesional visual field.

The primary motor cortex responsible for control of the arm (area B [**B**]) projects axons to the spinal cord, and activity within this region directly correlates with volitional movement. Damage to this region would result in an upper motor neuron lesion of the contralateral arm.

The primary somatosensory cortex is immediately adjacent to the central sulcus (area C [**C**]). Damage to this region would result in a loss of sensation (vibration, tactile, and pressure) of the contralateral body part. The precise location of the deficit would depend on the portion of sensory homunculus affected.

Area D (**D**), the superior parietal lobule, is involved in the attention. Damage to this region can cause a hemispatial neglect for contralesional visual space and other disorders of attention, such as tactile agnosia.

Area E (**E**) marks the dorsal border of the superior temporal gyrus, and in combination with adjacent portions of parietal cortex makes up Wernicke's area. This region is critical for the understanding of both written and spoken words.

Chapter 2
Meninges and CSF

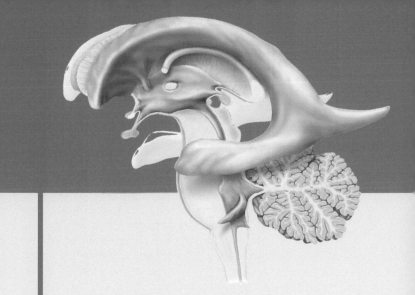

LEARNING OBJECTIVES

► Describe the disposition of the dural folds.

► Analyze the pathophysiology and the clinical features of meningitis. Distinguish between bacterial and viral meningitis.

► Describe the location and contents for the primary subarachnoid cisterns.

► Analyze the clinical features of uncal herniation.

► Describe the attachments for the dural folds.

► Describe the locations and blood supply for the choroid plexus.

► Analyze the etiopathogenesis of normal pressure hydrocephalus.

► Describe the location and contents for the primary subarachnoid cisterns.

► Describe the disposition of the dural folds.

► Identify the layers of the meninges.

► Localize the subdural space. Identify the layers of the meninges.

► Localize the subarachnoid space.

► Illustrate the pathway for the flow of CSF.

► Describe the disposition of the dural folds. Identify cerebral venous sinuses that are contained within folds of dura mater.

► Interpret CSF analysis and recognize values outside of the normal range.

► Analyze the etiologies for enlarged retrocerebellar space.

► Identify the clinical features associated with a subfalcial herniation.

► Describe the attachments for the dural folds.

► Illustrate the pathway for the flow of CSF. List the primary and secondary brain vesicles and trace their derivatives in human.

2.1 Questions

Easy	Medium	Hard

1. A 58-year-old man presents with a brain herniation involving the tentorium cerebelli. Which of the following structures are separated by this meningeal fold?

A. Cerebral hemispheres

B. Cerebellar hemispheres

C. Cerebellum and pons

D. Cerebellum and medulla

E. Cerebellum and cerebral hemisphere

2. A 14-year-old girl was brought to the emergency department following a day of worsening headache, fever, periods of confusion, and stiff neck. The patient's mother reported that she awoke at ~3 am with chills and body aches. By ~11 am, she was breathing quickly and had nausea and vomiting. Physical examination revealed a temperature of 101.5F, marked rigidity within the neck, and the appearance of nonblanching, purplish 2-mm-sized petechiae scattered on the arms, legs, and chest. A lumbar puncture was performed and CSF analysis showed normal opening pressure, elevated white blood cells, total protein, and lactate, and a low glucose level. What was the most likely cause of this patient's symptoms?

A. Ventricular stenosis

B. Viral meningitis

C. Beta-amyloid plaque deposits

D. Bacterial meningitis

E. Scarring of arachnoid granulations

3. A 6-month-old infant presents with medial deviation of his right eyeball. MRI indicates a huge cyst located within a subarachnoid cistern pressing on to the contained structures. Which of the following structures might also be involved?

A. Vertebral artery

B. Basilar artery

C. Posterior inferior cerebellar artery

D. Posterior communicating arteries

E. Middle cerebral arteries

4. A 33-year-old right-handed male presents with third cranial nerve palsy and weakness, affecting the same side of the body. Which of the following forms of brain herniation would you suspect in him?

A. Subfalcial

B. Uncal

C. Tonsillar-foramen magnum

D. Abducens herniation

5. A 51-year-old right-handed woman undergoes a CT scan, with the suspicion of having a tear in the dural fold at the point of its attachment to the crista galli of the ethmoid bone. Which of the following dural folds is affected?

A. Falx cerebri

B. Tentorium cerebelli

C. Falx cerebelli

D. Diaphragma sellae

6. A 2-month-old infant presents with hydrocephalus. He has been crying intermittently and has vomited several times in the past 24 hours. MRI reveals a choroid plexus papilloma in the roof of the third ventricle. Which of the following arteries is the principal feeder for the tumor?

A. Anterior choroidal artery

B. Medial posterior choroidal artery

C. Lateral posterior choroidal artery

D. Anterior inferior cerebellar artery

E. Posterior inferior cerebellar artery

7. An 81-year-old right-handed male presents to a neurologist accompanied by his wife. She says that her husband has become clumsier, resulting in several falls over the last few months. Additionally, he has been having periodic urinary incontinence. However, in recent days, he has become increasingly forgetful, and she now fears that he may be developing Alzheimer's disease, a condition that runs prevalent in his family. Physical examination reveals the patient has an abnormal gait. CSF analysis shows an opening pressure of 120 mm H_2O, total protein of 20 mg/dL, and WBC count < 5. It is determined that this patient is suffering from normal pressure hydrocephalus. Which of the following is the most likely cause for his symptoms?

A. Ventricular stenosis

B. Viral infection

C. Beta-amyloid plaque deposits

D. Bacterial meningitis

E. Scarring of arachnoid granulations

Consider the following image for questions 8 and 9:

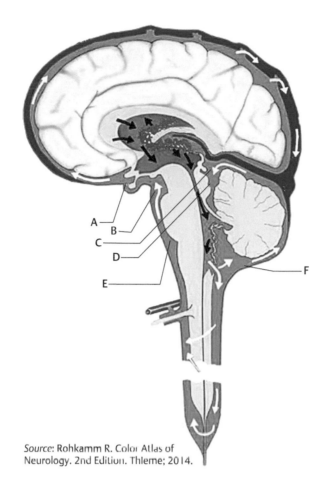

Source: Rohkamm R. Color Atlas of
Neurology. 2nd Edition. Thieme; 2014.

8. A 36-year-old man presents with a "down and out" right eye leading to diplopia, drooping of the right upper eyelid, and dilatation of the right pupil. Which of the following areas could be the location for a possible tumor?

A. Area A

B. Area B

C. Area C

D. Area D

E. Area E

F. Area F

9. A 58-year-old man presents with diplopia that is worse in downgaze. Physical examination hinted toward paralysis of the superior oblique muscle. Which of the following areas could be the location for a possible tumor?

A. Area A

B. Area B

C. Area C

D. Area D

E. Area E

F. Area F

10. A 63-year-old woman presents with headache and visual disturbances. MRI scan reveals a pituitary tumor that has outgrown the pituitary fossa. Which of the following structures might have initially been irritated by the tumor and cause headache for this patient?

A. Falx cerebri

B. Falx cerebelli

C. Tentorium cerebelli

D. Diaphragma sellae

E. Optic chiasma

11

Consider the following image for questions 11 to 13:

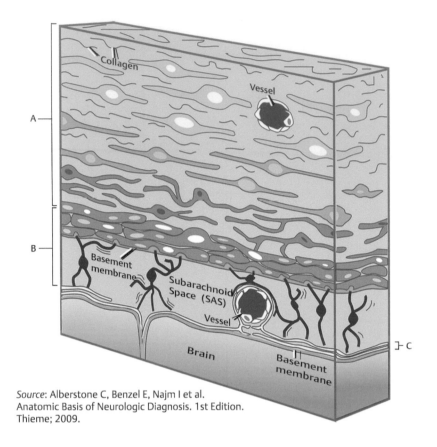

Source: Alberstone C, Benzel E, Najm I et al.
Anatomic Basis of Neurologic Diagnosis. 1st Edition.
Thieme; 2009.

11. A 24-year-old woman presented to your hospital with a 1-year history of headache and a single complex partial seizure 2 days earlier. Physical and neurological examination was unremarkable. Upon MRI, a dural-based 5 cm × 4 cm × 3 cm mass was found to be attached to the dura at the anterior side of the sylvian fissure. In the labeled image, which area best corresponds to the location of the tumor attachment?

A. Area A

B. Area B

C. Area C

12. A 76-year-old man presented to his physician with right-sided headaches and difficulty walking. The patient was in an automobile accident 2 months ago; his head was not hit or he did not lose consciousness, but he has felt tired and has had right-sided headaches ever since. Following a head CT scan, fluid hypodense relative to brain tissue was observed. At surgery, two burr holes were drilled into the skull. To release the buildup of fluid, which layer of meninges would the surgeon most likely have to open?

A. Area A

B. Area B

C. Area C

D. Areas A and B

E. Areas A, B, and C

13. A 19-year-old right-handed male received a T1-weighted MRI scan of the brain as part of participation in a research study at his university. During review, an incidental finding of a well-circumscribed mass within a subarachnoid cistern was found. Which area best corresponds to the location of the lower (deeper) extent of the cyst?

A. Area A

B. Area B

C. Area C

14. A 56-year-old woman presents to her ophthalmologist complaining of visual loss and headaches. She was found to have concentric loss of the peripheral visual fields in both eyes. Additionally, mild papilledema was observed in the right optic disk. An MRI scan was ordered. Lateral ventricles were markedly dilated, whereas the third and fourth ventricles were normal in appearance. A colloid cyst was found to be obstructing CSF flow. Where would you expect this cyst to have been located?

A. Foramen of Luschka

B. Foramen of Magendie

C. Cerebral aqueduct

D. Foramen of Monro

15. At autopsy of a 72-year-old man who died due to pulmonary embolism, the meningeal layer separating his two cerebellar hemispheres showed discoloration. A large thrombus and some sludge were found in the venous sinus contained within the dural fold. Which of the following, most likely, has been the direct source for the embolism in his case?

A. Superior sagittal sinus

B. Inferior sagittal sinus

C. Straight sinus

D. Cavernous sinus

E. Occipital sinus

16. A 32-year-old man presents to the emergency department with chronic headache. CSF analysis returned the following results: WBC count, 1 cell/μL; glucose, 53 mg/dL; total protein, 43 mg/dL; and pressure, 220 mm H_2O. Which of these values (if any) would warrant further investigation?

A. Cell count

B. Glucose

C. Total protein

D. Pressure

E. CSF analysis is normal

17. A 34-year-old woman, who was 22-week pregnant, underwent a routine transabdominal ultrasound examination to exclude any congenital fetal abnormalities. A triangular defect toward the posterior aspect of the fetal brain was observed, which was occupied by CSF. Measurements of the cisterna magna revealed a depth of 12 mm. Lateral ventricles appeared normal in size, and the fourth ventricle was normal in appearance. There were no cerebellar deformations observed. Which of the following is the most likely diagnosis?

A. Dandy–Walker complex

B. Cerebellar hypoplasia

C. Posterior fossa arachnoid cyst

D. Mega cisterna magna

E. Arnold–Chiari malformation

18. An 18-year-old right-handed woman undergoes an MRI scan for a suspected intracranial mass. The radiology report notes a subfalcial herniation. Which of the following clinical features would you expect in her due to such herniation?

A. Ipsilateral third nerve palsy

B. Respiratory collapse

C. Cardiovascular arrest

D. Contralateral hemiparesis

E. No clinical manifestation

19. A 22-year-old right-handed man undergoes an endoscopic endonasal transsphenoidal tumor resection. Complications comprised a tear in a dural fold resulting in the leaking of CSF. Which dural fold was most likely violated?

A. Falx cerebri

B. Tentorium cerebelli

C. Falx cerebelli

D. Diaphragma sellae

20. A neonate had suffered from a teratogenic insult during embryonic growth that has affected the mesencephalic part of his developing neural tube. In the presented cast of his ventricular system (left lateral view), which of the following areas might have suffered?

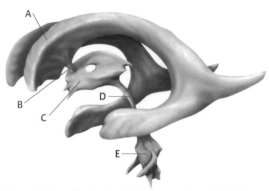

Source: Schünke M, Schulte E, Schumacher U et al. THIEME Atlas of Anatomy: Head, Neck, and Neuroanatomy. 2nd Edition. Thieme; 2016. Illustration by Karl Wesker/Markus Voll.

A. Area A
B. Area B
C. Area C
D. Area D
E. Area E

2.2 Answers and Explanations

Easy	Medium	Hard

1.   Correct: Cerebellum and cerebral hemisphere (E)

The tentorium cerebelli, a projection formed by the inner meningeal layer of the cranial dura, divides the cranial cavity into middle and posterior fossae and separates the occipital lobes of cerebral hemispheres (supratentorial) from the cerebellum (infratentorial).

The cerebral hemispheres (**A**) are separated by falx cerebri and cerebellar hemispheres (**B**) are separated by falx cerebelli.

The cerebellum is separated from the pons (**C**) and medulla (**D**) by the cavity of the fourth ventricle and not by dural folds.

2.   Correct: Bacterial meningitis (D)

This patient demonstrated clinical features strongly suggestive of meningeal irritation. Elevated protein and white blood cell count, and a low glucose level, is most consistent with bacterial meningitis.

Ventricular stenosis (**A**, as in obstructive hydrocephalus), β-amyloid deposit (**C**, as in Alzheimer's disease), or scarring of arachnoid granulation (**E**, as in normal pressure hydrocephalus) is unlikely to have such acute presentation with features of meningitis.

Viral meningitis (**B**) will most likely be associated with a normal, rather than reduced, glucose level in CSF.

3.   Correct: Basilar artery (B)

The infant is suffering from paralysis of his right lateral rectus muscle consequent to abducens nerve palsy. The subarachnoid cistern that contains the nerve is the prepontine cistern, which also contains the basilar artery, and the origins of the anterior inferior cerebellar and superior cerebellar arteries. A cyst located in the prepontine cistern, therefore, might affect any of these structures.

Vertebral (**A**) and posterior inferior cerebellar (**C**) arteries are contained within the cerebellomedullary cistern (cisterna magna). Posterior communicating arteries (**D**) are contained within the interpeduncular cistern. The sylvian cistern contains the middle cerebral arteries (**E**).

4.   Correct: Uncal (B)

Explanation: Uncal herniation refers to herniation of the uncus (anterior medial temporal gyrus) through the tentorial incisura. The uncus compresses the ipsilateral third cranial nerve (as it traverses the subarachnoid space). Lateral displacement of the midbrain may compress the contralateral cerebral peduncle (thereby causing ipsilateral weakness—a false localizing sign).

A subfalcial herniation (**A**) occurs when the cingulate gyrus is forced under the falx cerebri. No notable clinical features are associated with such herniation alone.

A tonsillar-foramen magnum herniation (**C**) is caused by the cerebellar tonsils being forced down into the foramen magnum, usually as a result of increased pressure within a small posterior fossa, as occurs in Chiari type I malformation.

Though not a herniation syndrome, the abducens nerve (**D**) can be forced downward and stretched due to its location within Dorello's canal during conditions of increased ICP.

5.   Correct: Falx cerebri (A)

The falx cerebri forms a partition along the vertical longitudinal fissure, separating the right and left cerebral hemispheres. The anterior aspect is attached to the crista galli of the ethmoid bone and the posterior portion is attached to the tentorium cerebelli.

The tentorium cerebelli (**B**) is attached along the periphery to the petrous portion of the temporal bone and the margins of the grooves for the transverse sinuses on the occipital bone.

The falx cerebelli (**C**) is anteriorly attached to the posterior part of the tentorium cerebelli and its posterior margin is attached to the lower division of the vertical crest on the inner surface of the occipital bone.

The diaphragma sellae (**D**) extends from the tuberculum sellae to the posterior clinoid processes and dorsum sellae.

6. Correct: Medial posterior choroidal artery (B)

The medial posterior choroidal artery usually arises from the posterior cerebral artery (PCA). It is the primary blood supply to the choroid plexus on the roof of the third ventricle.

The anterior choroidal artery (**A**) originates from the internal carotid artery and supplies the choroid plexus within the temporal horn of the lateral ventricle.

The lateral posterior choroidal artery (**C**), from the P2 segment of the PCA, supplies the choroid plexus within the atrium and the body of the lateral ventricle.

Anterior inferior cerebellar artery (**D**) arises from the basilar artery and supplies choroid plexus protruding from the foramen of Luschka.

The posterior inferior cerebellar artery (**E**) arises from the vertebral artery (~10% of cases arises from the basilar artery) and supplies choroid plexus within the fourth ventricle.

7. Correct: Scarring of arachnoid granulations (E)

As the name suggests, normal pressure hydrocephalus is a form of communicating hydrocephalus in which there is no increase in intracranial pressure (ICP). Despite the normal pressure values, the ventricular system appears dilated, and this condition often results in a triad of symptoms consisting of gait disturbance, urinary incontinence, and dementia.

The arachnoid granulations are projections of the arachnoid membrane into the dural sinuses that allow CSF to drain into the venous system. Although the exact mechanisms of normal pressure hydrocephalus is unknown, scarring of the arachnoid granulations may cause a reduction in the amount of CSF that can pass through, and hence be absorbed by, the arachnoid granulations, resulting in an increase in CSF in circulation.

Although a major cause of hydrocephalus includes ventricular stenosis (**A**), this would result in an increase in ICP, as well as dilation of the ventricles proximal to the obstruction.

Viral or bacterial infections (**B** and **D**) may result in cerebral edema, and would usually be associated with increased ICP. Additionally, CSF analysis is unlikely to return with normal results.

There is no known mechanism by which β-amyloid deposits (**C**) could result in normal pressure hydrocephalus.

Refer to the following image and image key for answers 8 and 9:

A, chiasmatic cistern; B, interpeduncular cistern; C, ambient cistern; D, quadrigeminal cistern; E, prepontine cistern; F, cerebellomedullary cistern.

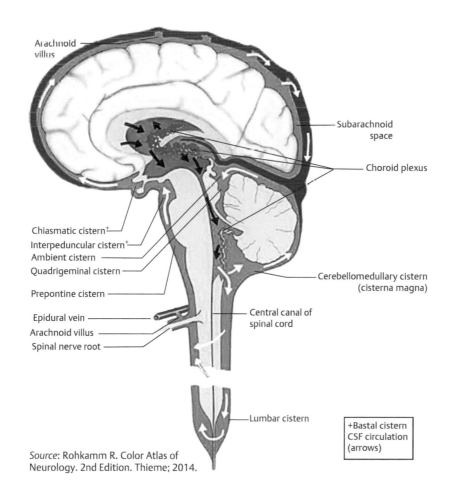

Source: Rohkamm R. Color Atlas of Neurology. 2nd Edition. Thieme; 2014.

8. Correct: Area B (B)

The patient presents with oculomotor nerve palsy. This can be inferred from a down and out eye (paralysis of superior rectus, inferior rectus, medial rectus, and inferior oblique muscles), drooping of upper eyelid (paralysis of levator palpebrae superioris muscle), and pupillary dilation (paralysis of sphincter pupillae muscle). The oculomotor nerve, being a content of the interpeduncular cistern, can be damaged by a tumor located in the cistern.

9. Correct: Area C (C)

The patient presents with superior oblique muscle palsy, which is supplied by the trochlear nerve. This nerve, being a content of the infratentorial portion of the ambient cistern, can be damaged by a tumor located in the cistern.

Major contents for the other listed cisterns:

Chiasmatic cistern (A): optic chiasma and optic nerves, hypophyseal stalk, and origin of the anterior cerebral arteries

Quadrigeminal cistern (D): great vein of Galen, posterior pericallosal arteries, and some parts and branches of the superior cerebellar and posterior cerebral arteries

Prepontine cistern (E): abducens nerve, basilar artery, and origin of the anterior inferior cerebellar and superior cerebellar arteries.

Cerebellomedullary cistern (F): vertebral artery, origin of the posterior inferior cerebellar artery, and the 9th, 10th, 11th, and 12th cranial nerves

10. Correct: Diaphragma sellae (D)

The diaphragma sellae, a dural fold attached anteriorly to the tuberculum sellae and posteriorly to the dorsum sellae, forms the roof of the sella turcica, the cavity in which the pituitary gland is lodged. A small gap in the sella allows for the passage of the pituitary stalk. Headache is a common symptom from irritation of cranial dura mater.

Falx cerebri (A), a dural fold, runs within the longitudinal cerebral fissure and separates the right and left cerebral hemispheres.

Falx cerebelli (B), a dural fold, separates the right and left cerebellar hemispheres within the posterior fossa.

Tentorium cerebelli (C), a dural fold, divides the cranial cavity into middle and posterior fossae and separates the occipital lobes of cerebral hemispheres (supratentorial) from the cerebellum (infratentorial).

Pressing on the optic chiasma (E), the meeting point of the right and left optic nerves, by the tumor would more likely result in visual disturbances (bitemporal hemianopia commonly) rather than a headache.

Refer to the following image for answers 11 to 13:

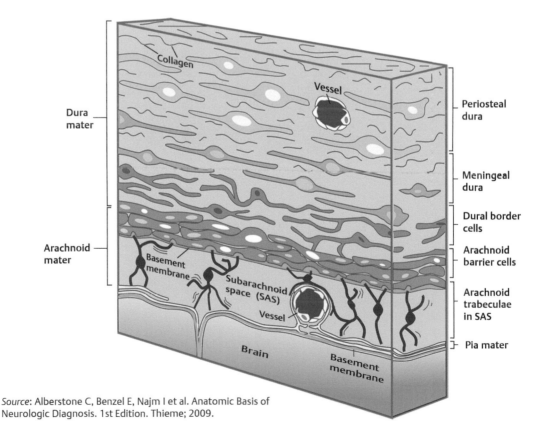

Source: Alberstone C, Benzel E, Najm I et al. Anatomic Basis of Neurologic Diagnosis. 1st Edition. Thieme; 2009.

11. Correct: Area A (A)

The meninges comprise three tissue types that encompass the central nervous system and separate it from the skull. The first layer, the dura mater (A), is tough and fibrous. It is composed of elongated fibroblasts and collagen fibrils.

12. Correct: Area A (A)

The patient's symptoms were a result of a subdural hematoma, the buildup of blood within the subdural space, between the dura and the arachnoid (B). To remove this fluid accumulation, the dura (A) would have to be opened. Neither arachnoid (B) nor pia (C) needs to be opened to drain a subdural hematoma.

13. Correct: Area C (C)

The pia mater adheres to the surface of the brain, closely following the gyri and sulci. In comparison, the arachnoid mater covers the superficial surface of the brain. In areas where the pia and arachnoid are separated, cavities called subarachnoid cisterns are formed. This mass would, therefore, be between the arachnoid mater (B) and the pia mater (C), with the lower (deeper) extent corresponding to the latter.

14. Correct: Foramen of Monro (D)

The lateral ventricles are dilated; however, the third and fourth ventricles appear normal in size. This would suggest a bilateral obstruction in the foramina of Monro, the passage by which CSF exits the lateral ventricles. A colloid cyst of the third ventricle is a common cause of obstruction of the foramina of Monro.

Obstruction of the foramina of Luschka (A) or Magendie (B) would present with dilated third and fourth ventricles. Obstruction of the cerebral aqueduct (C) would present with dilatation of the third ventricle.

15. Correct: Occipital sinus (E)

The occipital sinus lies within the falx cerebelli, which is the fold of dura mater that separates the cerebellar hemispheres. Thrombosis within the occipital sinus, therefore, might have been the source of embolism for him.

The superior sagittal sinus (A) runs along the superior margin of the falx cerebri, while the inferior sagittal sinus (B) runs along its inferior margin. The straight sinus (C) is carried in the attachment of the falx cerebri to the tentorium cerebelli. The cavernous sinus (D) is situated along the lateral surface of the body of sphenoid bone and extends from the superior orbital fissure to the petrous part of the temporal bone.

16. Correct: Pressure (D)

The normal pressure of CSF is within 70 to 180 mm H_2O.

The normal range is 0 to 5 for WBC count (A), 50 to 80 mg/dL for glucose (B), and 15 to 60 mg/dL for protein (C).

17. Correct: Mega cisterna magna (D)

Mega cisterna magna (D) is a normal variant characterized by focal enlargement of the subarachnoid space in the posterior and inferior portions of the posterior fossa.

Dandy–Walker complex (A) may result in an increased retrocerebellar space (posterior fossa); however, it usually involves atrophy of the cerebellar vermis.

Cerebellar hypoplasia (B), as the name suggests, is a condition in which the cerebellum is unusually small.

A posterior fossa arachnoid cyst (C) would commonly compress neighboring structures, including the cerebellum.

Chiari malformations (E) are associated with cerebellar herniation through the foramen magnum and a small posterior fossa.

18. Correct: No clinical manifestation (E)

During a subfalcial herniation, the cingulate gyrus is forced under the falx cerebri. Despite this shift, there are no associated clinical features.

Ipsilateral third nerve palsy (A) is typically observed in uncal herniation, when the uncus is forced through the tentorial incisura (opening for passage of brainstem) and compresses the midbrain. Contralateral hemiparesis (D) is also observed with such herniation.

Both respiratory collapse (B) and cardiovascular arrest (C) are associated with cerebellar and/or brainstem herniation through the foramen magnum, as occurs in Chiari malformations.

19. Correct: Diaphragma sellae (D)

The diaphragma sellae forms the roof of the sella turcica, which houses the pituitary gland. A small opening in the sellae allows the pituitary stalk to pass through to its point of attachment at the base of the brain. During a surgical resection of the pituitary gland, it is possible to tear this dural fold allowing for a leak in CSF.

The falx cerebri (A) forms a partition along the vertical longitudinal fissure, separating the right and left cerebral hemispheres. The anterior aspect is attached to the crista galli of the ethmoid bone and the posterior portion is attached to the tentorium cerebelli.

The tentorium cerebelli (B) is attached along the periphery to the petrous portion of the temporal bone and the margins of the grooves for the transverse sinuses on the occipital bone.

The falx cerebelli (C) is anteriorly attached to the posterior part of the tentorium cerebelli and its posterior margin is attached to the lower division of the vertical crest on the inner surface of the occipital bone.

20.   Correct: Area D (D)

Refer to the following image:

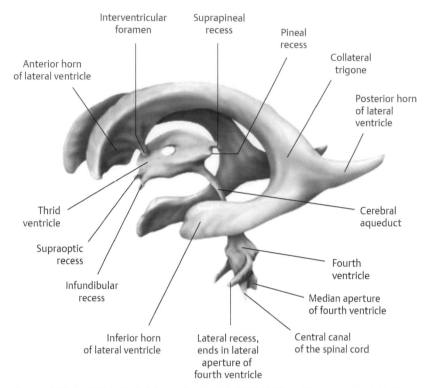

Source: Schünke M, Schulte E, Schumacher U et al. THIEME Atlas of Anatomy: Head, Neck, and Neuroanatomy. 2nd Edition. Thieme; 2016. Illustration by Karl Wesker/Markus Voll.

The cerebral aqueduct is the cavity of the midbrain that develops from the mesencephalon.

The lateral ventricle (**A**) is the cavity of telencephalon and the third ventricle (**C**) is the cavity of diencephalon. The interventricular foramen of Monro (**B**) serves as the communication between the two. The fourth ventricle (**E**) is the cavity of the rhombencephalon.

Chapter 3

Blood Supply of the Nervous System

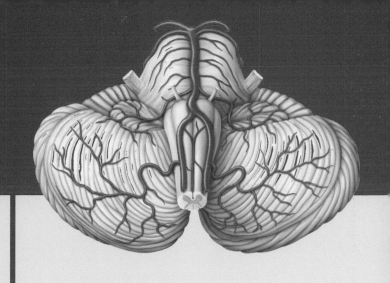

LEARNING OBJECTIVES

- ▶ Analyze the clinical features involving lesions of MCA and its branches.
- ▶ Identify the major sources of blood supply to the brain in an axial view.
- ▶ Describe the course, branches, and supply of the internal carotid artery.
- ▶ Describe the venous drainage of the cerebral hemispheres.
- ▶ Describe the etiopathogenesis and clinical features for trigeminal neuralgia. Describe the course and branches of the vertebrobasilar arterial system.
- ▶ Illustrate the branches and distribution of the ACA.
- ▶ Describe the venous drainage of the cerebral hemispheres. Describe the course, distribution, and functions of the glossopharyngeal and vagus nerves.
- ▶ Describe the course and distribution of the facial nerve.
- ▶ Recognize components of the circle of Willis.
- ▶ Describe the origin, course, and distribution for the oculomotor nerve. Analyze the clinical features resulting from oculomotor nerve palsy.
- ▶ Analyze the clinical features involving lesions of anterior choroidal artery.
- ▶ Analyze clinical features for facial, vagal, and hypoglossal nerve palsies.
- ▶ Analyze the clinical features involving occlusion of the PICA.
- ▶ Identify the major sources of blood supply to the brain in coronal view.

3.1 Questions

Easy	Medium	Hard

1. A 58-year-old man presents with right-sided face and arm paralysis. When asked about the onset of symptoms, he is unable to speak fluently but seems to understand what is being asked. Which of the following vessels might be affected in his case?

A. Right MCA, superior division

B. Right MCA, inferior division

C. Left MCA, superior division

D. Left MCA, inferior division

E. Right ACA

F. Left ACA

2. A 66-year-old right-handed male is suspected of having a blockage within the basilar artery. Which areas of the axial section of the brain in the following image would suffer from ischemia?

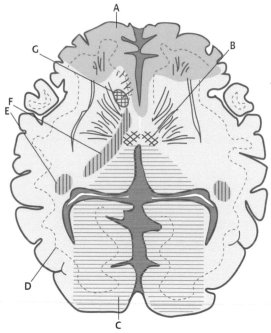

Source: Alberstone C, Benzel E, Najm I et al. Anatomic Basis of Neurologic Diagnosis. 1st Edition. Thieme; 2009.

A. Area A

B. Area B

C. Area C

D. Area D

E. Area E

3. A 48-year-old man presents with a tumor in the middle cranial fossa encroaching on the optic canal. Which of the following areas might suffer from vascular compromise?

A. Adenohypophysis

B. Neurohypophysis

C. Middle ear cavity

D. Middle ethmoidal sinus

E. Visual areas of cerebral cortex

4. A 26-year-old woman presents with a thrombus within the confluence of sinuses (torcular herophili). Which of the following might have a lesser chance of being affected, given that it lacks direct connection with the confluence?

A. Superior sagittal sinus

B. Inferior sagittal sinus

C. Straight sinus

D. Occipital sinus

E. Right transverse sinus

5. A 15-year-old girl presents with recurrent episodes of brief but stabbing right-sided facial pain that is triggered by chewing gum. Compression of the root of the involved nerve at its exit from the brainstem by aberrant branches of a blood vessel is an important cause for such pain. Which of the following vessels, most commonly, might have given off these branches?

A. Right PICA

B. Left PICA

C. Right SCA

D. Left SCA

E. Right AICA

F. Left AICA

Consider the following image for questions 6 and 7:

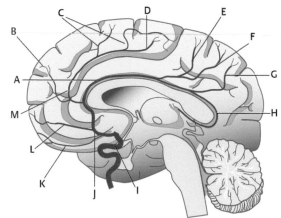

Source: Alberstone C, Benzel E, Najm I et al. Anatomic Basis of Neurologic Diagnosis. 1st Edition. Thieme; 2009.

6. A 52-year-old woman presents with symptomology consistent with an occlusion of the pericallosal artery. In which area would you expect the occlusion to be?

A. Area D

B. Area E

C. Area F

D. Area G

E. Area H

7. A 21-year-old male suffers an infarct of the posterior internal frontal artery. Which area of the image most closely matches the description of infarct?

A. Area D

B. Area E

C. Area F

D. Area G

E. Area H

8. A 30-year-old woman presents with milky discharge from her nipples, particularly on squeezing. She has history of frequently missing her menstrual periods, scanty amount and duration of bleeding during menstrual periods, and painful sexual intercourse due to vaginal dryness. Which of the following vessels is the source of the principal feeder for the dysfunctional cells/structure in her case?

A. Cervical part of internal carotid artery

B. Petrous part of internal carotid artery

C. Cavernous part of internal carotid artery

D. Cerebral part of internal carotid artery

E. Basilar artery

9. A 36-year-old woman presents with headache, nausea, vomiting, hoarseness of voice, and inability to shrug her left shoulder. Cerebral venous thrombosis was considered as a differential diagnosis. Which of the following structures, most likely, might lodge a thrombus in her case?

A. Cavernous sinus

B. Superior sagittal sinus

C. Right transverse sinus

D. Left transverse sinus

E. Terminal part of sigmoid sinus

10. A 56-year-old man presents with right-sided facial muscle weakness. He had difficulty in closing his right eye and whistling. Physical examination revealed no further neurodeficit. Which of the following arteries might be suffering from an ischemic stroke in his case?

A. Long circumferential branches of right basilar artery

B. Long circumferential branches of left basilar artery

C. Lateral striate branches of right MCA

D. Lateral striate branches of left MCA

E. Right AICA

F. Left AICA

Consider the following case for questions 11 and 12:

A 58-year-old man presents with right-sided homonymous hemianopia. When asked about the onset of symptoms, he speaks fluently but his answers are either meaningless or irrelevant, indicating his inability to comprehend what is being asked. He is unable to repeat single words or simple sentences.

11. Which of the following might be the site of lesion in his case?

A. Right MCA, superior division

B. Right MCA, inferior division

C. Left MCA, superior division

D. Left MCA, inferior division

E. Right PCA

F. Left PCA

12. Which of the following might be an additional finding for him?

A. Sensory loss in right arm

B. Sensory loss in left arm

C. Paralysis of right arm

D. Paralysis of left arm

E. Paralysis of right leg

F. Paralysis of left leg

13. A 73-year-old woman presents to the emergency department with a bitemporal heteronymous hemianopsia. It is determined that the visual field deficits were caused by an aneurysm within the anterior communicating artery. Which area in the following image corresponds to the location of the aneurysm?

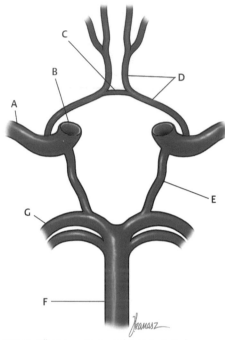

Source: Alberstone C, Benzel E, Najm I et al. Anatomic Basis of Neurologic Diagnosis. 1st Edition. Thieme; 2009.

A. Area A
B. Area B
C. Area C
D. Area D
E. Area E

14. A 42-year-old man presents with diplopia, inability to move his right eyeball medially, and a dilated right pupil. Which of the following might be the location of a causative aneurysm in his case?

A. Bifurcation of basilar artery
B. AICA
C. PICA
D. Pontine branches of basilar artery
E. Labyrinthine artery

15. A 60-year-old man presents with right-sided homonymous hemianopia, hemiplegia, and hemianesthesia. Which of the following arteries might have suffered from an ischemic stroke for his case?

A. Lateral striate branches of MCA
B. Superior division of the MCA
C. Inferior division of the MCA
D. PCA
E. Anterior choroidal artery

16. A 56-year-old man presents with left-sided lower facial muscle weakness. He, however, had no weakness in closing his left eye. His tongue deviated to the left on protrusion, and the uvula deviated to the right on an attempt to say "ah." Which of the following arteries might be suffering from an ischemic stroke for his case?

A. Long circumferential branches of right basilar artery
B. Long circumferential branches of left basilar artery
C. Lateral striate branches of right MCA
D. Lateral striate branches of left MCA
E. Right PICA
F. Left PICA

Consider the following case for questions 17 and 18:

A 72-year-old, right-handed male presents to the emergency department with loss of pain and thermal sense affecting the left side of his face and right side of his trunk. Although he was ataxic, his consciousness and vision were unaltered. A CT scan revealed a vascular lesion of the medulla oblongata.

17. Which of the following vessels might have been involved in this patient?

A. Anterior spinal artery
B. AICA
C. PICA
D. SCA
E. Basilar artery

18. Which of the following might be an additional finding in this patient?

A. Paralysis of left arm
B. Paralysis of right arm
C. Loss of vibration sense in left arm
D. Loss of vibration sense in right arm
E. Miosis of left eye
F. Miosis of right eye

Consider the following image of the coronal section of the brain for questions 19 and 20:

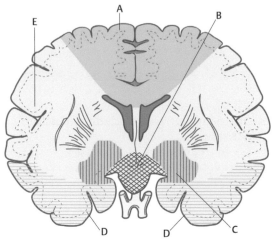

Source: Alberstone C, Benzel E, Najm I et al. Anatomic Basis of Neurologic Diagnosis. 1st Edition. Thieme; 2009.

19. A 66-year-old right-handed woman is suspected of having a stroke. She presented to the emergency department with hemiplegia and hemihypoesthesia. Suspecting the symptoms are a result of an occlusion of the anterior choroidal artery, in which area would one expect ischemic damage?

A. Area A

B. Area B

C. Area C

D. Area D

E. Area E

20. An 86-year-old right-handed male awakens one morning and has great difficulty recognizing familiar faces. Symptom onset was sudden, and there is minimal cognitive decline. CT scanning reveals a blockage in the distal portion of the left posterior cerebral artery. In which area would one expect ischemic damage?

A. Area A

B. Area B

C. Area C

D. Area D

E. Area E

3.2 Answers and Explanations

Easy	Medium	Hard

1. Correct: Left MCA, superior division (C)

The patient is suffering from a right-sided facial palsy and right upper limb paralysis. These indicate a lesion in his left primary motor cortex (area 4). His motor speech is also compromised, which indicates a lesion involving the left inferior frontal gyrus (Broca's area). Both of these areas are supplied by the superior division of the left MCA.

A lesion in the superior division of the right MCA (**A**) would result in weakness of the left arm and face. Also, Broca's area is only present in the dominant (left unless otherwise specified) hemisphere, so motor speech, most likely, would not be affected.

A lesion in the inferior division of the right MCA (**B**) would most likely cause a profound left hemineglect (involvement of parietal heteromodal association areas in nondominant hemisphere). Left visual field (visual association cortex) and somatosensory (primary somatosensory and parietal association cortices) deficits might be present, but motor weakness is unlikely.

A lesion in the inferior division of the left MCA (**D**) would most likely cause Wernicke's aphasia (left superior temporal gyrus), but motor speech would not be affected. Right-sided visual and somatosensory loss might also be present.

ACA (**E** and **F**) lesions often cause sensorimotor deficits affecting the lower limbs. Grasp reflex and frontal lobe behavior abnormalities might also be present.

2. Correct: Area C (C)

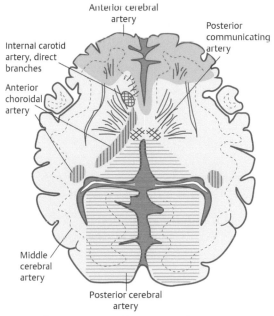

Source: Alberstone C, Benzel E, Najm I et al. Anatomic Basis of Neurologic Diagnosis. 1st Edition. Thieme; 2009.

The arteries of the brain are divided into two systems based on their branches of origin—the internal carotid and the vertebrobasilar systems. Area C in the image is supplied by the posterior cerebral arteries, which are the terminal branches from the basilar artery.

The internal carotid system (or anterior circulation) consists of the internal carotid artery and its terminal branches, the anterior (**A**) and middle cerebral (**D**) arteries. Prior to its terminal bifurcation, the internal carotid artery gives off the ophthalmic, the posterior communicating (**B**), and the anterior choroidal (**E**) arteries. The direct branches of the internal carotid artery can be seen in the region labeled G in the image.

3.   Correct: Middle ethmoidal sinus (D)

The optic canal is traversed by the optic nerve and the ophthalmic artery (branch from internal carotid artery). Important branches of the ophthalmic artery include central artery of retina (supplies optic nerve and retina), posterior ciliary arteries (supply choroid, iris, ciliary body, etc.), lacrimal artery (supplies lacrimal gland, eyelid, and conjunctiva), posterior ethmoidal artery (supplies posterior ethmoidal sinus), anterior ethmoidal artery (supplies anterior and middle ethmoidal air sinuses), and dorsal nasal artery (supplies external nose).

The adenohypophysis (**A**) is primarily supplied by the superior hypophyseal vessels that are given off the supraclinoid segment of internal carotid artery (segment that begins after penetration of dura until its bifurcation into anterior and middle cerebral arteries).

The neurohypophysis (**B**) is primarily supplied by the inferior hypophyseal arteries, which branch off the cavernous segment of the internal carotid artery (segment that passes through cavernous sinus).

The middle ear cavity (**C**) is supplied by tympanic branches of the internal carotid and several branches from the external carotid arteries.

Visual areas of the cerebral cortex (**E**) are primarily supplied by branches from posterior cerebral and middle cerebral arteries.

4.   Correct: Inferior sagittal sinus (B)

The inferior sagittal sinus occupies the posterior two-thirds of falx cerebri and drains into the straight sinus.

The confluence of sinuses is the dilated posterior end of the superior sagittal sinus (**A**).

The straight sinus (**C**) begins as a continuation of inferior sagittal sinus and drains into the confluence of sinuses and left transverse sinus.

The occipital sinus (**D**) is situated along attached margin of falx cerebelli and drains into the confluence of sinuses.

The right transverse sinus (**E**) is situated along the posterior attached margin of tentorium cerebelli. It begins from the confluence of sinuses as the continuation of superior sagittal sinus.

5.   Correct: Right SCA (C)

The patient seems to be suffering from trigeminal neuralgia, which presents with excruciating paroxysmal pain affecting sensory territories supplied by the trigeminal nerve. A frequent cause is compression of the root of the nerve at its exit from the brainstem by aberrant branches of the superior cerebellar artery, on the right side in this case, as determined by the patient's symptoms.

The PICA (**A** and **B**) are the largest branches from the vertebral arteries and are not related to the exit point of the trigeminal nerve at the level of the mid pons.

The AICA (**E** and **F**) are the caudal most branches from the basilar artery. These also are not related to the exit point of the trigeminal nerve at mid pons.

Aberrant branches of the left SCA (**D**) would compress the left trigeminal nerve, which would lead to left facial pain for the patient.

Refer to the following image for answers 6 and 7:

The sagittal section is displaying the anterior cerebral artery and its branches.

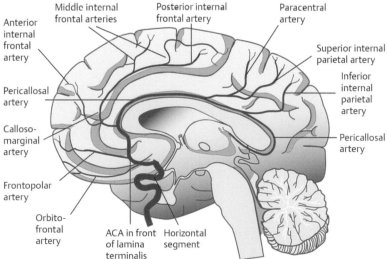

Anterior internal frontal artery

Middle internal frontal arteries

Posterior internal frontal artery

Paracentral artery

Superior internal parietal artery

Inferior internal parietal artery

Pericallosal artery

Pericallosal artery

Callosomarginal artery

Frontopolar artery

Orbitofrontal artery

ACA in front of lamina terminalis

Horizontal segment

Source: Alberstone C, Benzel E, Najm I et al. Anatomic Basis of Neurologic Diagnosis. 1st Edition. Thieme; 2009.

6. Correct: Area H (E)

The pericallosal artery (Areas A and H [**E**]) is a continuation of the anterior cerebral artery that courses over the superior aspect of the corpus callosum, readily identifiable in the image.

The posterior internal frontal artery (Area D [**A**]) supplies the anterior third of the internal surface of the superior frontal gyrus, as well as the anterior portion of the cingulate gyrus.

The paracentral artery (Area E [**B**]), a branch from the pericallosal artery, supplies the paracentral lobule.

The superior (Area F [**C**]) and the inferior (Area G [**D**]) internal parietal arteries supply the internal aspect of the parietal lobe. The superior internal parietal artery is often the largest branch of the anterior cerebral artery.

7. Correct: Area D (A)

The posterior internal frontal artery (Area D [**A**]) supplies the anterior third of the internal surface of the superior frontal gyrus, as well as the anterior portion of the cingulate gyrus.

The paracentral artery (Area E [**B**]), a branch from the pericallosal artery, supplies the paracentral lobule.

The superior (Area F [**C**]) and the inferior (Area G [**D**]) internal parietal arteries supply the internal aspect of the parietal lobe. The posterior aspect of the pericallosal artery (Area H [**E**]) travels along the pericallosal cistern giving off small branches to the corpus callosum, forming the pericallosal moustache (so named for its likeness to a poorly groomed moustache that outlines the superior surface of the corpus callosum).

8. Correct: Cerebral part of internal carotid artery (D)

Clinical features for the patient correspond to prolactinoma, which is a hormone-secreting pituitary tumor. This is characterized by excess synthesis and secretion of prolactin, a result of hyperactivity of lactotrophs within the anterior pituitary gland (adenohypophysis). The adenohypophysis is primarily supplied by the superior hypophyseal vessels that are given off the supraclinoid segment of the cerebral part of the internal carotid artery.

Normally, the cervical part of the internal carotid artery (**A**) has no branches, and would not supply the structure in question.

The petrous part of the internal carotid artery (**B**, within carotid canal) provides caroticotympanic branches and branches to the pterygoid canal.

The cavernous part of the internal carotid artery (**C**, within cavernous sinus) provides inferior hypophyseal and meningeal branches.

Major branches from the basilar artery (**E**) are the anterior inferior cerebellar, labyrinthine, pontine, superior cerebellar, and posterior cerebral arteries.

9. Correct: Terminal part of sigmoid sinus (F)

Hoarseness of voice and an inability to shrug her shoulders indicate vagus and accessory nerve involvement for this patient, respectively. Both of these nerves exit the skull through the jugular foramina. The sigmoid sinus also passes through the jugular foramina and is continuous with the superior bulb of the internal jugular vein. A thrombus lodged within the terminal part of the sigmoid sinus, therefore, has the maximum chance to involve structures passing through the jugular foramen.

The cavernous (**A**), superior sagittal (**B**), and right (**C**) and left (**D**) transverse sinuses are not related to the jugular foramen.

10. Correct: Long circumferential branches of right basilar artery (A)

Involvement of both upper and lower facial muscles indicate a lower motor neuron type of facial (Bell's) palsy. Lesion of the right facial motor nucleus (supplied by long circumferential branches of the right basilar artery) is a probable cause.

Involvement of similar branches for the left basilar artery (**B**) would cause left facial palsy.

Ischemic stroke of lateral striate branches of the MCA (**C** and **D**) would involve corticobulbar fibers for the facial nucleus. Such involvement would most likely present with contralateral lower face palsy with sparing of the upper face.

Compression of the facial nerve root by aberrant branches from the AICA (**E** and **F**) might cause ipsilateral facial palsy. However, these patients are likely to present with additional symptoms including vertigo, tinnitus, or hearing loss due to involvement of the adjacent vestibulocochlear nerve.

Consider the following explanation for answers 11 and 12:

The patient seems to be suffering from sensory aphasia, which is due to involvement of Wernicke's area (left superior temporal gyrus). This, along with right homonymous hemianopia, indicates an extensive lesion affecting the inferior division of the left MCA.

11. Correct: Left MCA, inferior division (D)

A lesion in the superior division of the right MCA (**A**) would result in weakness of the left arm and face due to involvement of primary motor cortex.

A lesion in the inferior division of the right MCA (**B**) would most likely cause a profound left hemineglect (parietal heteromodal association areas in nondominant hemisphere), constructional apraxia, and/or left visual field defects (visual association cortex). Additionally, somatosensory deficits (primary somatosensory and parietal association cortex) may be present.

A lesion in the superior division of the left MCA (**C**) would most likely result in weakness of the right arm and face (primary motor cortex). It might also be accompanied by motor (Broca's) aphasia due to involvement of the left inferior frontal gyrus.

A lesion in the right PCA (**E**) will most often cause left-sided homonymous hemianopia. In rare cases, visual or color anomia may be present.

Lesion in the left PCA (**F**) will cause right-sided homonymous hemianopia. Extensive involvement might cause transcortical aphasia, which might mimic Wernicke's aphasia except for the fact that repetition will be intact. In rare cases, alexia without agraphia may be present.

12.   Correct: Sensory loss in right arm (A)

Lesion in the inferior division of the left MCA will cause right-sided somatosensory deficits (due to involvement of primary somatosensory and parietal association cortices).

Sensory loss in left arm (**B**, involvement of right MCA inferior division), paralysis of arm (**C** and **D**, involvement of MCA superior divisions), and paralysis of leg (**E** and **F**, involvement of ACA) would not be usual findings in this case.

13.   Correct: Area C (C)

The circle of Willis shown in the following image is an anastomotic connection between the vertebrobasilar and internal carotid systems. Aneurysms of the anterior communicating artery are the most common circle of Willis aneurysms and can cause visual field defects such as bitemporal heteronymous hemianopsia (due to compression of the optic chiasm).

14.   Correct: Bifurcation of basilar artery (A)

The patient is suffering from oculomotor nerve palsy. Inhibition of medial and vertical gaze due to paralysis of superior, medial, and inferior rectus, and inferior oblique muscles is responsible for diplopia. Inhibition of preganglionic parasympathetic fibers originating from the Edinger–Westphal nucleus is responsible for mydriasis due to inhibition of the sphincter pupillae muscle, which acts as a constrictor of pupil. The oculomotor nerve (CN III) emerges between the posterior cerebral and superior cerebellar arteries within the interpeduncular fossa, at the junction of the midbrain and pons. It can be damaged by aneurysms affecting the basilar bifurcation, posterior communicating arteries, P1 segment of posterior cerebral arteries, or the origin of superior cerebellar arteries.

The other arteries listed are located inferior to the course of the oculomotor nerve and are therefore not related to its injuries.

15.   Correct: Anterior choroidal artery (E)

Hemiplegia and hemianesthesia affecting the same side of the body strongly suggests involvement of the posterior limb of the contralateral internal capsule. The additional symptom of homonymous hemianopia suggests involvement of the optic radiation, which passes through the retrolenticular limb of internal capsule. The anterior choroidal artery supplies both the posterior and retrolenticular limbs of the internal capsule.

Although the lateral striate branches (**A**) of the MCA supply the posterior limb of the internal capsule, their lesions would not be expected to cause homonymous hemianopia.

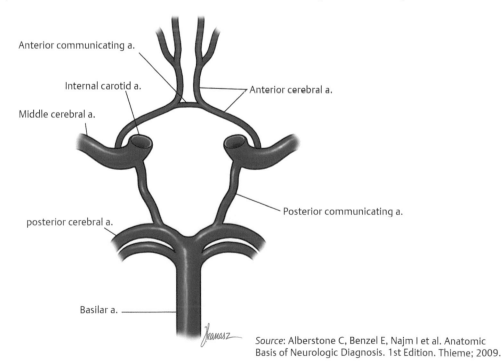

Source: Alberstone C, Benzel E, Najm I et al. Anatomic Basis of Neurologic Diagnosis. 1st Edition. Thieme; 2009.

A lesion of the superior division of the MCA (**B**, involvement of precentral gyrus) might cause hemiplegia but not hemianesthesia.

A lesion of the inferior division of the MCA (**C**, involvement of postcentral gyrus) might cause hemianesthesia but not hemiplegia.

Lastly, a lesion of the PCA (**D**, involvement of visual and parts of sensory association cortices) might cause homonymous hemianopia, rarely hemianesthesia, but never hemiplegia.

16. Correct: Lateral striate branches of right MCA (C)

Left-sided lower facial weakness indicates right UMN lesion of the facial nerve. Left deviation of tongue (paralyzed left genioglossus) indicates right UMN lesion of the hypoglossal nerve. Right deviation of uvula on attempt to say "ah" (paralyzed left levator veli palatini) indicates right UMN lesion of the vagus nerve. The combination of all three localizes the lesion to the genu of the right internal capsule (lesion of corticonuclear fibers, supplied by lateral striate branches of MCA and anterior choroidal artery).

Long circumferential branches of the basilar artery (**A** and **B**) supply the motor nucleus of facial nerve. Lesions of these branches would cause ipsilateral complete facial palsy. Lesions for the hypoglossal or vagus nerve would not be expected.

Lateral striate branches of the left MCA (**D**) supply the genu of the left internal capsule. Their lesions would likely result in right sided facial palsy, right deviation of tongue on protrusion, and left deviation of uvula on attempt to say "ah."

Posterior inferior cerebellar arterial lesion (**E** and **F**) would affect the nucleus ambiguus. The consequent vagal palsy would result in uvular deviation on attempt to say "ah." However, facial and hypoglossal palsies would not be seen.

Consider the following explanations for answers 17 and 18:

Loss of pain and thermal sense on the left side of the face (involvement of left trigeminal nucleus and tract) and right-sided trunk (involvement of left anterolateral system) suggests a left medullary lesion. Given the lateral location of these nuclei and fibers within the medulla, the diagnosis of left lateral medullary syndrome can be made.

17. Correct: PICA (C)

The affected vessel for such a lateral medullary syndrome is commonly the PICA.

The anterior spinal artery (**A**) primarily supplies the medial structures of the medulla (pyramids, medial lemniscus, medial longitudinal fasciculus, hypoglossal nucleus, and the inferior olivary nucleus). The AICA (**B**) primarily supplies the lateral part of the pons and the ventral and inferior surfaces of the cerebellum. The SCA (**D**) primarily supplies the rostral pons, caudal midbrain, and the superior surface of the cerebellum. Basilar artery (**E**) involvement would most commonly result in visual loss (due to involvement of visual cortex) and altered consciousness (due to involvement of the thalamus).

18. Correct: Miosis of left eye (E)

Lateral medullary syndrome often affects the left hypothalamospinal fibers causing left-sided Horner's syndrome (miosis, ptosis, anhidrosis, and flushing of face).

A paralysis of the arm (**A** and **B**) might occur with a lesion of the pyramidal tract, while a loss of vibratory sense (**C** and **D**) could occur due to involvement of the medial lemniscus. Given the medial location of these structures within the medulla, these are often involved in medial medullary syndrome, which often results from occlusion of the anterior spinal artery.

Miosis of the right eye (**F**) would be inconsistent with the laterality of symptoms reported in this case.

19. Correct: Area C (C)

The anterior choroidal artery originates from the internal carotid artery and supplies several brain structures including the choroid plexus, optic chiasm, optic tract, internal capsule, lateral geniculate body, globus pallidus, tail of the caudate nucleus, hippocampus, amygdala, and substantia nigra. Disruptions of blood flow affecting this artery often result in hemiplegia and hemihypoesthesia on the contralesional side of the body.

Areas A, B, D, and E (**A, B, D,** and **E**) are supplied by the anterior vertebral, PCommA, PCA and MCA, respectively.

20. Correct: Area D (D)

The posterior cerebral artery provides blood flow to the posterior aspect of the brain, such as the occipital and inferior temporal lobes. Depending on the location and extent of the blockage, clinical manifestations will vary. Distal occlusions often result in visual deficits, such as agnosia, prosopagnosia (as in this case), or cortical blindness.

Areas A, B, C, and E (**A, B, C,** and **E**) are supplied by the anterior vertebral, PCommA, anterior choroidal, and MCA, respectively.

Chapter 4

Development of the Nervous System

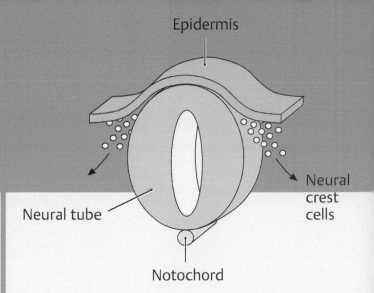

Epidermis

Neural tube

Neural crest cells

Notochord

LEARNING OBJECTIVES

- ▶ Describe the development and blood supply of the pituitary gland.
- ▶ Analyze the etiopathogenesis, clinical features, diagnosis, and complications of Chiari malformations.
- ▶ Trace the development of cranial nerve nuclei; correlate these with their functions.
- ▶ Formulate the pathway for the corneal reflex. Trace the development of motor and sensory components of cranial nerves.
- ▶ Analyze the etiopathogenesis, clinical features, and diagnosis of lissencephaly.
- ▶ Analyze the etiopathogenesis, clinical features, diagnosis, and complications of NTDs.
- ▶ Determine the distribution and fate of neural crest cells during development. Illustrate the structure and functions of central and peripheral glia.
- ▶ Analyze the etiopathogenesis, clinical features, and diagnosis of glossopharyngeal neuralgia. Trace the development of motor and sensory components of cranial nerves.
- ▶ Analyze the etiopathogenesis, clinical features, diagnosis, and complications of congenital aqueductal stenosis. List the primary and secondary brain vesicles and trace their derivatives in human.
- ▶ Formulate the pathway for taste sensation.
- ▶ Analyze the etiopathogenesis, clinical features, and diagnosis of holoprosencephaly.
- ▶ Analyze the etiopathogenesis, clinical features, and diagnosis of tethered cord syndrome.
- ▶ Trace the histogenesis of the developing neural tube.
- ▶ Evaluate the timeline of events or stages in embryology by identifying key stages and their unique vulnerabilities.
- ▶ Differentiate between developmental cortical malformations.

4.1 Questions

Easy	Medium	Hard

1. A 23-year-old pregnant woman shows up for a routine second-trimester checkup. Fetal ultrasonography reveals a cavernous sinus thrombosis, specifically affecting the inferior hypophyseal branch of the internal carotid artery. Which of the following is the embryonic source for the zone within the pituitary gland that will primarily be affected?

A. Endoderm

B. Surface ectoderm

C. Neuroectoderm

D. Neural crest cells

E. Somitic mesoderm

Consider the following case for questions 2 and 3:

A 6-year-old girl is brought to the physician because of headaches and neck pain. A CT scan shows herniation of the cerebellar tonsils through the foramen magnum, and a small posterior cranial fossa. No other structural abnormalities are present.

2. Which of the following best describes this finding?

A. Chiari type I malformation

B. Arnold–Chiari malformation

C. Dandy–Walker malformation

D. Holoprosencephaly

E. Lissencephaly

3. Which of the following is the underlying cause for her defects?

A. Defective somitogenesis

B. Lack of distension of embryonic ventricular system

C. Defective neural tube closure

D. Defective neural crest cell migration

E. Defective neuroblast migration

4. A 3-day-old male neonate presents with significant difficulty with suckling and swallowing. Physical findings are significant for absent facial and jaw movements. Eye and tongue movements appear normal for the age. Which of the following would explain this combination of deficits?

A. Defect in the motor nucleus of facial nerve

B. Defect in the motor nucleus of trigeminal nerve

C. Defect in the general somatic efferent cell columns

D. Defect in the general visceral efferent cell columns

E. Defect in the special visceral efferent cell columns

5. A 60-year-old woman is undergoing a follow-up neurological examination during her recovery from a stroke. When a wisp of cotton is touched to her left cornea, she blinks. Which of the following is the source of cell bodies involved in the primary afferent limb of this reflex?

A. Ectoderm

B. Neuroectoderm

C. Neural crest

D. A + B

E. A + C

6. A 6-month-old baby presents with microcephaly, hypotonia, profound mental retardation, and seizures. An MRI of the brain reveals grossly abnormal outline comprising reduced number of sulci, overall shallow sulci, and sylvian fissures, as well as gross cortical thickening. Which of the following fetal defects is consistent with these findings?

A. Failure of regression of Rathke's pouch

B. Failure of closure of the rostral neuropore

C. Failure of closure of caudal neuropore

D. Failure of migration of neural crest cells

E. Failure of migration of neuroblasts

7. A 23-year-old female presents with a dimple and a tuft of hair over the lower lumbar region of the vertebral column. She was asymptomatic and had shown up for regular checkup. There were no sensorimotor deficits noted during a detailed neurological examination. Plain radiograph revealed missing neural arches involving several lumbar vertebrae. Which of the following is a true statement regarding her?

A. MRI is most likely to detect incomplete dura and arachnoid mater covering the spinal cord

B. MRI is most likely to detect cystic dilatation of several segments of the spinal cord

C. Antenatal diagnosis of this condition could have been possible by noting decreased α-fetoprotein levels in maternal serum

D. Prevention of this condition might have been possible by maternal consumption of folic acid

E. Defective gastrulation is the primary cause for this defect in her

8. A 26-year-old first-time mother suffers from a viral illness during the third week of her pregnancy. The virus has a known inclination toward cells that form chromaffin cells of the adrenal medulla. Which of the following might also be defective in the fetus?

A. Scar formation during wound healing following injury to brain

B. Myelination of spinal cord tracts

C. Sensation from skin of the upper limb

D. Modulation of neuronal activities by buffering K^+ concentration in the extracellular space of the brain

E. Phagocytosis of microorganisms invading the brain

9. A 48-year-old man presents with a 2-year history of severe, transient, and stabbing pain that initiates in the right side of the throat. It gradually radiates to the base of his tongue, right ear, and occasionally beneath the angle of the right jaw. The paroxysmal attacks are frequently precipitated by swallowing of cold drinks. Which of the specific segments of the CNS does the affected structure in the individual connect to?

A. Telencephalon

B. Diencephalon

C. Mesencephalon

D. Metencephalon

E. Myelencephalon

Consider the following case for questions 10 and 11:

A 3-day-old girl presents with enlarging head size, bulging fontanelles, and gaping cranial sutures. Postnatal MRI is suggestive of congenital aqueductal stenosis.

10. Which of the following would be the least likely finding in this patient?

A. Headache

B. Sunset eye sign

C. Dilated lateral ventricles

D. Dilated third ventricle

E. Dilated fourth ventricle

11. Which of the following embryonic segments contributes to the development of the obstructed structure in her?

A. Diencephalon

B. Mesencephalon

C. Metencephalon

D. Myelencephalon

E. Telencephalon

12. A 39-year-old woman suffers a stroke involving the posterior inferior cerebellar artery that causes specific damage to the brainstem special somatic afferent column. Sensation from which of the following structures will be compromised?

A. Facial skin

B. Taste buds

C. Cochlea

D. Smooth muscle of esophagus

E. Striated muscle of face

13. A 48-year-old female presents with loss of taste sensation from the pharyngeal part of her tongue. Which of the following is the embryonic source for cell bodies of the involved primary afferent neurons?

A. Ectoderm

B. Neuroectoderm

C. Neural crest

D. A + B

E. A + C

14. A 28-week fetal ultrasound in a 20-year-old pregnant mother provided evidence of an absent interhemispheric fissure and corpus callosum, fused thalami, and fused cerebral hemispheres with one cerebral ventricle. The neonate, delivered preterm at 32 weeks, was born with cyclopia and macroglossia. Which of the following is a true statement regarding this anomaly?

A. Oligohydramnios, detected by antenatal ultrasound, is a common association

B. Maternal alcohol consumption is a frequent cause

C. Trisomy 21 is a common association

D. A + B

E. B + C

F. A + C

15. A second-trimester fetal ultrasound in a 28-year-old woman shows a midline cystic mass overlying the occipital bone that contains echoes from herniated brain tissue. Laboratory findings for her were within normal limits other than elevated serum α-fetoprotein. Which of the following fetal defects is consistent with these findings?

A. Failure of regression of Rathke's pouch

B. Failure of closure of the rostral neuropore

C. Failure of closure of caudal neuropore

D. Failure of migration of neural crest cells

E. Failure of migration of neuroblasts

16. An 18-year-old girl presents with overflow incontinence. On examination, she has decreased power around the ankle with absent reflex. Her sensation of pain and touch was lost in lateral side of foot with saddle type of perianal anesthesia. Lumbosacral bony defect was evident in X-ray spine. MRI identified extension of the conus medullaris to the disc between L3 and L4 vertebrae, and a thickened filum terminale. Which of the following is the most probable embryological basis for her problems?

A. Defective migration of neural crest cells

B. Defective histogenesis of the developing neural tube

C. Mechanical traction of spinal cord due to restricted mobility

D. Slower growth of spinal cord relative to vertebral column

E. Accelerated growth of thoracic spinal segments

17. A second-trimester ultrasound in a 42-year-old woman suggests a developmental defect affecting the neuroectoderm of the diencephalon segment of the neural tube. Which of the following organs might be at risk in the newborn, if the course of remaining of the pregnancy stays otherwise uneventful?

A. Cerebral cortex

B. Cerebellar cortex

C. Adenohypophysis

D. Neurohypophysis

E. Medulla oblongata

18. A 48-year-old female, being treated with colchicine (a drug that arrests mitosis) for chronic gout, finds out that she is 4-week pregnant. Cells within which of the following layers of the neural tube in the developing embryo would mostly be affected?

A. Marginal layer

B. Mantle layer

C. Ventricular layer

D. Marginal and mantle layers

E. Marginal, mantle, and ventricular layers

19. A 23-year-old pregnant woman shows up for a routine second-trimester checkup. Fetal ultrasonography reveals a neural mass protruding through arch defects in lower lumbar vertebrae. At what week of gestation did this defect most likely occur?

A. 1 to 3

B. 4 to 8

C. 9 to 11

D. 12 to 15

E. 16 to 19

20. A 7-month-old infant was brought in for growth retardation. He has vomited few times a week for the past 2 months. MRI of brain for the infant suggests a unilateral cortical cleft that has penetrated into the ventricular system. The cleft, as noted in the following image, is lined by cortical neurons.

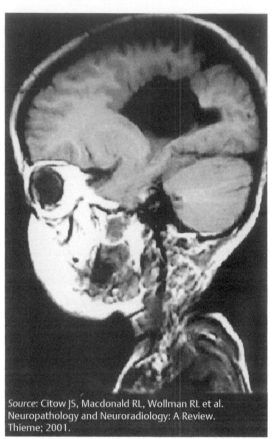

Source: Citow JS, Macdonald RL, Wollman RL et al. Neuropathology and Neuroradiology: A Review. Thieme; 2001.

Which of the following is the most likely diagnosis for him?

A. Lissencephaly

B. Schizencephaly

C. Holoprosencephaly

D. Anencephaly

E. Porencephaly

4.2 Answers and Explanations

Easy	Medium	Hard

1.   Correct: Neuroectoderm (C)

The inferior hypophyseal artery, off the cavernous part of the internal carotid artery, primarily supplies the pars nervosa of the neurohypophysis. This zone of the pituitary gland develops from neuroectoderm (as an outgrowth from the diencephalon).

The ectoderm of Rathke's pouch (**B**) contributes for the development of adenohypophysis (primarily supplied by superior hypophyseal branch off the cerebral part of internal carotid artery).

Endoderm (**A**), neural crest (**D**), and mesoderm (**E**) do not contribute toward the formation of pituitary gland.

Consider the following for answers 2 and 3:

Chiari malformations refer to a group of congenital hindbrain abnormalities affecting the structural relationships between the cerebellum, brainstem, upper cervical cord, and the skull base.

2.   Correct: Chiari type I malformation (A)

In type I, the cerebellar tonsils displace into the upper cervical canal through the foramen magnum.

Displacement of the medulla, fourth ventricle, and cerebellar vermis through the foramen magnum occur in type II (**B**, Arnold–Chiari malformation).

Dandy–Walker malformation (**C**) is characterized by agenesis or hypoplasia of the cerebellar vermis, cystic dilatation of the fourth ventricle, and enlargement of the posterior fossa.

Holoprosencephaly (**D**) occurs when the prosencephalon fails to cleave down the midline such that the telencephalon contains a single ventricle.

Lissencephaly (**E**) is a heterogeneous group of disorders of cortical formation characterized by a smooth brain, with absent or hypoplastic sulci.

3.   Correct: Defective somitogenesis (A)

In type I Chiari malformation, an underdeveloped occipital bone, possibly due to underdevelopment of the occipital somite originating from the paraxial mesoderm, induces overcrowding in the posterior cranial fossa, which contains the normally developed hindbrain.

The cause of Chiari II malformation in children born with a myelomeningocele can be explained by the lack of distention of the embryonic ventricular system (**B**). Defective neural tube closure (**C**) precludes the accumulation of fluid and pressure within the ventricles. This distention is critical to normal brain development. Decompression of the brain vesicles causes overcrowding in the posterior fossa and changes in the fetal skull.

Failure of migration of neural crest cells (**D**, neurocristopathies) or neuroblasts (**E**, causing agyria, pachygyria, heterotopia, etc.) are not known to contribute to Chiari malformations.

4.   Correct: Defect in the special visceral efferent cell columns (E)

The neonate presents with absent facial (muscles innervated by motor nucleus of facial nerve) and jaw (muscles innervated by motor nucleus of trigeminal nerve) movements, and difficulty in swallowing (muscles innervated by nucleus ambiguous). These nuclei belong to the special visceral efferent (branchiomotor) cell columns.

A defect in the motor nucleus of the facial (**A**) nerve would not cause absent jaw movements or difficulty in swallowing.

A defect in the motor nucleus of the trigeminal (**B**) nerve would not cause absent facial movements or difficulty in swallowing.

The general somatic efferent column (**C**) includes oculomotor, trochlear, abducens, and hypoglossal nuclei. Normal eye and tongue movements in this patient preclude their involvement.

The general visceral efferent column (**D**) innervates glands and smooth muscles. This includes the Edinger–Westphal, superior and inferior salivatory, and dorsal vagal nuclei. No indications for their involvement are present in this case.

5.   Correct: A + C (E)

The corneal reflex is initiated by the free nerve endings in the cornea and involves the trigeminal nerve and ganglion, the spinal trigeminal tract and nucleus, interneurons in the reticular formation, motor neurons in the facial nucleus and nerve, and the orbicularis oculi. The cell body of the primary afferent neuron lies in the trigeminal (semilunar) ganglia, which develop from both neural crest (**C**) and trigeminal placode (localized regions of columnar epithelium that develop from ectoderm, **A**). No known direct contribution from the neuroectoderm (**B and D**) exists.

6.   Correct: Failure of migration of neuroblasts (E)

The neonate is suffering from lissencephaly (absence of cortical gyri) and possibly from neuronal heterotopia (normal neurons in abnormal locations), both of which are caused due to neuroblast migration defects.

Rathke's pouch is an ectodermal outpouching of stomodeum which forms the adenohypophysis of the pituitary gland. The lumen of the pouch narrows to form a Rathke's cleft that normally regresses. Persistence of this cleft is believed to cause Rathke's cleft cyst and/or craniopharyngioma (**A**).

Failure in the closure of the rostral (**B**) or caudal (**C**) neuropore causes NTDs; failure of migration of neural crest cells (**D**) is termed neurocristopathy—none of these defects contribute toward lissencephaly.

7.   Correct: Prevention of this condition might have been possible by maternal consumption of folic acid (D)

She is suffering from spina bifida occulta, the most common and least severe of NTDs. This occurs due to failure of closure of one or several vertebral arches posteriorly; the meninges and spinal cord are normal. A dimple or small lipoma may overlie the defect. Most cases are asymptomatic and discovered incidentally. Folic acid supplements at the time of conception and in the first 12 weeks of pregnancy reduce the incidence of NTDs in the fetus by ~70%.

Incomplete cover of dura and arachnoid mater (**A**, meningocele) or cystic dilatation of several segments of the spinal cord (**B**, syringomyelia) is highly unlikely to be asymptomatic.

Antenatal diagnosis of NTDs is possible by finding elevated levels of α-fetoprotein levels in maternal serum or amniotic fluid (**C**).

Gastrulation (**E**) is the process of forming three definitive germ layers in the embryo. Spina bifida is the result of failure of closure of the posterior neuropore, which indicates defective neurulation. Less severe forms, such as spina bifida occulta, are result of failure of secondary neurulation (debatable in human).

8. Correct: Sensation from skin of the upper limb (C)

The virus targets the neural crest cells (truncal), which gives rise to chromaffin cells of adrenal medulla. Truncal neural crest cells also form dorsal root ganglia (cell bodies of somatic sensory nerves). Disruption of these truncal neural crest cells, therefore, might also lead to somatosensory loss.

Scar formation during wound healing following injury to the brain (**A**) and K+ spatial buffering (**D**) are important functions of astrocytes that develop from the neuroepithelium (neuroectoderm).

Myelination of the CNS (**B**) is a function of oligodendrocytes. These cells also develop from neuroepithelium (neuroectoderm).

Phagocytosis of microorganisms invading the brain (**E**) is a function of microglia. These cells develop from mesenchymal progenitors within the bone marrow.

9. Correct: Myelencephalon (E)

The patient is suffering from glossopharyngeal neuralgia. Clusters of unilateral attacks of sharp, stabbing, and shooting pain localized in the throat radiating to the ear or vice versa are characteristic of glossopharyngeal neuralgia. The distribution of pain is diagnostic: it usually starts in the pharynx, tonsil, and tongue base, and then rapidly involves the eustachian tube and inner ear or spreads to the mandibular angle. Swallowing of cold liquids is the most common trigger factor. The glossopharyngeal nerve (CN IX) is attached to the medulla oblongata, which is derived from the myelencephalon.

CN I and II are attached to the forebrain (derived from the telencephalon [**A**] and diencephalon [**B**], respectively). CN III and IV attach to the midbrain (derived from the mesencephalon, **C**). CN V is attached to the pons (derived from the metencephalon, **D**). CN VI, VII, and VIII attach to the pontomedullary junction. CN IX, X, XI, and XII attach to the medulla.

Consider the following for answers 10 and 11:

This patient has clinical features of congenital aqueductal stenosis, which commonly presents with obstructive hydrocephalus.

10. Correct: Dilated fourth ventricle (E)

Since the obstruction lies at the level of the aqueduct of Sylvius, the fourth ventricle is usually of normal size. The lateral (**C**) and third (**D**) ventricles are often dilated consequent to the obstruction. The usual symptoms and signs of raised intracranial pressure and hydrocephalus are headache (**A**), vomiting, decreased conscious state, and sunset eye sign (**B**, upgaze paresis with the eyes appearing driven downward).

11. Correct: Mesencephalon (B)

The obstruction lies at the level of the aqueduct of Sylvius, which is the cavity of the midbrain. A developmental defect in the mesencephalon, therefore, would cause the condition reported.

The diencephalon (**A**) and telencephalon (**E**) give rise to forebrain structures. The metencephalon (**C**) and myelencephalon (**D**) give rise to hindbrain structures.

12. Correct: Cochlea (C)

The special somatic afferent column in the brainstem includes the vestibulocochlear nuclei. Hence, hearing and balance sensation from the inner ear will most likely be affected.

Sensation from the skin (**A**) and striated muscle (**E**, proprioception) of the face relay to the general somatic afferent column (trigeminal sensory nuclei).

Sensation from the taste buds (**B**, special visceral afferent) and smooth muscles of esophagus (**D**, general visceral afferent) relays back to the nucleus solitarius.

13. Correct: Ectoderm (A)

The glossopharyngeal nerve supplies the pharyngeal part (posterior one-third) of the tongue. Cell bodies for the primary afferent neurons lie in the inferior glossopharyngeal (petrosal) ganglia, which develop from the second epibranchial placode. These placodes are localized regions of columnar epithelium that develop from ectoderm.

No direct contribution from the neuroectoderm (**B** and **D**) or neural crest (**C** and **E**) to the inferior glossopharyngeal ganglion is known to exist.

Note that the cell bodies for second-order sensory neurons are located in the nucleus of the solitary tract, and those for third-order neurons are located in the VPM of thalamus. The VPM projects to the ipsilateral gustatory cortex.

14. Correct: Maternal alcohol consumption is a frequent cause (B)

The neonate is suffering from holoprosencephaly (alobar).

The fundamental problem is a failure of the developing prosencephalon to divide into left and right halves (which normally occur at the end of the fifth week of gestation). This results in variable loss of midline structures of the brain and face as well as fusion of lateral ventricles and the third ventricle.

Environmental factors such as maternal diabetes mellitus, alcohol use, and retinoic acid have been implicated in the pathogenesis of holoprosencephaly, as has mutation of several genes including sonic hedgehog.

On antenatal ultrasound, there may be evidence of polyhydramnios (not oligohydramnios—**A**, **D**, and **F**), a secondary feature due to impaired fetal swallowing.

Trisomy 13 (most common) and trisomy 18 have been frequently associated with holoprosencephaly, but not trisomy 21 (**C**, **E**, and **F**).

15. Correct: Failure of closure of the rostral neuropore (B)

The fetus is suffering from an occipital encephalocele. This is an NTD caused due to defective closure of the rostral neuropore, where brain tissue encased in meninges herniates out through a defect in the cranium.

Rathke's pouch is an ectodermal outpouching of stomodeum, which forms the adenohypophysis of the pituitary gland. The lumen of the pouch narrows to form a Rathke's cleft that normally regresses. Persistence of this cleft is believed to cause Rathke's cleft cyst and/or craniopharyngioma (**A**).

Failure of closure of caudal neuropore (**C**) causes spinal dysraphism (meningocele, meningomyelocele, etc.) commonly involving lumbosacral segments.

Failure of migration of neural crest cells (**D**, neurocristopathies) or neuroblasts (**E**, causing agyria, pachygyria, heterotopia, etc.) does not contribute to encephalocele.

16. Correct: Mechanical traction of spinal cord due to restricted mobility (C)

The girl is suffering from tethered cord syndrome, in which the thickened filum tethers the cord to the sacrum. Diagnosis is made by low-lying conus (below the L2 vertebral level) and a thick filum, when accompanied by neurogenic bladder with sensorimotor deficits of the lower limb.

At week 8 of gestation, the spinal cord extends the length of the spinal canal. For the remainder of gestation, the bony spinal elements outgrow the spinal cord (**D**). This results in ascension of the conus to the normal position (lower border of L1 in adults and L3 in infants). Tethering prevents this rostral ascension. Partial traction on the cord can result in progressive ischemia, leading to lumbosacral neuronal dysfunction, which is manifest in neurological, musculoskeletal, and urological abnormalities.

Defective migration of neural crest cells (**A**), defective histogenesis of neural tube (**B**), or accelerated growth of thoracic spinal segments (**E**) does not contribute to the syndrome.

17. Correct: Neurohypophysis (D)

Neurohypophysis, or posterior pituitary, develops from the infundibulum, which is a downward extension of neural ectoderm from the floor of the diencephalon.

Cerebral cortex (**A**) develops from telencephalon; cerebellar cortex (**B**) develops from metencephalon; adenohypophysis (**C**), or anterior pituitary, develops from Rathke's pouch (upward extension of oral ectoderm from roof of stomodeum); and medulla oblongata (**E**) develops from myelencephalon.

18. Correct: Ventricular layer (C)

Colchicine, a microtubule growth inhibitor, affects mitosis and other microtubule-dependent functions of cells. With the beginning of cellular differentiation in the neural tube, the layer of cells closest to the lumen of the neural tube remains epithelial and is called the ventricular zone. This zone, which still contains mitotic cells, ultimately becomes the ependyma.

Farther from the ventricular zone is the intermediate (formerly called mantle) zone, which contains the cell bodies of the differentiating postmitotic neuroblasts (**B**, future gray matter). As the neuroblasts continue to produce axonal and dendritic processes, these processes form a peripheral marginal zone (**A**, future white matter).

19. Correct: 4 to 8 (B)

The embryonic period (weeks 4–8) is most vulnerable to teratogens and structural defects. The fetus is suffering from myelomeningocele consequent to defective closure of neural tube. The rostral and caudal neuropores normally close during late fourth week.

The germinal period (**A**, weeks 1–3) is characterized by high rate of spontaneous abortions, chromosomal abnormalities being the leading cause.

Weeks 9 through 19 (**C**, **D**, and **E**) are not considered as vulnerable to teratogens as the embryonic period. These are times when most organ systems grow and mature, rather than form.

20. Correct: Schizencephaly (B)

Schizencephaly can be diagnosed by cortical clefts that penetrate to the ventricular system, often occurring in areas of polymicrogyria. Severity of symptoms is related to the size of the cleft and a patent cleft opening.

Lissencephaly (**A**) can be diagnosed by reduced number of enlarged gyri (pachygyria), consequent to neuronal migration defects. It might be associated with mutations of the doublecortin gene (X-linked) or LIS-1 gene (autosomal dominant).

Holoprosencephaly (**C**) refers to a failure of prosencephalon to cleave down the midline resulting in a single ventricle for the prosencephalon. A smooth cortical surface without gyri or sulci is the usual finding.

Anencephaly (**D**) refers to nondevelopment of brain tissue due to defective closure of the anterior neuropore.

Porencephaly (**E**) mimics schizencephaly except for the facts that clefts tend to be symmetric and bilateral, and gray matter does not extend into the cleft.

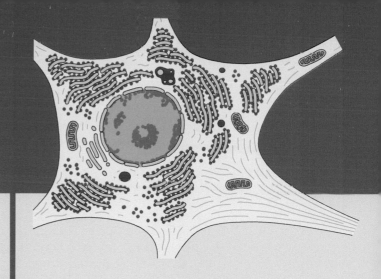

Chapter 5

Histology of the Nervous System

LEARNING OBJECTIVES

▶ Illustrate anterograde and retrograde axonal transport. Determine the needs for slow and fast axonal transports.

▶ Analyze the role of Schwann cells, with respect to both myelinated and unmyelinated neurons. Determine the pathophysiology of Charcot–Marie–Tooth disease and predict the clinical outcomes.

▶ Illustrate the microscopic structure of central and peripheral glia (astrocytes, oligodendrocytes, microglia, ependyma, Schwann cells, and satellite cells); correlate their ultrastructure to their development and functions.

▶ List the cells within the cerebellar cortex and analyze how they fit in the microscopic circuitry.

▶ Analyze neural responses to injury in the CNS and PNS; illustrate axonal and perikaryal changes in response to such injury.

▶ Illustrate the microscopic structure of spinal and autonomic ganglia; correlate their structure with their development and function.

▶ Analyze the clinical symptoms of alcoholic cerebellar degeneration with an emphasis on the cells and zones of cerebellum involved.

▶ Illustrate the organization of connective tissue in a nerve; correlate their structure with the functions.

▶ Illustrate the microscopic structure of neurons; correlate their ultrastructure to their development and functions.

▶ Illustrate the composition and properties of nerve tissue; correlate their ultrastructure to their development and function.

▶ Illustrate the histological layers of the neocortex; correlate structure of cortical tissue with distribution and functions.

5.1 Questions

Easy | Medium | Hard

1. A 26-year-old sexually active woman presents with vesicular lesions on the cervix and bilateral painful vesicles on the external genitalia. Following laboratory studies, she was diagnosed with genital herpes. She was treated with oral antivirals and was counselled carefully for prevention of recurrence. Virions travel from the initial site of infection on the mucosa to the dorsal root ganglion (DRG), where latency is established. Which of the following mechanisms is responsible for such movement of the virus?

A. Positive to negative terminal; molecular motor kinesin

B. Positive to negative terminal; molecular motor dynein

C. Negative to positive terminal; molecular motor kinesin

D. Negative to positive terminal; molecular motor dynein

E. Negative to positive terminal; molecular motor actin

Consider the following case for questions 2 and 3:

A 60-year-old man presents with a history of lower extremity weakness that began in his second decade. Weakness had progressed over time and was associated with significant muscle wasting of both lower extremities and hands. Review of the patient's family history revealed two similarly affected relatives in an autosomal dominant pattern of inheritance. Physical examination revealed severely decreased vibration sense and proprioception. A nerve conduction velocity test performed on the median nerve confirmed markedly reduced conduction velocity.

2. Which of the following cells is responsible for synthesizing the defective protein in this patient?

A. Fibroblasts

B. Schwann cells

C. Satellite cells

D. Skeletal muscle cells

E. Oligodendrocytes

3. Which of the following additional finding(s) might be expected in this patient?

A. Exaggerated deep tendon reflexes (DTR)

B. Intact pain and temperature sensation

C. "Onion bulb" appearance in nerve biopsy

D. A + B + C

E. B + C

4. A biopsy obtained from the lower brainstem of a 26-year-old male is examined under the microscope. Which of the following is true about the cell labeled "1" in the micrograph?

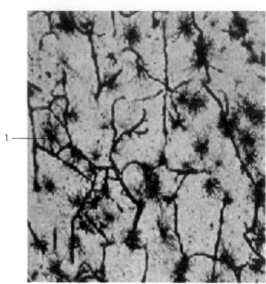

1 ———

Source: Kühnel W. Color Atlas of Cytology, Histology, and Microscopic Anatomy. 4th Edition. Thieme; 2003.

A. It is instrumental in synthesizing and secreting CSF

B. It is instrumental in forming glia limitans

C. It is instrumental in laying down the myelin sheath for neurons in the PNS

D. It is instrumental in laying down the myelin sheath for neurons in the CNS

E. It expresses neurofilament as the intermediate filament

5. Medulloblastoma is a common malignant tumor in children that involves the cerebellar vermis. Precursors of an excitatory neuron and the molecular mechanisms involved in controlling their proliferation have been implicated in its pathogenesis. The predecessor of which of the following cells seems to be involved in the etiopathogenesis of the tumor?

A. Basket cells

B. Golgi cells

C. Granule cells

D. Purkinje cells

E. Stellate cells

6. A 39-year-old woman presents with weakness in right shoulder abduction 2 weeks following a right-sided axillary lymph node resection. Physical examination reveals decreased sensation over the upper and outer side of her right shoulder. Which of the following histological changes might be noted in a right anterior horn cell of her fourth cervical spinal segment?

A. Increased cytoplasmic basophilia

B. Increase in number of cellular organelles

C. Decrease in volume (shrinkage)

D. Increase in Nissl granules

E. Peripheral movement of the nucleus

7. Mutations in genes coding for proteins responsible for transporting neurotransmitters synthesized in the cell body to the axon terminal have been identified as etiological factors for certain motor neuron diseases. Which of the following proteins might be a target for such mutation?

A. Kinesin

B. Dynein

C. Actin

D. Myosin

E. Tropomyosin

8. A 35-year-old man presents with a spastic type of paralysis in the right lower extremity, visual impairment in his right eye, and fatigue. MRI confirms areas of patchy demyelination in specific areas of the left cerebral hemisphere. Which of the following cells are specifically targeted in his condition?

A. Astrocytes

B. Oligodendrocytes

C. Ependymal cells

D. Schwann cells

E. Satellite cells

9. A 72-year-old man presents with severe peripheral vascular disease unsuitable for vascular reconstruction. Neurosurgery was advised and proved beneficial. The H&E stained slide, obtained from routine biopsy of the tissue procured during the procedure, is shown in the accompanying image. Which of the following is/are true of the photomicrograph?

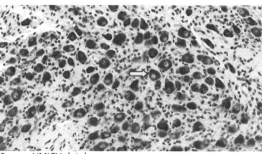

Source: UMICH database

A. The chief source of the indicated cells is neuroectoderm

B. The chief source of the indicated cells is neural crest

C. The micrograph has probably been obtained from a dorsal root ganglion (DRG)

D. The micrograph has probably been obtained from a sympathetic ganglion

E. A + C

F. A + D

G. B + C

H. B + D

10. The cell in the following photomicrograph would have a role in which of the following?

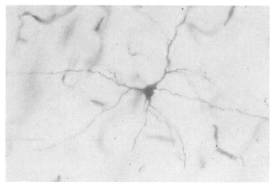

Source: Kühnel W. Color Atlas of Cytology, Histology, and Microscopic Anatomy. 4th Edition. Thieme; 2003.

A. Produce myelin in CNS

B. Line ventricles in CNS

C. Produce scar tissue in CNS

D. Macrophage activity in CNS

E. Produce CSF in CNS

11. A chronic alcoholic presents with truncal instability and an uncoordinated gait. MRI confirms alcoholic degeneration of the cerebellar vermis. Which of the following cells is most notably destroyed in this patient?

A. Basket cells

B. Golgi cells

C. Granule cells

D. Purkinje cells

E. Stellate cells

12. A 20-year-old male presents with progressive weakness of both legs developing over several hours. A nerve biopsy confirmed immune-mediated damage to the blood–nerve barriers in his lower limbs. Which of the following is instrumental in establishing these barriers for the affected nerves?

A. Astrocytes

B. Endoneurium

C. Perineurium

D. Epineurium

E. Satellite cells

13. Unmyelinated axons are more vulnerable to degeneration than the myelinated ones in neurodegenerative disorders. Which of the following cell types supports unmyelinated axons in the PNS?

A. Ganglion cells

B. Satellite cells

C. Schwann cells

D. Astrocytes

E. Ependymal cells

14. A 2-month-old infant presents with poor muscle tone, muscle weakness, and feeding and breathing difficulty. A spinal cord biopsy (shown in the accompanying photomicrograph) was obtained to confirm a diagnosis. Which of the following is/are true of the area indicated by the arrow?

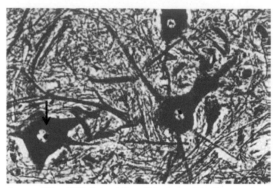

Source: Kühnel W. Color Atlas of Cytology, Histology, and Microscopic Anatomy. 4th Edition. Thieme; 2003.

A. The chief source of the indicated structure is neuroectoderm

B. The chief source of the indicated structure is neural crest

C. It expresses neurofilament as the intermediate filament

D. It expresses GFAP as the intermediate filament

E. A + C

F. A + D

G. B + C

H. B + D

15. A 45-year-old female presents with recent-onset dizziness and nausea. The symptoms are followed by vertigo, nystagmus, limb ataxia, and dysarthria. She has no history of hypertension, diabetes, stroke, or alcoholism. CSF sampling reveals autoantibodies against the chief output cells for the cerebellum and a diagnosis of paraneoplastic cerebellar degeneration was made. Which of the following cells is the target for the antibodies?

A. Basket cells

B. Golgi cells

C. Granule cells

D. Purkinje cells

E. Stellate cells

16. A biopsy (shown in the accompanying photomicrograph) was obtained from the ventral horn of the spinal cord of a 16-year-old male. Which of the following is/are true of the composition of the area indicated by the arrow?

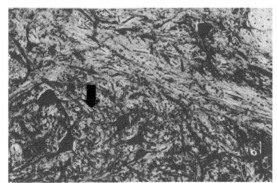

Source: Kühnel W. Color Atlas of Cytology, Histology, and Microscopic Anatomy. 4th Edition. Thieme; 2003.

A. Cell bodies of glia

B. Processes of glial cells

C. Cell bodies of neurons

D. Processes of neurons

E. Capillaries

F. A + B + C + D + E

G. A + B + D + E

H. A + B + E

17. A section from the sciatic nerve is shown in the accompanying photomicrograph. Which of the following layers would have been affected by a teratogenic insult during embryogenesis if the newborn suffered from a defect in synthesis of area "1"?

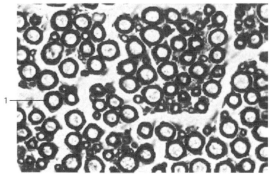

Source: Kühnel W. Color Atlas of Cytology, Histology, and Microscopic Anatomy. 4th Edition. Thieme; 2003.

A. Surface ectoderm

B. Mesoderm

C. Endoderm

D. Neural crest cells

E. Neuroectoderm

Consider the following case for questions 18 to 20:

A 68-year-old man was admitted with sudden onset of severe neck pain. CT scan of the brain revealed a ventricular hematoma and acute hydrocephalus. Despite several attempts to resuscitate, he died on the sixth day from complications of the subarachnoid hemorrhage. The accompanying image demonstrates normal cortical (cerebral) tissue, which was obtained from him at autopsy.

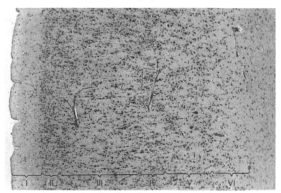

Source: Kühnel W. Color Atlas of Cytology, Histology, and Microscopic Anatomy. 4th Edition. Thieme; 2003.

18. Which of the following cortical areas is most likely to be the source of the tissue?

A. Primary motor cortex

B. Primary sensory cortex

C. Primary visual cortex

D. Primary auditory cortex

E. Prefrontal association cortex

19. How would the image be different if it was obtained from the anterior paracentral lobule?

A. Disproportionately larger layer II

B. Disproportionately larger layer III

C. Disproportionately larger layer IV

D. Disproportionately larger layer V

E. Disproportionately larger layer VI

20. How would the image be different if it was obtained from the posterior paracentral lobule?

A. Disproportionately larger layer II

B. Disproportionately larger layer III

C. Disproportionately larger layer IV

D. Disproportionately larger layer V

E. Disproportionately larger layer VI

5.2 Answers and Explanations

Easy	Medium	Hard

1. Correct: Positive to negative terminal; molecular motor dynein (B)

The movements of the virus described can be identified as retrograde, occurring from the mucosa (peripheral axonal process, positive terminal) to the DRG (neuronal cell body, negative terminal). Dynein is the molecular motor for such transport.

Kinesin (**A** and **C**) is the molecular motor for anterograde axonal transport. This occurs from the cell body to the periphery. Actin (**E**) is not directly involved in either retrograde or anterograde axonal transport.

Consider the following for answers 2 and 3:

The patient is suffering from Charcot–Marie–Tooth disease (member of the group hereditary motor and sensory neuropathies (HMSN)), the most commonly inherited neurological disorder characterized by progressive motor weakness, decreased nerve conduction velocities, and nerve root enlargement. About 70 to 80% of these cases are caused by a mutation in the *PMP22* gene that results in abnormal myelin, which is unstable and spontaneously breaks down. Demyelination leads to uniform slowing of nerve conduction velocity, as well as abnormal axon structure and function, thereby causing weakness and numbness.

2. Correct: Schwann cells (B)

Schwann cells are responsible for synthesis of PMP22, a component protein of myelin for the peripheral nerves. Fibroblasts (**A**), satellite cells (**C**), or skeletal muscle cells (**D**) are not involved in the process, while oligodendrocytes (**E**) are responsible for myelin synthesis for the CNS, as opposed to the peripheral nerves.

3. Correct: B + C (E)

In response to demyelination, Schwann cells proliferate and form concentric arrays of myelin. Repeated cycles of demyelination and remyelination result in a thick layer of abnormal myelin around the peripheral axons. These changes cause the onion bulb appearance (**C**) evident in nerve biopsies. As expected with lower motor neuron lesions, DTRs are markedly diminished or are absent (**A**). Pain and temperature sensations usually are not affected (**B**) because they are carried by unmyelinated (type C) nerve fibers.

4. Correct: It is instrumental in forming glia limitans. (B)

The cell labeled "1" is a protoplasmic astrocyte. It can be identified by the large number of processes radiating from the perikaryon, resembling spiders. Astrocyte foot processes form glia limitans (outermost layer of nervous tissue of the brain and spinal cord, lying directly under the pia mater) that serve as a functional barrier at the interface between non-neural tissue and CNS neural parenchyma.

Ependymal cells secrete CSF (**A**), Schwann cells are responsible for myelination of the PNS (**C**), and oligodendrocytes are responsible for myelination of the CNS (**D**). Astrocytes express glial fibrillary acidic protein (GFAP), while neurons express neurofilament as intermediate filaments (**E**).

5. Correct: Granule cells (C)

From the list, granule cells are the only excitatory neurons within the cerebellar cortex. The microscopic circuitry of the cerebellum is shown in the accompanying image.

The excitatory inputs carried by mossy fibers (from cerebral cortex, brainstem, and spinal cord) and climbing fibers (from the contralateral inferior olivary nuclear complex) synapse directly (climbing) or indirectly (mossy) onto Purkinje cells, which carry the

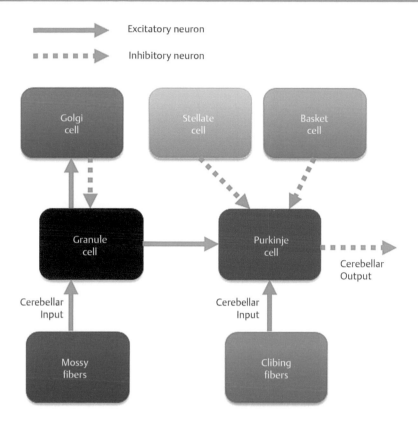

Excitatory neuron

Inhibitory neuron

outputs to the deep cerebellar and vestibular nuclei. Mossy fiber afferents project to the cerebellar glomerulus in the granular layer. In the cerebellar glomerulus, the mossy fiber afferents synapse with granule cells. After this first processing stage, the granule cells convey this afferent information to the Purkinje cells and the Golgi cells (through the excitatory parallel fibers). The Golgi (**B**) cells exert an inhibitory (feedback) influence on the synapse between the mossy fiber and the granule cells, within the glomerulus. The Purkinje cells also receive direct afferent information (excitatory) through the climbing fibers. Further synapses with the Purkinje cells are from stellate (**E**) cells and basket (**A**) cells (both inhibitory). The Purkinje (**D**) cells then send their efferent projections (inhibitory) to the deep cerebellar nuclei. The deep cerebellar nuclei serve as relay and processing stations for information coming from the cerebellar cortex to targets outside the cerebellum.

6. Correct: Peripheral movement of the nucleus (E)

The clinical features point toward an axillary nerve injury during the surgical procedure. Cell bodies of the motor axons (peripheral nerve) lie in the ventral horn cells of the third, fourth, and fifth segments of the cervical cord. The histological changes that occur within a neuronal cell body following an axonal injury are referred to as chromatolysis. The features of chromatolysis are a dissolution of the Nissl granules (rough endoplasmic reticulum) and hence decreased basophilia (**A** and **D**), cellular swelling (**C**), death of cell organelles (**B**), and peripheral displacement of the nucleus (**E**).

7. Correct: Kinesin (A)

The microtubule-associated protein families of kinesins and dyneins serve as the molecular motors that distribute intracellular cargo along microtubules, with kinesins working in the anterograde direction (from the cell body [-ve terminal] to the periphery [+ve terminal]) and dyneins (**B**) working in the retrograde direction. Actin (**C**), myosin (**D**), and tropomyosin (**E**) are not directly involved in anterograde axonal transport.

8. Correct: Oligodendrocytes (B)

Oligodendrocytes are responsible for myelination in the CNS. Schwann cells (**D**) are responsible for myelination in the PNS. Astrocytes (**A**), ependymal cells (**C**), and satellite cells (**E**) are not responsible for myelination.

9. Correct: B + D (H)

The micrograph has been obtained from a sympathetic ganglion. Autonomic ganglia can be distinguished from DRGs by presence of multipolar ganglion cells (as opposed to pseudounipolar neurons in DRGs), eccentric nuclei of the ganglion cells (as opposed to central nuclei in DRG neurons), and loosely packed satellite cells. While the multipolarity of the neurons is not best demonstrated in the image (because of nonstaining of neuronal processes), the eccentricity of the nuclei and spreading out of satellite cells are the stand-out features. The arrow indicates satellite cells, which are peripheral glia that support ganglionic neurons. These cells (along with the ganglionic cells) are derived from the neural crest.

10. Correct: Produce scar tissue in CNS (C)

The cell in the micrograph is a fibrous astrocyte. It can be identified by long and rarely branched processes of the perikaryon. Gliosis is the focal proliferation of glial cells in the CNS in response to insult. Astrocytes and the microglia are the glial cells predominantly responsible for tissue response to injury. Proliferation and hypertrophy of astrocytes play a huge role in formation of scar tissue within the CNS.

Oligodendrocytes are responsible for myelination within the CNS (**A**). Ependymal cells line the ventricles (brain) and the central canal (spinal cord), and are responsible for the production of CSF (**B** and **E**). Microglia are neuroglia that perform the role of macrophages within the CNS (**D**), specifically involved in active immune defense.

11. Correct: Purkinje cells (D)

Alcohol is toxic to the cerebellum, causing degeneration of the anterior superior vermis and hemispheres. Chronic alcoholism results in a risk of significant loss of Purkinje cells. This is worsened by vitamin B1 deficiency often associated with chronic alcoholism, resulting from both a poor diet and a direct toxic effect on vitamin B1 metabolism. Alcohol impairs thiamine uptake from the gastrointestinal tract, reduces thiamine-dependent enzyme activity, and depletes liver thiamine stores.

The Golgi (**B**) cells exert an inhibitory influence on the synapse between the mossy fiber and the granule cells, within the cerebellar glomerulus. Basket (**A**) and stellate (**E**) cells provide direct inhibitory influences on the Purkinje cells. In the cerebellar glomerulus, the mossy fiber afferents synapse with granule cells (**C**). After this first processing stage, the granule cells convey this afferent information to the Purkinje cells and the Golgi cells (through excitatory parallel fibers).

12. Correct: Perineurium (C)

The perineurium is a specialized connective tissue surrounding a nerve fascicle that contributes to the formation of the blood–nerve barrier. Cells in this layer possess receptors, transporters, and enzymes that provide for the active transport of substances.

Astrocytes (**A**) help maintain a blood–brain barrier in the CNS. Endoneurium (**B**) comprises loose connective tissue wrapping around an individual nerve fiber. Macrophages in this layer phagocytose debris following nerve injury. The epineurium (**D**) comprises dense irregular connective tissue that binds nerve fascicles into a common bundle. It contains the larger blood vessels that supply the nerve. Satellite cells (**E**) provide support for ganglionic neurons and are not involved in forming the blood–nerve barrier.

13. Correct: Schwann cells (C)

Schwann cells wrap around and support the unmyelinated axons in the PNS. Ganglion cells (**A**) are neuronal cell bodies that are involved in conduction of impulses. Satellite cells (**B**) are peripheral glial cells that surround and support the ganglion cells. Astrocytes (**D**) are glial cells found in the CNS that support neurons. Ependymal cells (**E**) line the ventricles (brain) and the central canal (spinal cord), and are functional in production of CSF.

14. Correct: A + C (E)

The indicated structure is a multipolar neuron located in the ventral horn of the spinal cord. It is therefore derived from neuroectoderm and not the neural crest (**B**). Also, neurons express neurofilaments as the intermediate filament and not GFAP (**D**) like some of the glial cells.

15. Correct: Purkinje cells (D)

The excitatory inputs carried by mossy fibers (from cerebral cortex, brainstem, and spinal cord) and climbing fibers (from the contralateral inferior olivary nuclear complex) synapse directly (climbing) or indirectly (mossy) onto Purkinje cells, which carry the outputs to the deep cerebellar and vestibular nuclei. The deep cerebellar nuclei serve as relay and processing stations for information coming from the cerebellar cortex to targets outside the cerebellum.

Golgi (**B**) cells exert an inhibitory influence on the synapse between the mossy fiber and the granule cells, within the cerebellar glomerulus. Basket (**A**) and stellate (**E**) cells provide direct inhibitory influences on the Purkinje cells. In the cerebellar glomerulus, the mossy fiber afferents synapse with granule cells (**C**). After this first processing stage, granule cells convey this afferent information to the Purkinje and Golgi cells (through the excitatory parallel fibers).

Paraneoplastic cerebellar degeneration is a complication of a malignancy (usually undetected), typically mediated by antibodies generated against tumor antigens. Similar proteins are also expressed on Purkinje cells leading to their immunologic destruction. This should be suspected in patients who present with acute or subacute cerebellar degeneration and no risk factors for cerebellar disorders (e.g., stroke, alcoholism).

16. Correct: A + B + D + E (G)

The arrow indicates neuropil—structure that fills the spaces between perikarya (**C**, neuronal cell bodies). Neuropils comprise glial cells (**A**) with their processes (**B**), processes of nerve cells (**D**) (mainly unmyelinated axons), and capillaries (**E**).

17. Correct: Neural crest cells (D)

Area "1" is myelin. Since this is a peripheral nerve (sciatic), Schwann cells are responsible for myelin synthesis. Schwann cells are derived from neural crest cells. Neuroectoderm (**E**) gives rise to oligodendrocytes, which are responsible for myelination within the CNS. Surface ectoderm (**A**), mesoderm (**B**), and endoderm (**C**) do not produce cells related to myelin synthesis.

Refer to the following table for answers 18 to 20:

The histological organization of the neocortex can be summarized as:

18. Correct: Prefrontal association cortex (E)

The larger size of layer III compared with that of layers IV and V, in the accompanying image, indicates it to be from an association area rather than from a primary motor or a primary sensory area. Primary motor cortex (**A**) would have a disproportionately larger layer V (internal pyramidal layer) with minimal layer IV (internal granular layer) representation (agranular cortex), while each of the primary sensory (**B**), primary visual (**C**), and primary auditory (**D**) areas would have a larger layer IV (internal granular layer, granular cortex).

19. Correct: Disproportionately larger layer V (D)

The anterior area of the paracentral lobule is a primary motor area that controls movements of the contralateral lower limbs. This area would therefore represent agranular cortex, with maximum thickness of layer V (internal pyramidal layer), with pyramidal cells predominating.

20. Correct: Disproportionately larger layer IV (C)

The posterior area of the paracentral lobule is primarily sensory and involves sensation from the contralateral lower limbs. This area would therefore represent granular cortex, with maximum thickness of layer IV (internal granular layer).

Cell Layers of the Neocortex

Layer	Name	Description	Major connections
I	Molecular layer	Cell sparse	Dendrites and axons from other layers
II	External granular layer	Scattered granular cells	Intra and inter cortical connections
III	External pyramidal layer	Scattered pyramidal cells	Intra and inter cortical connections
IV	Internal granular layer	Densely packed granual cells	Receives inputs from thalamus
V	Internal pyramidal layer	Densely packed pyramidal cells	Sends outputs to subcortical structures
VI	Multiform layer	Polymorphic layer	Sends output to thalamus

Chapter 6

Spinal Cord

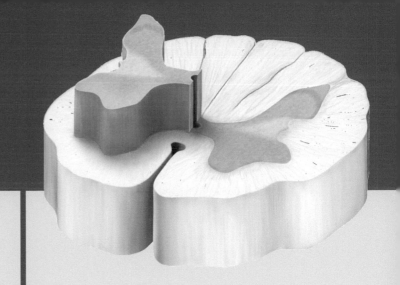

LEARNING OBJECTIVES

- ▶ Compare the clinical effects of a complete section and hemisection of the spinal cord.
- ▶ Describe the clinical features of radiculopathy; contrast these with peripheral neuropathies.
- ▶ Identify gray and white matter structures on an axial spinal cord slice, and relate tract function to clinical symptoms.
- ▶ Identify spinal cord features on an axial spinal cord slice, and relate tract function to clinical symptoms.
- ▶ Describe the clinical features of lesion of the anterolateral system or spinothalamic tract. Describe the Babinski's sign and its clinical significance.
- ▶ Describe the clinical features of syringomyelia.
- ▶ Describe the clinical features of central disk herniation at the lower lumbosacral cord.
- ▶ Describe the clinical features of Guillain-Barre Syndrome (GBS).
- ▶ Compare the clinical features of femoral nerve lesion with L4 radiculopathy.
- ▶ Identify laminar structures within an axial spinal cord segment. Establish the link between substance P and first-order sensory afferent fibers.
- ▶ Identify the symptoms and the location of damage associated with tabes dorsalis.
- ▶ Describe the pathophysiology of subacute combined degeneration.
- ▶ Analyze the implications of spinal cord development on a lumbar puncture procedure.
- ▶ Describe the supply for spinal nerve roots. Describe spinal nerve root involvement with disc herniation.
- ▶ Identify the information contained within the dorsal column at the level of the neck.
- ▶ Describe the pathophysiology of spinal muscular atrophy.
- ▶ Describe the blood supply of the spinal cord.

6.1 Questions

Easy   Medium   Hard

1. A 24-year-old man was brought to the ER following a driving accident. Neurological testing revealed paraplegia and loss of all sensory modalities in bilateral lower limbs. Sensation for the upper limbs and the trunk was intact. Which of the following might be the nature and location of the lesion in this patient?

A. Complete section of spinal cord at C8 level

B. Hemisection of spinal cord at C8 level

C. Complete section of spinal cord at T8 level

D. Hemisection of spinal cord at T8 level

E. Central cord syndrome

2. A 60-year-old man presents with left-sided low back pain radiating down all the way to his big toe. Neurological examination reveals weakness in inversion, eversion, and dorsiflexion of his left foot, and extension of his left big toe. Sensation is decreased in his anterolateral calf and dorsum of the foot, but is intact in the sole. A straight-leg raising test worsens the pain radiating to the left big toe. Which of the following is the most likely diagnosis in him?

A. Left superficial fibular nerve injury

B. Left deep fibular nerve injury

C. Left common fibular nerve injury

D. Left sciatic nerve injury

E. Left L5 radiculopathy

Consider the following image for questions 3 to 5:

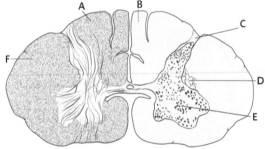

Source: Schünke M, Schulte E, Schumacher U et al. THIEME Atlas of Anatomy: Head, Neck, and Neuroanatomy. 2nd Edition. Thieme; 2016. Illustration by Karl Wesker/Markus Voll.

3. A 42-year-old right-handed male arrives to the emergency department and is intoxicated. At the time of presentation, he is unable to move his hands and arms. The following day, once he is sober, a more thorough neurological examination reveals a complete flaccid paralysis of the upper limbs and severely diminished-to-absent reflex activity. What is the most likely area of spinal damage?

A. Area A

B. Area B

C. Area C

D. Area D

E. Area E

F. Area F

4. A 21-year-old man is rushed to the emergency department following an altercation outside of a night club, where it is discovered he has suffered a knife wound to his spine. A neurological examination reveals a profound ataxia as he attempts to walk. Further neurological testing of other movements appears normal. What is the most likely area of spinal damage?

A. Area A

B. Area B

C. Area C

D. Area E

E. Area F

5. An 82-year-old left-handed woman is found unconscious on her floor by her family. An ambulance takes her to the emergency department and she regains consciousness ~2 hours following her admission. As she awakes, she reports that she cannot move her dominant arm or hand. Additional neurological testing reveals she has both hyperreflexia and hypertonia in her left limb. What is the most likely area of spinal damage?

A. Area A

B. Area B

C. Area C

D. Area D

E. Area E

F. Area F

Consider the following case for questions 6 and 7:

A 26-year-old man presents with spinal cord injury. Neurological examination reveals motor weakness of his left lower limb and loss of pinprick sensation on the right side of his body from the C8 dermatome downward.

6. Which of the following might be an associated finding in this patient?

A. Plantar flexion of right great toe on plantar stimulation

B. Plantar flexion of left great toe on plantar stimulation

C. Dorsiflexion of right great toe on plantar stimulation

D. Dorsiflexion of left great toe on plantar stimulation

7. Which of the following might be the location of lesion in this patient?

A. Right C6 cord

B. Right C8 cord

C. Left C6 cord

D. Left C8 cord

8. A 31-year-old right-handed woman presents to the emergency department with a progressive weakness of all limbs. She also reports suffering from headaches and a loss of pinprick sensation over both shoulders and right arm. Vibration sensation, however, of the affected regions was intact. Which of the following might be the initial location of a pathology in her?

A. Left dorsal horn of spinal cord

B. Left lateral funiculus

C. Spinal canal

D. Spinal reticular formation

E. Left fasciculus gracilis

Consider the following case for questions 9 and 10:

A 48-year-old man presents with severe bilateral gluteal pain following a trauma while lifting weights. Neurological testing revealed no motor loss for his lower limbs. A spinal CT revealed a central L5–S1 disk herniation.

9. Which of the following reflexes is likely to be abnormal in this patient?

A. Cremasteric reflex

B. Knee jerk

C. Ankle jerk

D. Babinski's reflex

E. Perineal reflex

10. Which of the following might be an associated finding in this patient?

A. Anesthesia involving anterolateral leg

B. Anesthesia involving posterior leg

C. Anesthesia involving dorsum of foot

D. Anesthesia involving the sole

E. Anesthesia involving the genitals

11. A 55-year-old right-handed woman spends several weeks as an inpatient with a severe gastro-intestinal infection. Following the infection, she displays a prominent weakness and myalgia in her feet and hands. Further examination reveals a subtle loss of muscle tone and diminished tendon reflexes. Neurological testing reveals demyelination. At a follow-up examination, ~1 week later, muscle weakness of the face is noticed. These symptoms persist for ~9 months, after which they begin to subside. Which of the following diagnoses would be most likely?

A. Lumbar disk prolapse

B. Poliomyelitis

C. Amyotrophic lateral sclerosis

D. Multiple sclerosis (MS)

E. Guillain–Barre Syndrome (GBS)

12. A 52-year-old presents with weak hip flexion and knee extension. Abduction and adduction movements of his hip were unaffected, but his knee jerk was lost. He also had sensory deficits along the anterior thigh and anteromedial leg. Which of the following is the most likely diagnosis for him?

A. L2 radiculopathy

B. L3 radiculopathy

C. L4 radiculopathy

D. Femoral nerve lesion

E. Sciatic nerve lesion

13. A pharmaceutical company looking to provide an analgesic for pain associated with neuropathies is in the process of developing a novel antagonist for substance P. If these efforts are successful, in which area of the following image would you expect the therapeutic effects of the drug to act?

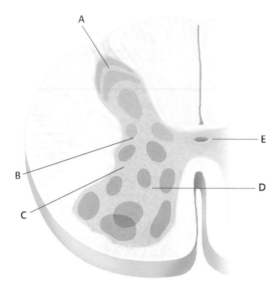

Source: Schünke M, Schulte E, Schumacher U et al. THIEME Atlas of Anatomy: Head, Neck, and Neuroanatomy. 2nd Edition. Thieme; 2016. Illustration by Karl Wesker/Markus Voll.

A. Area A

B. Area B

C. Area C

D. Area D

E. Area E

14. A 55-year-old man presents to his family physician complaining of generalized paresthesia, paroxysmal episodes of shooting pain, and bladder dysfunction. Neurological examination reveals an ataxia of the lower limbs and pinpoint pupils that are not responsive to light, but that constrict with accommodation. A venereal disease research laboratory test comes back positive for syphilis. Which structure would you expect to be abnormal if a CT scan of the spinal cord were performed?

A. Ventral horn

B. Ventral column

C. Dorsal horn

D. Dorsal column

E. Lateral column

15. A 39-year-old man was referred to the outpatient neurology clinic with a 1-month history of limb numbness and fine motor movement difficulties. Neurological testing revealed a substantial loss of position and vibration sensation. Romberg's sign was positive, and the patient displayed clinical signs of ataxia. His personality had not changed, and his ocular examination was normal. Over the next few weeks, his condition worsened to include a spastic paresis. Based on these symptoms, what is the most likely diagnosis?

A. Syringomyelia

B. Amyotrophic lateral sclerosis

C. Neurosyphilis

D. Subacute combined degeneration

E. Spinal muscular atrophy

16. A 5-day-old child has been treated in the intensive care unit since birth. A sample of cerebral spinal fluid is required. Where would be the safest place to perform a lumbar puncture?

A. Between C7 and T1 vertebrae

B. Between T12 and L1 vertebrae

C. Between L1 and L2 vertebrae

D. Between L3 and L4 vertebrae

E. Between L4 and L5 vertebrae

17. A 20-year-old woman presents with sensory loss affecting her left thumb. There was weakness noted for her elbow flexion, forearm supination, and wrist extension. Which of the following might be the cause for her symptoms?

A. C3–C4 disc herniation

B. C4–C5 disc herniation

C. C5–C6 disc herniation

D. C6–C7 disc herniation

E. C7–C8 disc herniation

18. A 14-year-old right-handed girl is injured in a skateboarding accident. Although she was wearing a helmet, she hit the back of her neck on an obstacle at the skate park. An MRI reveals that a bony fragment has invaded the lateral portion of the dorsal columns. What symptoms would most likely occur with this injury?

A. Loss of motor control of the contralateral foot

B. Loss of vibratory sense of the ipsilateral arm

C. Loss of sweating of the ipsilateral face

D. Fine motor control of the ipsilateral fingers

E. Loss of proprioception of the ipsilateral leg

19. An inpatient at the local hospital presents with flaccid paralysis consistent with a lesion at the C7–T2 level. While his motor losses are restricted to an LMN type, sensation in the affected areas is intact. Which of the following is the most likely diagnosis for this patient?

A. Spinal muscular atrophy

B. Multiple sclerosis (MS)

C. Syringomyelia

D. Amyotrophic lateral sclerosis

E. Neurosyphilis

20. A 42-year-old man presents with an inability to feel extremes of temperature in both lower limbs. He also had a spastic type of paralysis affecting his right lower limb muscles. If this is consequent to a vascular injury, which of the following might be an additional feature in this patient?

A. Loss of vibration sensation from right lower limb

B. Loss of fine touch sensation from right lower limb

C. Flexor plantar response from left lower limb

D. Extensor plantar response from left lower limb

E. Loss of vibration sensation from left lower limb

F. Loss of fine touch sensation from left lower limb

6.2 Answers and Explanations

Easy	Medium	Hard

1. Correct: Complete section of spinal cord at T8 level (C)

The patient is suffering from neurodeficits of the bilateral lower limbs. His sensory lesions can be accounted for by involvement of bilateral posterior columns and anterolateral system/spinothalamic tracts at T8 spinal cord level. His motor lesions can be accounted for by involvement of bilateral corticospinal tracts at the same cord level.

Complete section of the cord at C8 level (**A**) would produce additional sensory deficits for the upper limbs and trunk, which is not reported in our patient.

Hemisection of the spinal cord (**B** and **D**) would produce ipsilateral motor loss (corticospinal tract) and contralateral loss of pain and temperature sensation. This is also not the case in our patient.

Central cord syndrome (**E**) generally spares the posterior column sensations, and hence can be excluded in our patient.

2. Correct: Left L5 radiculopathy (E)

Weakness in inversion (tibialis anterior muscle), eversion (fibularis longus and brevis muscles), dorsiflexion of foot (tibialis anterior, extensor digitorum, and extensor hallucis longus muscles), and extension of the big toe (extensor hallucis longus muscle) indicate

L5 root involvement. Sensory loss over the anterolateral calf and dorsum of foot (superficial fibular nerve, L5) supports this diagnosis. Worsening of the pain on straight-leg raising test strongly suggests radiculopathy.

Superficial fibular nerve injury (**A**) does not explain the weakness in inversion, foot dorsiflexion, and extension of the great toe in the patient.

Deep fibular nerve injury (**B**) does not explain the sensory loss over the anterolateral calf and dorsum of the foot.

Common fibular nerve injury (**C**) closely resembles the clinical scenario of motor and sensory deficits. However, the fact that the pain is reproduced on straight-leg raising test tilts the diagnosis toward radiculopathy.

Sciatic nerve injury (**D**) does not explain intact sensation in the sole (medial and lateral plantar nerves) of the patient's foot.

3. Correct: Area E (E)

The anterior horn (**E**) is the final common path for descending corticospinal pathways, as they directly innervate skeletal muscle. Damage to this region would result in an LMN type of lesion and present with flaccid paralysis and diminished reflexes.

The fasciculus cuneatus (**A**) contains information pertaining to fine touch, vibration, and proprioception from C1–T6 spinal nerves, whereas the fasciculus gracilis (**B**) carries same information from the lower spinal nerves.

The posterolateral tract (**C**) contains centrally projecting axons from dorsal root ganglion cells carrying pain and temperature information (location, intensity, and quality) and eventually joins the spinothalamic tract (**F**) to ascend to the thalamus.

The spinal reticular formation (**D**) is involved in the maintenance of balance, tone, and posture through bidirectional fibers to coordinate and modulate motor, sensory, and other signals.

Lesion of the lateral funiculus (**F**) could produce paralysis of limbs due to involvement of the lateral corticospinal tract. However, it would produce an upper motor lesion with spastic paralysis of limbs and exaggerated deep tendon reflexes.

4. Correct: Area B (B)

The fasciculus gracilis (**B**) conveys information from the joint capsules of the lower limbs to the brain. Therefore, damage to this pathway will block positional information from the lower limbs required for sensory feedback related to proprioception. To compensate for this lack of sensory information, a compensatory ataxic gait is adopted.

The fasciculus cuneatus (**A**) contains information pertaining to fine touch, vibration, and proprioception from C1–T6 spinal nerves, and therefore damage to this tract would not account for an ataxic gait.

The posterolateral tract (**C**) contains centrally projecting axons from dorsal root ganglion cells carrying pain and temperature information (location, intensity, and quality) and eventually joins the spinothalamic tract to ascend to the thalamus.

The anterior horn (area E [**D**]) is the final common path for descending corticospinal pathways, as they directly innervate skeletal muscle. Damage to this region would result in an LMN type of lesion and present with flaccid paralysis and diminished reflexes.

Lesion of the lateral funiculus (area F [**E**]) could produce UMN type of paralysis of limbs due to involvement of the lateral corticospinal tract. It would also produce contralateral loss of pain and temperature sensation due to involvement of the spinothalamic tact.

5. Correct: Area F (F)

Hyperreflexia and hypertonia are consistent with a UMN syndrome. The lateral funiculus transmits corticospinal and spinothalamic tracts. Therefore, lesion of the lateral funiculus results in paralysis of limbs of the UMN type.

The fasciculus cuneatus (**A**) contains information pertaining to fine touch, vibration, and proprioception from C1–T6 spinal nerves, whereas the fasciculus gracilis (**B**) carries same information from the lower spinal nerves.

The posterolateral tract (**C**) contains centrally projecting axons from dorsal root ganglion cells carrying pain and temperature information (location, intensity, and quality) and eventually joins the spinothalamic tract to ascend to the thalamus.

The spinal reticular formation (**D**) is involved in the maintenance of balance, tone, and posture through bidirectional fibers to coordinate and modulate motor, sensory, and other signals.

The anterior horn (**E**) is the final common path for descending corticospinal pathways, as they directly innervate skeletal muscle. Damage to this region would result in an LMN type of lesion and present with flaccid paralysis and diminished reflexes.

6. Correct: Dorsiflexion of left great toe on plantar stimulation (D)

The clinical scenario is consistent with left hemisection of the spinal cord involving the left corticospinal tract (producing left-sided weakness) and the left anterolateral system (producing right-sided loss of pain sensation). This is a UMN type of lesion and hence would produce dorsiflexion of left great toe on plantar stimulation (positive Babinski's sign).

Plantar flexion of great toe (**A** and **B**) is considered a negative Babinski's sign and is found with LMN-type lesions.

Dorsiflexion of right great toe on plantar stimulation (**C**) would be found with right hemisection of the cord, but not the left.

7. Correct: Left C6 cord (C)

Loss of pain sensation indicates a lesion involving the anterolateral system. Since the fibers of this pathway ascend a couple of spinal segments before crossing to the opposite side of the cord, involvement of anterolateral system presents with sensory deficits that begin about two levels caudal to the level of the lesion on the contralateral side. Hence, left C6 cord is most likely damaged in our patient.

Right-sided cord lesions (**A** and **B**) would produce loss of pinprick sensations on the left side of the body, which is not the case in our patient.

Left C8 cord lesion (**C**) would produce a right-sided sensory deficit from C10 dermatome downward.

8. Correct: Spinal canal (C)

Syringomyelia is a disorder in which a cyst forms within the spinal cord, with first evidence appearing within the central canal. Bilateral motor and sensory losses reported in this patient are highly suggestive of effects of gradual widening of the cyst and compressing neighboring structures.

The dorsal horn (**A**) contains centrally projecting axons from dorsal root ganglion cells carrying pain and temperature information (location, intensity, and quality) and eventually joins the spinothalamic tract to ascend to the thalamus. Its lesion will fail to explain limb weakness and bilateral sensory loss.

Lesion in the left lateral funiculus (**B**) will result in left limb paralysis and right-sided loss of pain and temperature sensation. Again, bilateral losses could not be accounted for.

The spinal reticular formation (**D**) is involved in the maintenance of balance, tone, and posture through bidirectional fibers to coordinate and modulate motor, sensory, and other signals. A lesion of the area could produce ataxia but not paralysis of limbs.

The fasciculus gracilis (**E**) conveys information related to fine touch, vibration, and proprioception from the lower limbs. Damage to this pathway does not explain the paralysis and pattern of sensory loss in our patient.

9. Correct: Perineal reflex (E)

The perineal reflex or the anal wink is contraction of the external anal sphincter in response to a sharp stimulus in the perineal area. The spinal roots involved are S2–S4, which are likely damaged due to a central disk herniation at L5–S1.

The cremasteric (**A**) and knee (**B**) reflexes involve spinal nerve roots L1 and L3–L4, respectively. Such roots would not be involved in an L5–S1 disk herniation.

The ankle jerk (**C**) involves the spinal root S1. While this root can be commonly involved in a lateral L5–S1 disk herniation, injury to this root would cause significant weakness in plantar flexion of the foot (which is not the case in our patient).

Babinski's reflex (**D**) would be abnormal (positive) in the case of a UMN lesion. Herniation of intervertebral disks compresses on spinal nerve roots and is considered as LMN lesion.

10. Correct: Anesthesia involving the genitals (E)

S2–S4 root lesion would produce saddle anesthesia that involves the genitals and buttocks.

Anesthesia over the anterolateral leg (**A**), posterior leg (**B**), dorsum of foot (**C**), and sole of the foot (**D**) primarily involves L5, S1, L5, and S1 nerve roots, respectively. Involvement of such nerve roots are highly unlikely without associated motor deficits of the lower limb.

11. Correct: GBS (E)

GBS is classically thought to follow a gastrointestinal or respiratory infection. This syndrome results in a form of ascending paralysis, which begins with myalgia of the lower limbs and a loss of muscle tone and tendon reflexes. It is also possible to observe flaccidity of the lower limb. As the condition progresses, it may include the trunk, arms, bulbar muscles, and the facial nerve. Interestingly, as GBS is an acute polyneuropathy, it resolves without intervention.

A lumbar disk prolapse (**A**) may result in similar symptoms, but would not include demyelination.

Although poliomyelitis (**B**) can have a similar presentation, it would progress at a substantially faster rate (on the order of days) than what was observed with this patient once it has entered the CNS.

Amyotrophic lateral sclerosis (**C**) may present with similar symptoms and progression; however, this is a progressive disorder where recovery is not known to occur.

Lastly, MS (**D**) primarily affects the CNS, and would present primarily with features of UMN disease. Also, spontaneous recovery is highly unusual.

12. Correct: Femoral nerve lesion (D)

This patient had weakness in hip flexion (iliopsoas muscle) and knee extension (quadriceps muscles). These movements are produced by muscles that are supplied by the femoral nerve. Sensations along the anterior thigh (L2) and anteromedial leg (saphenous branch, L4) are also provided by the femoral nerve. Finally, integrity of the knee jerk (L4) is dependent on femoral nerve function. Therefore, a femoral nerve lesion best describes the clinical scenario for our patient.

L2 (**A**) and L3 (**B**) radiculopathies can closely resemble the clinical features seen with our patient, but will fail to explain any sensory deficits below the knee.

L4 radiculopathy (**C**) would produce an almost identical clinical scenario, except for the fact that the patient would also have weakness in hip adduction (obturator nerve).

Sciatic nerve injury (**E**) would produce weakness in knee flexion (hamstrings), and sensory loss in the anterolateral and posterior leg, and foot. This is not the case in our patient.

13. Correct: Area A (A)

Substance P is a neuropeptide (capable of acting as both a neuropeptide and neuromodulator) that is known to be prevalent within laminar I (**A**) and II of the dorsal horn of the spinal cord, and is also thought to be directly associated with first-order sensory afferent fibers, making it a viable target for analgesic development.

Neurons within laminae VI (**B**), VII (**C**), VII (**D**), and X (**E**) have no known association with substance P.

14. Correct: Dorsal column (D)

The patient has tabes dorsalis, which is a form of neurosyphilis seen many years following the primary disease. Argyll Robertson pupils (bilateral small pupils that respond to changes in focus but not changes in light) are diagnostic for neurosyphilis. Characteristically, the dorsal columns, which contain the ascending tracts for sensory information, become atrophic.

The ventral horn (**A**) contains LMNs, the dorsal gray horn (**C**) contains sensory neurons, and the ventral (**B**) and lateral (**E**) columns contain both ascending and descending tracts. Neither of these are affected in tabes dorsalis and their lesions do not correspond with the combination of symptoms in our patient.

15. Correct: Subacute combined degeneration (D)

Subacute combined degeneration of the cord is characterized by initial involvement of the dorsal columns, followed subsequently by degeneration of the corticospinal tract. Clinically, this manifests early as loss of position and vibration sensation, ataxia, and positive Romberg's sign (due to degeneration of the dorsal columns), and then a spastic paresis (due to the degeneration of the corticospinal tracts).

Syringomyelia (**A**) is a disorder in which a cyst forms within the spinal cord, with first evidence appearing within the central canal. Bilateral motor and sensory losses are found due to gradual widening of the cyst and compressing neighboring structures. Posterior column sensations (position, vibration, and fine touch) are usually spared.

Amyotrophic lateral sclerosis (**B**) is characterized by selective degeneration of the lateral corticospinal tract in conjunction with damage to the anterior horn cells. Therefore, typical symptomology includes flaccid paralysis at the level of the lesion as well as spastic paralysis below the level of the lesion due to involvement of the corticospinal tracts.

Neurosyphilis (**C**) is most often associated with the emergence of tabes dorsalis, a selective destruction of the dorsal columns. Loss of position and vibration sense can resemble the clinical presentation of our patient, but neurosyphilitic patients frequently feature personality changes (mania, paranoia, etc.) and pupillary changes (anisocoria, Argyll Robertson pupil, etc.).

Spinal muscular atrophy (**E**) results in selective destruction of the anterior horn cells, resulting in flaccid paralysis of the muscles innervated by the destroyed anterior horn cells. Therefore, LMN signs are present in the involved muscles. As damage is restricted to the anterior horn, sensation remains intact.

16. Correct: Between L4 and L5 vertebrae (E)

In newborns and infants, the conus of the spinal cord lies at the level of L3 vertebra, so a lower level such as between the L4 and L5 vertebrae is required for a lumbar puncture.

In adults, where the conus lies at the level of L1, the space between L3 and L4 vertebrae (**D**) is considered appropriate for lumbar punctures. In infants and neonates, a lumbar puncture at such a level, and anything higher up (**A, B,** and **C**) would carry the risk of cord damage.

17. Correct: C5–C6 disc herniation (C)

Clinical features for the woman are typical for C6 radiculopathy. This presents with motor weakness of biceps brachii (elbow flexor and forearm supinator) and wrist extensors (extensor carpi radialis longus and brevis), sensory loss over first and second digits and lateral forearm, and compromised biceps and brachioradialis (more specific) reflex. This is commonly caused by C5–C6 disc herniation.

Cervical nerve roots exit above the correspondingly numbered vertebra (except C8, since there is no corresponding vertebra). These have a fairly horizontal course as they emerge from the dural sac near the intervertebral disc and exit through the intervertebral foramen. Cervical discs are usually constrained by the posterior longitudinal ligament to herniate laterally toward the nerve root, rather than centrally toward the spinal cord. In cervical cord, therefore, the nerve root involved usually corresponds to the lower vertebral bone of the disc space.

C3–C4 disc herniation (**A**) would cause C4 radiculopathy, which might present as sensorimotor deficits in the neck region.

C4–C5 disc herniation (**B**) would cause C5 radiculopathy. Motor weakness of deltoid, sensory loss over shoulder and upper lateral arm, and compromised biceps reflex would be characteristic.

C6–C7 disc herniation (**D**) would cause C7 radiculopathy. This would present with motor weakness of triceps brachii, sensory loss over the middle finger, and compromised triceps reflex.

C7–C8 disc herniation (**E**) would cause C8 radiculopathy. This will result in weakness of digit flexors and sensory loss affecting the ring and little fingers.

18. Correct: Loss of vibratory sense of the ipsilateral arm (B)

At the level of the neck, the lateral portion of the dorsal columns (funiculus) is composed of the fasciculus cuneatus. Damage to the fasciculus cuneatus would result in a deficit in tactile, proprioceptive, and vibratory sense in the ipsilateral arm.

Motor control of the contralateral foot (**A**) is carried by the ipsilateral corticospinal tract.

Hemianhidrosis (lack of sweating) of the face (**C**) could be produced by interruption of sympathetic innervation to the face, which would be carried in the lateral funiculus.

Fine motor control of the fingers (**D**) would be carried principally by the ipsilateral lateral corticospinal tract.

Proprioception from the ipsilateral leg (**E**) is carried by the fasciculus gracilis in the medial part of the dorsal columns.

19. Correct: Spinal muscular atrophy (A)

Spinal muscular atrophy results in selective destruction of the anterior horn cells, resulting in flaccid paralysis of the muscles innervated by the destroyed anterior horn cells. Therefore, LMN signs are present in the involved muscles. As damage is restricted to the anterior horn, sensation remains intact.

MS (**B**) primarily affects the neurons within the CNS. UMN type of features (e.g., spastic muscle paralysis) and sensory abnormalities are frequently encountered in the disease.

Syringomyelia (**C**) is a disorder in which a cyst forms within the spinal cord, with first evidence appearing within the central canal. Bilateral motor and sensory losses are found due to gradual widening of the cyst and compressing neighboring structures.

Amyotrophic lateral sclerosis (**D**) is characterized by selective degeneration of the lateral corticospinal tract in conjunction with damage to the anterior horn cells. Therefore, typical symptomology includes flaccid paralysis at the level of the lesion as well as spastic paralysis below the level of the lesion due to involvement of the corticospinal tracts.

Neurosyphilis (**E**) is most often associated with the emergence of tabes dorsalis, a selective destruction of the dorsal columns. Loss of position and vibration sense below the level of the lesion, among other findings, is a significant feature.

20. Correct: Extensor plantar response from left lower limb (D)

The clinical features in this patient are consistent with bilateral involvement of the anterolateral system, which occurs due to anterior spinal artery occlusion. Bilateral corticospinal tracts are also commonly involved, and therefore bilateral spastic paralysis and extensor (but not flexor, **C**) plantar responses are often observed (UMN type of lesion).

Posterior column sensations such as fine touch and vibration (**A, B, E,** and **F**) are not involved in anterior spinal artery occlusion.

Chapter 7
Medulla

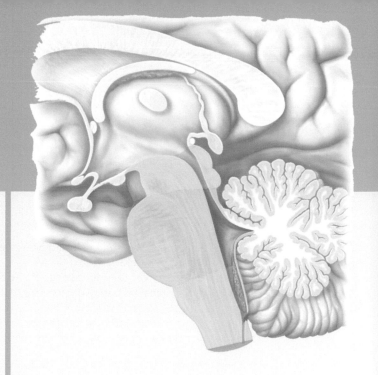

LEARNING OBJECTIVES

- ► Identify the major sources of blood supply to the medulla.
- ► Identify the role of the medulla in emesis.
- ► Identify the role of the medulla in breathing.
- ► Identify the location and role of the trigeminal nucleus and tract within the medulla.
- ► Identify the location and function of the nucleus gracilis within the medulla.
- ► Identify the location and function of the medial lemniscus within the medulla.
- ► Recognize the symptoms of medial medullary syndrome and identify regions of medulla oblongata affected.
- ► Identify the role of the medullary reticular formation in the modulation of the sleep–wake cycle.
- ► Describe the innervation of larynx.
- ► Predict functional outcomes that might result from injury to the structures passing through the jugular foramen.
- ► Describe the afferent and efferent limbs of the gag reflex.
- ► Describe the functions of superior and inferior salivatory nuclei located within the medulla.
- ► Identify lateral medullary syndrome based on symptoms, and recognize the affected region of medulla oblongata.

7.1 Questions

Easy | Medium | Hard

1. A 71-year-old man presents to the emergency department after displaying signs of a stroke. The medical team suspects damage to the corticospinal tract and medial lemniscus at the upper level of the medial medulla. Which of the following arteries would you expect to find occluded?

A. Posterior inferior cerebellar artery

B. Vertebral artery

C. Anterior spinal artery

D. Superior cerebellar artery

E. Anterior inferior cerebellar artery

2. A long-time patient presents to the family practice complaining of severe nausea. The 48-year-old male was recently diagnosed as having an acute lymphoblastic leukemia, and recently began chemotherapy. Which area in the medulla is the most likely cause of nausea in this patient?

A. Pyramids

B. Olivary bodies

C. Medial lemniscus

D. Postrema

E. Tuberculum cinereum

3. A 22-year-old male presents to the emergency room following unspecified trauma. Of particular concern is an irregular pattern of breathing consisting of irregular pauses and periods of apnea. The patient is immediately placed on mechanical ventilation to regulate breathing. Based on this information alone, where would you expect damage?

A. Forebrain

B. Midbrain

C. Rostral pons

D. Ventrolateral medulla

E. Dorsal medulla

Consider the following image for questions 4 to 6:

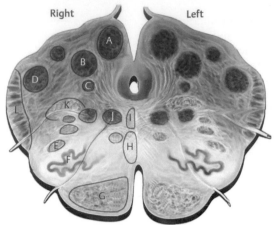

Source: Schünke M, Schulte E, Schumacher U et al. THIEME Atlas of Anatomy: Head, Neck, and Neuroanatomy. 2nd Edition. Thieme; 2016. Illustration by Karl Wesker/Markus Voll.

4. A 68-year-old female presents to the emergency department, with deficits in sensation on the right side of her face. Diagnostic imaging reveals damage to the caudal medulla. Based on this information alone, in which area would you expect the damage to be?

A. Area A

B. Area B

C. Area C

D. Area D

E. Area E

5. A 77-year-old left-handed male is found unconscious on his bathroom floor. Upon arriving at the emergency department, he has regained consciousness; however, he has diminished-to-absent proprioception, vibration, and tactile sensation on the lower half of his body on the right side. Based on this information alone, where is the most likely location of medullary damage?

A. Area A

B. Area B

C. Area C

D. Area D

E. Area E

6. A 66-year-old male presents with stroke affecting the ventral region of H of the given image. Which of the following might be a presenting symptom for him?

A. Loss of proprioception from right arm

B. Loss of proprioception from right leg

C. Loss of pain sensation from right arm

D. Loss of pain sensation from right leg

E. Loss of proprioception from left arm

F. Loss of proprioception from left leg

G. Loss of pain sensation from left arm

H. Loss of pain sensation from left leg

Consider the following case for questions 7 and 8:

An 81-year-old left-handed woman is brought to the emergency department after she lost consciousness at her granddaughter's birthday party. When she awakes, a neurological exam is performed; it is determined she has a deviation of the tongue toward the right side on attempted protrusion. Neuroimaging revealed caudal medullary infarction involving the territory of a specific artery.

7. Which of the following arteries is most likely affected by her stroke?

A. Right posterior inferior cerebellar artery

B. Left posterior inferior cerebellar artery

C. Right anterior spinal artery

D. Left anterior spinal artery

E. Right vertebral artery

F. Left vertebral artery

8. Which of the following might be an additional symptom found in her?

A. Loss of pain sensation from right arm

B. Loss of pain sensation from left arm

C. Loss of proprioception from right arm

D. Loss of proprioception from left arm

E. Loss of pain sensation from right face

F. Loss of pain sensation from left face

9. A 16-year-old right-handed male is involved in a motorcycle collision. Following the accident, he develops severe daytime sleepiness. Believing the excessive tiredness may be a result of a mild traumatic brain injury resulting in concussive symptoms, further diagnostic imaging is ordered. Surprisingly, a lesion within the medulla is discovered. Where is this lesion most likely to be within the medulla?

A. Pyramidal tract

B. Inferior cerebellar peduncle

C. Nucleus ambiguus

D. Medullary reticular formation

E. Medial longitudinal fasciculus

10. A 39-year-old woman presents with hoarseness of voice. Examination reveals a paralyzed (paramedian) left vocal cord with normal motion of the right cord. Sensation from her epiglottis also seems to be intact. Touching her posterior pharyngeal wall with a tongue blade leads to symmetrical elevation of the palate and constriction of pharyngeal muscles. Which of the following might be a possible cause for her symptoms?

A. Lesion in the right nucleus ambiguus

B. Lesion in the left nucleus ambiguus

C. Fracture of the skull through the left jugular foramen

D. Lesion of the vagus nerve in neck immediately after it exits through the left jugular foramen

E. Mediastinal tumor

11. A 20-year-old man presents with a fracture affecting his skull base that passes through the left jugular foramen. During neurologic testing, which of the following will be an unlikely finding in him?

A. Right palatal elevation on an attempt to say "ah"

B. Uvular deviation to the right on an attempt to say "ah"

C. Inability to shrug left shoulder

D. Inability to rotate head toward left side

E. Hemianesthesia of soft palate

Consider the following case for questions 12 and 13:

A 45-year-old female presents for a neurological follow-up 6 months after she suffered from a stroke affecting her lower medulla. The physician uses a tongue blade to touch her pharyngeal wall and the tonsillar area, to which she responded by retracting her tongue. Constriction of her pharyngeal muscles, as a reflexive act, was also noted.

12. Which of the following nuclei needs to be functional for an intact sensory limb for the reflex?

A. Nucleus ambiguus

B. Dorsal vagal nucleus

C. Nucleus of the spinal tract of trigeminal

D. Rostral part of nucleus solitarius

E. Caudal part of nucleus solitarius

13. Which of the following nuclei needs to be functional for an intact motor limb for the reflex?

A. Nucleus ambiguus

B. Dorsal vagal nucleus

C. Nucleus of the spinal tract of trigeminal

D. Rostral part of nucleus solitarius

E. Caudal part of nucleus solitarius

14. A 36-year-old male presents with a paramedian mass that affects his rostral medulla. Which of the following functions will most likely be affected in him?

A. Secretion from the lacrimal gland
B. Secretion from the parotid gland
C. Secretion from the submandibular gland
D. Secretion from the palatine glands
E. Secretion from the nasal glands

15. A 56-year-old male presents with a mass that affects the lower part of his dorsomedial medulla. Which of the following nuclei is most likely to be affected in him?

A. Medial vestibular nucleus
B. Lateral vestibular nucleus
C. Dorsal nucleus of vagus
D. Superior salivatory nucleus
E. Caudal part of the solitary nucleus

16. A 68-year-old man presents with left-sided hemiplegia. Imaging reveals a mass that is pressing onto the rostral medulla. Which of the following locations is most likely being affected?

A. Ventromedial part of his right medulla
B. Dorsomedial part of his right medulla
C. Lateral part of his right medulla
D. Ventromedial part of his left medulla
E. Dorsomedial part of his left medulla
F. Lateral part of his left medulla

17. A 54-year-old female presents with a tumor pressing onto the tuberculum cinereum of her left medulla. Which of the following might be a presenting symptom in her?

A. Right-sided hemiplegia
B. Left-sided-hemiplegia
C. Loss of pain sensation from the right lower limb
D. Loss of pain sensation from the left lower limb
E. Loss of pain sensation from the right cheek
F. Loss of pain sensation from the left cheek

Consider the following case for the questions 18 to 20:

A 58-year-old man is found unconscious in the break room of the factory where he worked. Co-workers rushed him to the nearest hospital where he was immediately seen by the attending emergency department physician. He awakes ~2 hours after he is admitted, and displays clinical symptoms including ataxia and unilateral hypalgesia on the right side of his face and the left side of his body. Neuroimaging revealed rostral medullary infarction involving the territory of a specific artery.

18. Which of the following arteries is most likely affected by his stroke?

A. Right posterior inferior cerebellar artery
B. Left posterior inferior cerebellar artery
C. Right anterior spinal artery
D. Left anterior spinal artery
E. Right posterior spinal artery
F. Left posterior spinal artery

19. Which of the following might be an additional symptom in him?

A. Right hemiplegia
B. Left hemiplegia
C. Right miosis
D. Left miosis
E. Right deviation of tongue on attempted protrusion
F. Left deviation of tongue on attempted protrusion

20. Neurological testing might reveal which of the following signs in him?

A. Positive Babinski's sign
B. Negative gag reflex
C. Negative corneal reflex
D. Negative jaw jerk
E. Limb astereognosis

7.2 Answers and Explanations

Easy	Medium	Hard

1. Correct: Vertebral artery (B)

The upper medial portion of the medulla, including the corticospinal tract and the medial lemniscus, is supplied by the vertebral artery (**B**). Although the anterior spinal artery (**C**) also supplies the medial medulla, this is at lower levels. The posterior inferior cerebellar artery (**A**) also supplies the medulla, but rather the lateral portion including the spinothalamic tract, descending sympathetic fibers, and the nucleus of the trigeminal nerve. The superior cerebellar artery (**D**) and anterior inferior cerebellar artery (**E**) both supply the spinothalamic tract, descending sympathetic fibers, and the nucleus of the trigeminal nerve, but at the level of the pons.

2. Correct: Postrema (D)

The postrema (**D**) is a small structure on the dorsal surface of the medulla, caudal to the fourth ventricle. Importantly, it is highly vascularized, but lacks the tight junctions between endothelial cells that normally protect the brain from toxins within the bloodstream. Therefore, the postrema is able to sense toxins in the bloodstream and trigger vomiting when concentrations of toxins are high. This specific portion of the postrema is known as the chemoreceptor trigger zone. The pyramids (**A**) house the pyramidal tract containing the corticospinal and corticobulbar tracts and would not be involved in emesis. The olivary bodies (**B**) are a pair of swellings between the anterolateral and posterolateral sulcus in the upper aspect of the medulla, and contain the inferior olivary nucleus (involved in cerebellar motor-learning and function) and the superior olivary nucleus (first major site of convergence of auditory information from the ear). The medial lemniscus (**C**) is important for somatosensation from the skin and joints (from the limbs and trunk), and also would not be involved in the nausea reported. The tuberculum cinereum (**E**) is the raised area, between the rootlets of the posterolateral sulcus and the accessory nerve, overlaying the spinal tract of trigeminal nerve (related to pain and temperature sensation from face).

3. Correct: Ventrolateral medulla (D)

Damage to all of the listed regions may result in atypical breathing patterns. Importantly, irregular breathing patterns consisting of irregular pauses and periods of apnea is known as ataxic breathing, commonly a result of damage to a respiratory group of neurons located within the ventrolateral medulla (**D**) that are crucial in the formation of respiratory patterns. Damage to the forebrain (**A**) can result in Cheyne–Stokes respiration, in which breathing becomes shallower with each successive breath, leading to apnea, at which point the cycle repeats with breaths starting as deep but becoming shallower with each inspiration. Midbrain (**B**) lesions are most likely to result in central neurogenic hyperventilation, characterized by deep and rapid (typically above 25 breaths per minute) breaths. Damage to the rostral pons (**C**) is more often associated with apneustic respiration, in which the patient has brief 2- to 3-second pauses in respiration at full inspiration. Lastly, the dorsal medulla (**E**) conveys inputs from hypoxia-sensitive peripheral chemoreceptors and mechanoreceptors to the other nuclei of the network involved in respiration, via the nucleus of the solitary tract, and damage is not often associated with ataxic breathing.

Refer to the following image for answers 4 to 6:

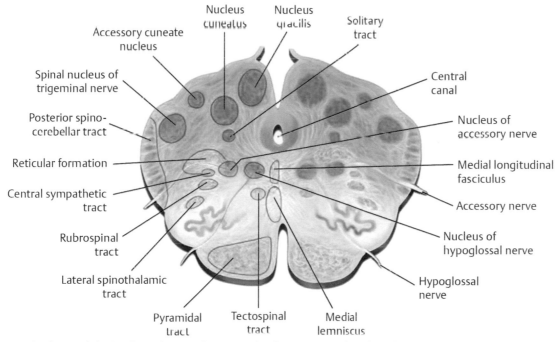

Source: Schünke M, Schulte E, Schumacher U et al. THIEME Atlas of Anatomy: Head, Neck, and Neuroanatomy. 2nd Edition. Thieme; 2016. Illustration by Karl Wesker/Markus Voll.

4. Correct: Area D (D)

The spinal trigeminal nucleus and tract receive descending projections of cranial nerve V and therefore would include facial pain and temperature sensation ipsilateral to the lesion.

Nuclei gracilis (**A**) and cuneatus (**B**) convey proprioception, vibration, and tactile sensation for the body from below and above spinal cord T6 level, respectively. The solitary nucleus (**C**) is related to taste sensory fibers (rostral half) and sensory inputs from cardiovascular, respiratory, and GI functions (caudal half). The lateral spinothalamic tract (**E**) is involved in conveying nociceptive information from the body, but not face.

5. Correct: Area A (A)

The nucleus gracilis receives large fiber sensory input from below spinal cord level T6 and contains information related to proprioception, vibration, and tactile sensitivity from the ipsilateral side of the body when at the level of the medulla.

Nucleus cuneatus (**B**) carries similar sensory information for spinal levels C2–T6. The solitary nucleus (**C**) is related to taste sensory fibers (rostral half) and sensory inputs from cardiovascular, respiratory, and GI functions (caudal half). The spinal trigeminal nucleus and tract (**D**) carry pain and temperature sensation from the face. The lateral spinothalamic tract (**E**) is involved in conveying nociceptive information from the body.

6. Correct: Loss of proprioception from left leg (F)

The medial lemniscus is formed by crossed axons of the nuclei gracilis and cuneatus that carry information related to proprioception, vibration, and tactile sensitivity from the contralateral limbs. Within the medullary segment of the medial lemniscus, the body is represented in an upright somatotopy, with the legs in the most ventral portion and the arms at the most dorsal portion.

Pain sensation from the limbs (**C, D, G,** and **H**) is carried within the lateral spinothalamic tract and spinal lemniscus on its way to the thalamus. Proprioception from arms (**A** and **E**) would be involved with a dorsally located lesion of the medial lemniscus. Proprioception from right leg (**B**) would be involved with a left-sided medial lemniscal lesion.

7. Correct: Right anterior spinal artery (C)

Deviation of the tongue to the right indicates ipsilateral muscle weakness due to a lower motor lesion (since damage is at the level of the medulla) of the right-sided hypoglossal nucleus or the nerve. These are supplied by branches of the right, not the left (**D**), anterior spinal artery.

Posterior inferior cerebellar (**A** and **B**) and vertebral (**E** and **F**) arteries supply the dorsolateral and anterolateral part of medulla, respectively. None of these will include the hypoglossal nucleus or the nerve.

8. Correct: Loss of proprioception from left arm (D)

Occlusion of the anterior spinal artery, as seen in medial medullary syndrome, typically damages the pyramid, the hypoglossal nerve fibers, and the medial lemniscus. This results in hemiplegia and loss of discriminative touch, proprioception, and vibration on the contralateral side of the body, and ipsilateral deviation of the tongue on attempted protrusion.

Pain sensation from the limbs (**A** and **B**) and face (**E** and **F**) is carried by the spinothalamic tract and spinal nucleus and tract of the trigeminal nerve, respectively. These could be affected in lateral medullary involvement.

Loss of proprioception from the right arm (**C**) would be seen in lesions of the left medial lemniscus.

9. Correct: Medullary reticular formation (D)

Lesions within the medullary reticular formation may result in downstream loss of orexin peptides, which results in excessive daytime sleepiness.

Damage to the pyramidal tract (**A**), which includes the corticospinal and corticobulbar tracts, would result in deficit in the motor control of the body. The inferior cerebellar peduncle (**B**) carries many types of input and output fibers, mostly conveying information necessary to integrate proprioceptive sensory input with vestibular functions. The nucleus ambiguus (**C**) is a group of motor neurons that innervate muscles primarily involved with speech and swallowing. The medial longitudinal fasciculus (**E**) contains information for the position and movement of eyes in response to changes in position of head and body.

10. Correct: Mediastinal tumor (E)

The patient is suffering from left recurrent laryngeal nerve palsy, which commonly occurs within the tracheoesophageal groove due to compression of the nerve by mediastinal tumors (e.g., bronchogenic carcinoma). The recurrent laryngeal nerve supplies all muscles of larynx except the cricothyroid, and its palsy leads to a paralyzed vocal cord with hoarseness of voice. The left recurrent laryngeal nerve has a much longer course than the right, making it much more susceptible to damage.

Lesion of the nucleus ambiguus (**A** and **B**) would result in loss of the palatal reflex with asymmetrical elevation of the palate, since this nucleus supplies all skeletal muscles of palate, larynx, and pharynx.

Fracture of the skull through the jugular foramen (**C**) or lesion of the vagus nerve in the neck immediately after it exits through the jugular foramen (**D**) would injure both the main trunk and the superior laryngeal branch of vagus. Neither the palatal reflex nor sensation of the epiglottis (by internal laryngeal branch of superior laryngeal nerve) would be intact in such cases.

11. Correct: Inability to rotate head toward left side (D)

A fracture line passing through the left jugular foramen would likely affect the left glossopharyngeal, vagus, and accessory nerves. An inability to rotate head toward the left side indicates paralysis of the right sternocleidomastoid muscle, which could be paralyzed in cases involving the right, but not the left, accessory nerve.

Damage to the left vagus nerve would paralyze the left levator veli palatini. The intact muscle from the right side will deviate the palate and the uvula to the right side (**A** and **B**) on attempted elevation.

Paralysis of the left trapezius consequent to left accessory nerve palsy would result in an inability to shrug the left shoulder (**C**).

Anesthesia of the left side of the soft palate will result from left glossopharyngeal palsy (**E**).

Consider the following explanation for answers 12 and 13:

The physician was testing the pharyngeal (gag) reflex that can be elicited by tapping the posterior pharyngeal wall, tonsillar area, or the base of the tongue. The normal reaction is retraction of the tongue along with elevation and constriction of pharyngeal muscles. The afferent limb of the reflex is formed by the glossopharyngeal nerve that relays to the caudal part of the solitary nucleus (**E**). The efferent limb of the arc is formed by the vagus nerve, the cell bodies of which are located within the nucleus ambiguus (**A**).

Dorsal nucleus of vagus (**B**), a member of the general visceral efferent group, contains preganglionic parasympathetic fibers for vagus nerve. Nucleus of the spinal tract of trigeminal (**C**) contains cell bodies of second-order neurons involved in pain and temperature sensation from the ipsilateral face. The rostral part of the solitary nucleus (**D**) contains cell bodies of second-order neurons involved in taste sensation.

12. Correct: Caudal part of nucleus solitarius (E)

13. Correct: Nucleus ambiguus (A)

14. Correct: Secretion from the parotid gland (B)

A paramedian mass that affects the rostral medulla is likely to involve the inferior salivatory nucleus, which comprises cell bodies of preganglionic parasympathetic neurons for the parotid gland (axons to be carried in the glossopharyngeal nerve).

Secretion from lacrimal (**A**), submandibular (**C**), palatine (**D**), and nasal (**E**) glands could be affected by involvement of the superior salivatory nucleus, which is located in the caudal pons. Recall that preganglionic parasympathetic fibers for these are carried in facial nerve branches.

15. Correct: Dorsal nucleus of vagus (C)

The dorsal nucleus of vagus, which is a member of the general visceral efferent group, contains preganglionic parasympathetic fibers for the vagus nerve and is located in the dorsomedial part of lower medulla.

Vestibular nuclei (**A** and **B**) and the solitary nucleus (**E**) are all located lateral to the dorsal nucleus of vagus in the caudal medulla.

The superior salivatory nucleus (**D**) is located in the caudal pons.

16. Correct: Ventromedial part of his right medulla (A)

Hemiplegia indicates compression of corticospinal fibers, which are contained within the pyramids in the ventromedial medulla. Since the mass is affecting the rostral medulla, it is rostral to the level of pyramidal decussation. A lesion of the corticospinal tract at this level would, therefore, cause contralateral hemiplegia—hence, the ventromedial part of the right medulla is most likely affected (**A**).

The dorsomedial rostral medulla (**B** and **E**) contains the hypoglossal nucleus, inferior salivatory nucleus, etc. Lesions of these would not be expected to cause hemiplegia.

The lateral part of medulla (**C** and **F**) contains the vestibular group of nuclei, spinal tract of trigeminal, solitary nucleus, etc. Lesions of these would also not be expected to cause hemiplegia.

Compression of the ventromedial part of the left medulla (**D**) would cause right hemiplegia, not left, as was reported in this case.

17. Correct: Loss of pain sensation from the left cheek (F)

Tuberculum cinereum overlies the spinal tract of trigeminal that contains pain and temperature fibers from the ipsilateral face. Ipsilateral hemianesthesia of the cheek, therefore, would be a probable finding in this patient.

Hemiplegia (**A** and **B**) is consequent to corticospinal tract palsy, which is contained within the pyramids. Pain sensation from the lower limbs (**C** and **D**), at the level of medulla, are carried within the fibers of the anterolateral system. Loss of pain sensation from the right cheek (**E**) would be consequent to compression of the right spinal tract of trigeminal, not the left one.

Consider the following explanation for answers 18 to 20:

Ataxia (damage to restiform body and spinocerebellar tracts) and unilateral hypalgesia on the right side of face (damage to right spinal nucleus and tract of trigeminal) and the left side of body (damage to right spinothalamic tract) indicate involvement of the lateral medulla, as occurs in lateral medullary (Wallenberg's) syndrome.

18. Correct: Right posterior inferior cerebellar artery (A)

Lateral medullary syndrome occurs from occlusion of the posterior inferior cerebellar artery ipsilateral to the facial deficits and contralateral to the trunk and extremities, not contralateral to the facial deficits and ipsilateral to the trunk and extremity deficits (**B**).

Anterior (**C** and **D**) and posterior (**E** and **F**) spinal arteries supply the medial and posterior caudal aspects of the medulla, respectively. Lesions of these would not include all the damaged structures indicated for this patient.

19. Correct: Right miosis (C)

The descending hypothalamospinal fibers are an important structure involved in lateral medullary syndrome that result in ipsilateral Horner's syndrome. These will include miosis, ptosis, anhidrosis, and flushing of the face.

Hemiplegia (**A** and **B**) and deviation of the tongue on attempted protrusion (**E** and **F**) occur due to damage to corticospinal fibers and hypoglossal nuclei, respectively. Both are medial structures and are not involved in Wallenberg's syndrome. Left miosis (**D**) will occur due to left lateral medullary syndrome.

20. Correct: Negative gag reflex (B)

Other structures included in lateral medullary syndrome are the nucleus ambiguus and the caudal parts of the solitary nucleus. These form parts of the afferent and efferent limbs of the gag reflex, respectively.

A positive Babinski's sign (**A**) is indicative of an upper motor neuron lesion and might result from a lesion within the corticospinal tract. This is a medial structure and is not involved in lateral medullary syndrome.

The corneal reflex (**C**) comprises bilateral forced eye closure in response to stimulation of either cornea. Its afferent limb consists of the ophthalmic branch of the trigeminal nerve relaying to the chief sensory nucleus of trigeminal. The efferent limb consists of the facial nerve fed by the motor nucleus of facial. These structures reside in the pons and are not involved in lateral medullary syndrome.

Afferent and efferent limbs for the jaw jerk (**D**) involve the mesencephalic and motor nuclei of trigeminal, respectively. These, too, are pontine structures and are not involved in lateral medullary syndrome.

Astereognosis for the limbs (**E**) could result from a lesion of the medial lemniscus at the level of the rostral medulla. This is a medial structure and is not involved in lateral medullary syndrome.

Chapter 8
Pons

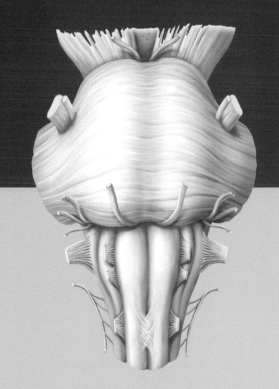

LEARNING OBJECTIVES

▶ Predict clinical outcomes of lesions involving the lower pons.

▶ Diagnose ataxic-hemiparesis syndrome based on symptomology; predict clinical outcomes of damage to major structures within the pons.

▶ Differentiate the clinical features between abducens nerve and nucleus palsy.

▶ Describe blood supply for lower pons.

▶ Identify cerebellar peduncles on a gross specimen of brainstem; correlate their functions with clinical features resulting from their lesions.

▶ Describe the function and location of the vestibulocochlear nerve within the pons.

▶ Describe the function and location of the abducens nuclei within the pons.

▶ Describe classic symptoms of locked-in symptoms, and relate symptoms to major structures within the pons.

▶ Describe the signs and symptoms of Foville's syndrome, and correlate symptomology with damage to the pons.

▶ Describe blood supply for rostral pons.

▶ Describe locations and functions of cranial nerve nuclei in brainstem sections; analyze clinical features of brainstem lesions at different levels.

▶ Describe the role of fluoxetine as an SSRI. Recognize the role of the paramedian raphe nuclei in the release of serotonin and locate the paramedian raphe nuclei on a cross-sectional diagram of the mid pons.

▶ Describe the three fasciculi of the middle cerebellar peduncle (MCP) and locate the MCP at the level of the mid pons.

▶ Describe the structures forming the floor of the fourth ventricle on a gross specimen of brainstem; correlate their functions with clinical features resulting from their lesions.

▶ Predict clinical outcomes of lesions involving rostral pons.

8.1 Questions

Easy	Medium	Hard

1. A 38-year-old right-handed male presented to the emergency department with complaint of acute headache. A CT scan of the brain at the level of the caudal pons seen in the accompanying image shows an infarct (shaded area in red). Which of the following might be a presenting symptom for him?

Right   Left

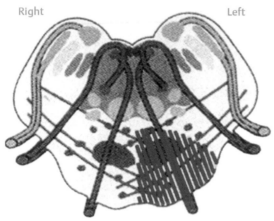

Source: Borsody M. Comprehensive Board Review in Neurology. 2nd Edition. Thieme; 2009.

A. Right-sided facial weakness
B. Left-sided facial weakness
C. Left hemiplegia
D. Left-sided conjugate horizontal gaze palsy
E. Ataxia

Consider the following case for questions 2 and 3:

A 62-year-old woman presents to the emergency department with unilateral ataxia, weakness, dysarthria, and nystagmus. Upon neurological examination, it is found that while weakness is worse in the lower extremity, ataxia is worse in the upper affected limb.

2. Which of the following might be the diagnosis for her?

A. Ataxic-hemiparesis syndrome
B. Ventral pontine (Millard–Gubler) syndrome
C. Ventromedial pontine (Raymond's) syndrome
D. Pseudobulbar/supranuclear palsy
E. Pontine locked-in syndrome

3. Which of the following structures within the pons might be damaged in her?

A. Pontine reticular formation + transverse pontine fibers
B. Pontine reticular formation + pyramidal tract
C. Transverse pontine fibers + pyramidal tract
D. Medial lemniscus + pyramidal tract
E. Lateral lemniscus + pyramidal tract

4. A 66-year-old woman presents with the complaint of double vision. Movements of her eyeball during the physical examination are noted in the accompanying images. Which of the following is the likely cause for her defect?

A. Paramedian lesion, right midbrain
B. Paramedian lesion, left midbrain
C. Paramedian lesion, right pons
D. Paramedian lesion, left pons
E. CN VI lesion, right superior orbital fissure
F. CN VI lesion, left superior orbital fissure

Rightward gaze   Look straight ahead   Leftward gaze

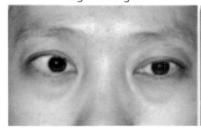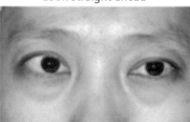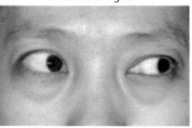

Source: Han SB, Kim JH, Hwang JM. Presumed metastasis of breast cancer to the abducens nucleus presenting as gaze palsy. Korean J Ophthalmol; 2010.

5. A 62-year-old male presents with stroke affecting his caudal pons. The area affected is designated by the shaded area in red on the accompanying image. Which of the following blood vessels is most likely to be involved in the stroke?

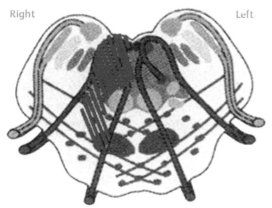

Source: Borsody M. Comprehensive Board Review in Neurology. 2nd Edition. Thieme; 2009.

A. Anterior inferior cerebellar artery
B. Posterior inferior cerebellar artery
C. Superior cerebellar artery
D. Paramedian branches of basilar artery
E. Long circumferential branches of basilar artery
F. Short circumferential branches of basilar artery

6. A 48-year-old man presents with appendicular ataxia. The circuit that connects the cerebral cortex to the cerebellum is being investigated for a possible lesion. Which of the areas in the following image contains fibers that serve as a direct communication between the pons and cerebellum?

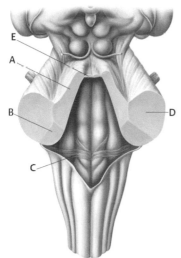

Source: Schünke M, Schulte E, Schumacher U et al. THIEME Atlas of Anatomy: Head, Neck, and Neuroanatomy. 2nd Edition. Thieme; 2016. Illustration by Karl Wesker/Markus Voll.

A. Area A
B. Area B
C. Area C
D. Area D
E. Area E

Consider the following image for questions 7 to 11:

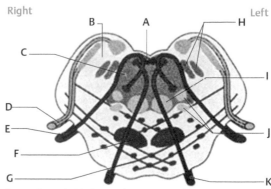

Source: Borsody M. Comprehensive Board Review in Neurology. 2nd Edition. Thieme; 2009.

7. A 55-year-old right-handed male presents to the emergency department. He reported that he awoke at 4 in the morning, and was very dizzy. The dizziness subsided when he turned on the lights, but he still described the room as moving around him. He also reported having a hard time hearing on his right side. Rinne and Weber tests revealed loss in both bone and air conduction on the right side. In which area of the image would you expect to see damage?

A. Area A
B. Area B
C. Area C
D. Area D
E. Area E

8. A 48-year-old woman presents to the emergency department after noticing a feeling of numbness on the left side of her face. Both sides of her body have intact sensation. Damage to which of the following areas is most likely responsible for her symptoms?

A. Area G
B. Area H
C. Area I
D. Area J
E. Area K

9. A 91-year-old right-handed woman is found unresponsive in her bed at an assisted-care facility by staff. Upon arrival at the emergency department, a thorough neurological exam reveals she is conscious and aware, though she cannot move or communicate, with the exception of vertical eye movements and blinking. Which of the following is the possible diagnosis for her?

A. Ataxic-hemiparesis syndrome
B. Ventral pontine (Millard–Gubler) syndrome
C. Ventromedial pontine (Raymond's) syndrome
D. Pseudobulbar/supranuclear palsy
E. Pontine locked-in syndrome

10. A 91-year-old right-handed woman is found unresponsive in her bed at an assisted-care facility by staff. Upon arrival at the emergency department, a thorough neurological exam reveals she is conscious and aware, though she cannot move or communicate, with the exception of vertical eye movements and blinking. Which areas of the image could explain the combination of symptoms for her?

A. Areas A and B

B. Areas B and C

C. Areas E and F

D. Areas F and K

E. Areas E and K

11. A 33-year-old right-handed male presented to the emergency department complaining of the "worst headache of his life," pain in his right eye, and weakness and numbness on left side of his body. Results of ophthalmic examination showed paralysis of conjugate eye movements when attempting to look right; however, vertical eye movements were intact. Neurological exam revealed moderate facial paralysis on the right. Which of the following areas might be damaged in him?

A. Area E

B. Area H

C. Area I

D. Area J

E. Area K

12. A 68-year-old female presents with dizziness and hearing loss. The area affected within her rostral pons is designated by the shaded area in red in the accompanying image. Which of the following blood vessels are more likely to be involved in the stroke?

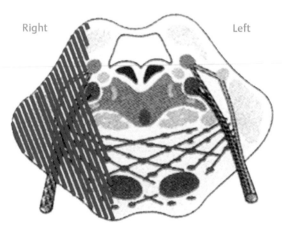

Source: Borsody M. Comprehensive Board Review in Neurology. 2nd Edition. Thieme; 2009.

A. Paramedian branches of basilar artery + posterior inferior cerebellar artery

B. Long circumferential branches of basilar artery + posterior inferior cerebellar artery

C. Long circumferential branches of basilar artery + anterior inferior cerebellar artery

D. Short circumferential branches of basilar artery + posterior inferior cerebellar artery

E. Anterior inferior cerebellar artery + posterior inferior cerebellar artery

13. A 2-year-old male baby presents with corneal ulceration consequent to dry eyes. A CT scan reveals a tumor affecting his brainstem to be responsible for his symptoms. If the tumor mass extends medially, which of the following could be an associated finding in this patient?

A. Inability to adduct the ipsilateral eyeball

B. Inability to abduct the ipsilateral eyeball

C. Inability of intorsion, depression, and abduction of ipsilateral eyeball

D. Anesthesia over the ipsilateral cheek

E. Deafness affecting ipsilateral ear

Consider the following image for questions 14 and 15:

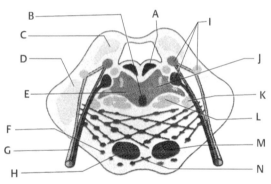

Source: Borsody M. Comprehensive Board Review in Neurology. 2nd Edition. Thieme; 2009.

14. Following diagnosis of severe depression, a 26-year-old woman is prescribed fluoxetine, an antidepressant that acts by selective inhibition of serotonin reuptake. Which of the following areas is most likely related to the mechanism of action for the antidepressant?

A. Area A

B. Area B

C. Area G

D. Area K

E. Area L

15. A 72-year-old left-handed male is admitted to the emergency department following a brief loss of consciousness. Diagnostic radiology reveals a probable lesion to the superior fasciculus that contains upper transverse fibers from the pons to the lobules on the inferior surface of the cerebellar hemisphere. Which area of the image is most related to the damage observed?

A. Area A

B. Area B

C. Area C

D. Area D

E. Area E

16. A 54-year-old right-handed male presented to the emergency department with ataxia. CT scan of the brain at the level of the caudal pons seen in the accompanying image shows an infarct (shaded area in red in the accompanying image). Which of the following might be an additional symptom for him?

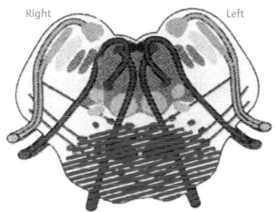

Right　　　　　　　　　　Left

Source: Borsody M. Comprehensive Board Review in Neurology. 2nd Edition. Thieme; 2009.

A. Right-sided facial weakness

B. Left-sided facial weakness

C. Right-sided conjugate horizontal gaze palsy

D. Left-sided conjugate horizontal gaze palsy

E. Paralysis of left lower limb

F. Paralysis and loss of touch sensation of left lower limb

Consider the following image for questions 17 to 19:

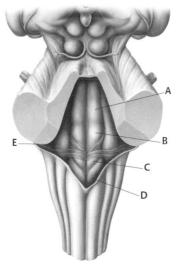

Source: Schünke M, Schulte E, Schumacher U et al. THIEME Atlas of Anatomy: Head, Neck, and Neuroanatomy. 2nd Edition. Thieme; 2016. Illustration by Karl Wesker/Markus Voll.

17. A 58-year-old male presents with horizontal diplopia and inability to abduct his right eyeball. Which of the following areas might be affected by a tumor in his case?

A. Area A

B. Area B

C. Area C

D. Area D

E. Area E

18. Which of the following might be the presenting symptom for a patient with a lesion involving area D?

A. Horizontal diplopia

B. Facial palsy

C. Tachycardia

D. Dysphagia

E. Tongue atrophy

19. Which of the following might be the presenting symptom for a patient with a lesion involving area C?

A. Loss of taste sensation from anterior two-thirds of tongue

B. Loss of taste sensation from posterior third of tongue

C. Spastic paralysis of tongue musculature

D. Deviation of tongue to the right on attempted protrusion

E. Deviation of tongue to the left on attempted protrusion

20. A 60-year-old man presents with left-sided facial numbness. A CT scan of the brain at the level of the rostral pons seen in the accompanying image shows a huge infarct (shaded area in red). Which of the following might be an additional symptom in him?

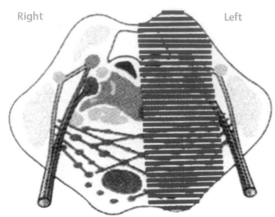

Right   Left

Source: Borsody M. Comprehensive Board Review in Neurology. 2nd Edition. Thieme; 2009.

A. Right-sided ataxia
B. Right-sided paralysis of temporalis muscle
C. Left-sided ataxia
D. Left-sided hemianesthesia of lower limb
E. Left-sided hemiplegia

8.2 Answers and Explanations

Easy	Medium	Hard

1. Correct: Ataxia (E)

As evident from the following image, structures within the lesion are left pyramidal tract, left abducens nerve, and pontine nuclei and tracts. Transverse pontine fibers (tracts) arise from the pontine nuclei, traverse the contralateral MCPs, and convey cortical information to cerebellum. These are critical components of the cortico-ponto-cerebellar pathway and their lesions result in ataxia.

Facial weakness (**A** and **B**) would result from facial nerve or nucleus involvement—neither of which is included in the presented lesion.

Involvement of the left pyramidal tract would cause right, but not left, hemiplegia (**C**).

Left-sided conjugate horizontal gaze palsy (**D**) would result either from involvement of left abducens nucleus or from involvement of the right MLF and the left abducens nerve—not from lesion of the left abducens nerve in isolation.

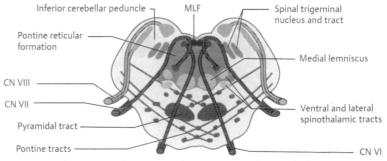

Inferior cerebellar peduncle — MLF — Spinal trigeminal nucleus and tract

Pontine reticular formation —

Medial lemniscus

CN VIII —

CN VII —

Pyramidal tract —

Ventral and lateral spinothalamic tracts

Pontine tracts — CN VI

Source: Borsody M. Comprehensive Board Review in Neurology. 2nd Edition. Thieme; 2009.

2. Correct: Ataxic-hemiparesis syndrome (A)

The patient is displaying the classic signs of an ataxic-hemiparesis syndrome, in which contralateral ataxia and hemiparesis predominate. As noted for the patient, ataxia primarily involves the upper limbs, while hemiparesis primarily involves the lower limbs. Dysarthria and nystagmus are variable, but suggestive signs. Although this is classically a result of a lesion of the basis pontis, this syndrome can also occur with internal capsule involvement.

Ventral pontine (Millard–Gubler) syndrome (**B**), a result of caudal pontine lesion, includes ipsilateral facial weakness, horizontal diplopia, and contralateral hemiplegia. It results from involvement of the facial and abducens motor nuclei, and the pyramidal tract.

Ventromedial pontine (Raymond's) syndrome (**C**), also a result of pontine lesion, is similar to Millard–Gubler syndrome, but will classically include ipsilateral ataxia (MCP involvement) and ipsilateral facial hemisensory loss (CN V root involvement).

Pseudobulbar palsy (**D**) typically presents with spastic dysarthria, dysphagia, and weakness of the face and extremities. Perhaps most unique, pseudobulbar palsy may include emotional behaviors without the patient experiencing the feeling associated with the emotion.

Pontine locked-in syndrome (**E**), a lesion of bilateral ventral pons, typically includes weakness in all extremities (lesion of bilateral corticospinal fibers), aphonia (lesion of bilateral corticobulbar fibers), and bilateral loss of horizontal eye movements (lesion of bilateral CN VI fibers).

3. Correct: Transverse pontine fibers + pyramidal tract (C)

Hemiparesis would most likely be a result of damage to the pyramidal tract (corticospinal fibers), as it is the aggregation of upper motor neuron nerve fibers that terminate at the spinal cord and is involved in motor functions of the body. Transverse pontine fibers arise from the pontine nuclei, traverse the contralateral MCPs, and convey cortical information to cerebellum. These are critical components of the cortico-ponto-cerebellar pathway and their lesions result in ataxia.

The pontine reticular formation (**A** and **B**) influences somatic motor pathways, cardiovascular responses, perception of pain, and sleep and consciousness. Its damage will not lead to hemiparesis or ataxia.

The medial lemniscus (**D**) is the pathway that ascends from the skin to the thalamus and is involved in conveying somatic sensation of pressure, vibration, and touch. The lateral lemniscus (**E**), in comparison, carries auditory information from the cochlear nuclei to a multitude of brainstem nuclei and ultimately the inferior colliculus.

4. Correct: Paramedian lesion, right pons (C)

The patient is suffering from right conjugate horizontal gaze palsy that results from lesion of the right abducens nucleus. Right abducens nucleus damage results in dysfunction of the right lateral rectus and left medial rectus on attempted right gaze. Since the abducens nucleus is located in the paramedian area of caudal pons, it could be affected by lesion involving this area.

Paramedian lesions of midbrain (**A** and **B**), depending on the level, could affect the oculomotor or the trochlear nucleus. However, neither of those would produce ipsilateral conjugate horizontal gaze palsy. Similarly, CN VI lesions (**E** and **F**) would produce isolated lateral rectus palsies, but not conjugate gaze palsy. A paramedian lesion of the left pons (**D**) could affect the left abducens nucleus, which would result in left conjugate horizontal gaze palsy.

5. Correct: Paramedian branches of basilar artery (D)

Primary arterial supply to the shaded area within the caudal pons is by the right paramedian branches of the basilar artery.

Long circumferential branches of basilar (**E**) and the anterior inferior cerebellar (**A**) arteries chiefly supply the posterolateral, while the short circumferential branch of basilar artery (**F**) supplies the anterolateral parts of the caudal pons.

The posterior inferior cerebellar (**B**) and superior cerebellar (**C**) arteries have no significant supply for the lower pons.

6. Correct: Area D (D)

Pontocerebellar fibers contain sensory information from the cerebral cortex (conveyed by corticopontine fibers to pontine nuclei) and travel to contralateral cerebellum via the middle cerebellar peduncle (MCP) (**D**).

The superior (**A**) and inferior (**B**) cerebellar peduncles serve to communicate between the cerebellum and the midbrain and medulla, respectively.

The stria medullaris of the fourth ventricle (**C**) contains fibers travelling to the cerebellum from the arcuate nuclei (medulla) via the inferior cerebellar peduncle.

The roof of the rhomboid fossa is formed by the superior medullary velum (**E**). The trochlear nerve decussates in the rostral aspect of the velum.

Refer to the following image for answers 7 to 11:

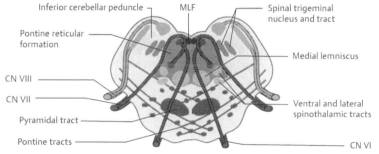

Source: Borsody M. Comprehensive Board Review in Neurology. 2nd Edition. Thieme; 2009.

7. Correct: Area D (D)

In this case, the patient is complaining of vertigo and dizziness which is worse in the dark, and a false sense of motion along with right-sided hearing loss. Rinne and Weber tests confirmed a right-sided sensorineural deficit. Combined, these symptoms strongly suggest damage to the vestibulocochlear system. Area D (**D**) in the image corresponds to the vestibulocochlear nerve (CN VIII).

Area A (**A**) represents the MLF, which is primarily responsible for eye movements, connecting CN III, CN IV, and CN VI. A lesion of this area would result in internuclear ophthalmoplegia—a slowed or absent adduction of the ipsilateral eye and nystagmus in the contralateral eye.

Area B (**B**) is the location of the inferior cerebellar peduncle. Although damage here may result in symptoms consistent with the reported disorders of the vestibular system, such damage would not explain the reported auditory deficits.

Area C (**C**) corresponds to the pontine reticular formation, with damage resulting in a range of deficits, most identifiable being deficits in eye movements and loss of consciousness.

Area E (**E**) corresponds to CN VII, the facial nerve, with damage most likely including facial paralysis.

8. Correct: Area H (B)

Area H (**B**) corresponds to the spinal trigeminal nucleus and tract, and is responsible for information about pain, temperature, and crude touch from face.

Area G (**A**) corresponds to the transverse pontine fibers (tracts). These arise from the pontine nuclei, traverse the contralateral MCPs, and convey cortical information to the cerebellum. These are critical components of the cortico-ponto-cerebellar pathway and their lesion could result in ataxia and other cerebellar signs.

Area I (**C**) corresponds to the medial lemniscus, which is important for somatosensation from the skin and joints (from body but not face).

Area J (**D**) represents the ventral and lateral spinothalamic tracts, involved in temperature and pain sensation (lateral) and crude touch (ventral) from the body, but not the face.

Area K (**E**) corresponds to cranial nerve VI, with damage resulting in horizontal diplopia (paralyzed lateral rectus muscle), with the affected eye being pulled toward the midline due to unopposed action of the medial rectus muscle.

9. Correct: Pontine locked-in syndrome (E)

The patient is displaying the classic signs of pontine locked-in syndrome, a lesion of bilateral ventral pons, which typically includes paralysis/weakness in all extremities, aphonia, and bilateral loss of horizontal eye movements.

Ataxic-hemiparesis syndrome (**A**), a lesion of basis pontis, results in contralateral ataxia and hemiparesis. Ataxia primarily involves the upper limbs, while hemiparesis primarily involves the lower limbs.

Ventral pontine (Millard–Gubler) syndrome (**B**), a result of caudal pontine lesion, includes ipsilateral facial weakness, horizontal diplopia, and contralateral hemiplegia. It results from involvement of the facial and abducens motor nuclei, and the pyramidal tract.

Ventromedial pontine (Raymond's) syndrome (**C**), also a result of pontine lesion, is similar to Millard–Gubler syndrome, but will classically include ipsilateral ataxia (MCP involvement) and ipsilateral facial hemisensory loss (CN V root involvement).

Pseudobulbar palsy (**D**) typically presents with spastic dysarthria, dysphagia, and weakness of the face and extremities. It may include emotional behaviors without the patient experiencing the feeling associated with the emotion.

10. Correct: Areas F and K (D)

In pontine locked-in syndrome, quadriplegia (damage to corticospinal fibers) and aphonia (damage to corticobulbar fibers) result from lesion of bilateral pyramidal tracts (area F), and loss of horizontal eye movements results from lesion of bilateral abducens nerves (area K).

Area A (**A**) represents the MLF, which is primarily responsible for eye movements, connecting CN III, CN IV, and CN VI. A lesion of this area would result in internuclear ophthalmoplegia—a slowed or absent adduction of the ipsilateral eye and nystagmus in the contralateral eye.

Area B (**A** and **B**) is the location of the inferior cerebellar peduncle. Damage here may result in disorders of the vestibular system (balance and equilibrium), since it conveys fibers connecting the cerebellum with the vestibular nuclei.

Area C (**B**) corresponds to the pontine reticular formation, with damage resulting in a range of deficits, most identifiable being deficits in eye movements (PPRF) and loss of consciousness.

Area E (**C** and **E**) corresponds to CN VII, the facial nerve, with damage most likely including facial paralysis.

11. Correct: Area E (A)

This patient is showing the classic symptoms of Foville's syndrome, a condition resulting from a lesion within the caudal pontine tegmentum, in this case on the right side. Symptoms commonly include ipsilateral facial paralysis, due to involvement of the facial nucleus/nerve (CN VII—area E), a paralysis of conjugate gaze toward the side of the lesion, due to involvement of the abducens nerve (CN VI) and/or the paramedian pontine reticular formation (PPRF), and contralateral hemiplegia due to involvement of the corticospinal tract.

Area H (**B**) represents left spinal nucleus of trigeminal—a lesion will cause hemianesthesia (involving crude touch, pain, temperature, etc.) of the left face.

Area I (**C**) represents left medial lemniscus—a lesion will cause right-sided hemianesthesia (involving discriminate touch, conscious proprioception, etc.) of the body, not left-sided.

Area J (**D**) represents left spinothalamic tracts—a lesion will cause right hemianesthesia (involving crude touch, pain, temperature, etc.) of body, not left.

Area K (**E**) represents left the abducens nerve—a lesion will cause paralysis of conjugate eye movements when attempting to look left, not right.

12. Correct: Long circumferential branches of basilar artery + anterior inferior cerebellar artery (C)

Arterial supply to the shaded area within the rostral pons is provided by the long and short circumferential branches of the basilar arteries, and the anterior inferior and superior cerebellar arteries.

Paramedian branches of basilar artery (**A**) chiefly supply the midline of rostral pons, while posterior inferior cerebellar artery (**B, D,** and **E**) has no supply to the rostral pons.

13. Correct: Inability to abduct the ipsilateral eyeball (B)

Lacrimation is controlled by the superior salivatory nucleus, which is located in the caudal pons. If a tumor mass affecting the area extends medially, it will affect the abducens nucleus with consequent loss of abduction for the ipsilateral eyeball (due to paralysis of the ipsilateral lateral rectus muscle).

Inability to adduct the ipsilateral eyeball (**A**) could be consequent to involvement of the ipsilateral oculomotor nucleus (due to paralyzed ipsilateral medial rectus muscle). The oculomotor nucleus is located in the rostral midbrain and not at the level of caudal pons.

Intorsion, depression, and abduction of ipsilateral eyeball (**C**) are the actions of the superior oblique muscle. This muscle is innervated by the ipsilateral trochlear nerve that arises from the contralateral trochlear nucleus. This nucleus, located at the caudal midbrain, would not be affected by medial extension of a tumor involving the caudal pons.

Anesthesia over the cheek (**D**) could result from lesion of the principal pontine (rostral pons) or spinal trigeminal (caudal pons) nucleus, but these nuclei are lateral to the superior salivatory nucleus.

Deafness (**E**) could result from a lesion of the vestibulocochlear nuclei at the level of the caudal pons, but these nuclei are also located laterally to the superior salivatory nucleus.

Refer to the following image for answers 14 and 15:

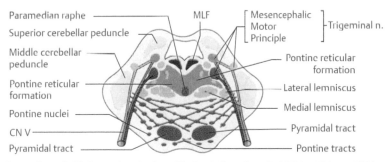

Source: Borsody M. Comprehensive Board Review in Neurology. 2nd Edition. Thieme; 2009.

14. Correct: Area B (B)

The paramedian raphe nucleus is a narrow layer of cells within the pontine reticular formation. It has a large number of serotonergic cells and is known for its role in the release of serotonin. Selective serotonin reuptake inhibitors (SSRIs), such as fluoxetine, therefore, would be expected to influence this area.

The other labeled areas (A, medial longitudinal fasciculus [MLF]; G, trigeminal nerve; K, lateral lemniscus; and L, medial lemniscus [**A, C, D,** and **E**]) are not directly involved in the serotonergic system of the brain, and are relatively unaltered through the use of SSRIs.

15. Correct: Area D (D)

The superior fasciculus is one of the three fasciculi of the MCP. The MCP (area D [**D**]) carries pontocerebellar fibers from pontine nuclei to primarily the posterior lobes of the cerebellar hemispheres.

Areas A, median longitudinal fasciculus (**A**); B, paramedian raphe nucleus (**B**); C, superior cerebellar peduncle(**C**); and E, pontine reticular formation (**E**) are not related to the superior fasciculus of pontocerebellar fibers.

16. Correct: Paralysis of left lower limb (E)

As evident from the following image, areas within the lesion are bilateral pyramidal tracts, bilateral abducens nerves, and pontine nuclei and tracts. Involvement of both pyramidal tracts would result in paralysis of all limbs (quadriplegia).

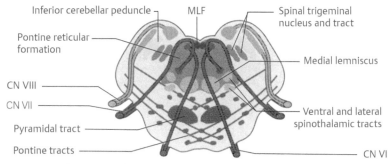

Source: Borsody M. Comprehensive Board Review in Neurology. 2nd Edition. Thieme; 2009.

Facial weakness (**A** and **B**) would result from facial nerve or nucleus involvement—neither of which is included in the lesion.

Conjugate horizontal gaze palsy (**C** and **D**) would result either from involvement of the abducens nuclei or from involvement of the MLF and the abducens nerve—not from lesion of the abducens nerve in isolation.

Loss of touch sensation in the left lower limb (**F**) would occur due to lesion of the right medial lemniscus, which evidently is not involved.

17. Correct: Area B (B)

This patient is suffering from paralysis of his right lateral rectus muscle consequent to right abducens nucleus palsy. Area B is the facial colliculus in the floor of the fourth ventricle that overlies motor fibers of the facial nerve arching around the abducens nucleus. Compressing the area, therefore, will result in loss of motor function associated with both abducens and facial nerves.

Compression of the medial eminence rostral to the facial colliculus (**A**), hypoglossal trigone (**C**), vagal trigone (**D**), or the vestibular area (**E**) by a tumor will not produce horizontal diplopia.

18. Correct: Tachycardia (C)

Area D represents the vagal trigone that overlies the Dorsal nucleus of vagus (DVN), which contains cell bodies of preganglionic parasympathetic fibers carried by the vagus nerve. Vagal stimulation to the heart causes bradycardia; therefore, a lesion of DVN could cause tachycardia by uninhibited sympathetic activity.

Horizontal diplopia (**A**) and facial palsy (**B**) could result from compression of the facial colliculus (area A) which overlies motor fibers of facial nerve arching around the abducens nucleus. Dysphagia (**D**) could result from a lesion of the nucleus ambiguus, which is not related to the vagal trigone. Tongue atrophy (**E**) could result from a lesion of the hypoglossal nucleus, which lies beneath the hypoglossal trigone (area C).

19. Correct: Deviation of tongue to the right on attempted protrusion (D)

Area C represents the right hypoglossal trigone, which overlies the right hypoglossal nucleus. Lesion of this nucleus will produce lower motor neuron type paralysis (atrophy, fasciculations, etc.) of the tongue and a deviation of the tongue to the right side (by action of the functional left genioglossus muscle) on attempted protrusion.

Loss of taste sensation from anterior two-thirds of tongue (**A**) could result from lesion of any of the components of the ascending pathway from tongue to gustatory cortex (chorda tympani, geniculate ganglion, rostral part of solitary nucleus, etc.), but not the hypoglossal nucleus.

Loss of taste sensation from posterior third of tongue (**B**) could result from lesion of any of the components of the ascending pathway from tongue to gustatory cortex (glossopharyngeal nerve, inferior glossopharyngeal ganglion, rostral part of solitary nucleus, etc.), but not the hypoglossal nucleus.

Spastic type of paralysis (**C**) could result from lesion of the upper motor neuron (corticobulbar fibers) that feeds the hypoglossal nucleus.

Deviation of tongue to the left on attempted protrusion (**E**) can result from damage to the left hypoglossal nucleus, but would not be expected with damage to the right hypoglossal nucleus.

20. Correct: Left-sided ataxia (C)

This patient is suffering from a stroke affecting his left pons. Hemianesthesia of the face results from involvement of the left chief sensory nucleus of trigeminal. The following image will help identify structures that are involved in the stroke.

Ipsilateral, but not contralateral ataxia (**A**), results from damage to the superior and middle cerebellar peduncles.

Associated symptoms for this patient would be left-sided paralysis of muscles of mastication (not right-sided, B) due to involvement of left motor nucleus of trigeminal, right hemiplegia (not left, E) due to involvement of left corticospinal tract, and hemianesthesia of right lower limb (not left, D) due to involvement of left medial lemniscus.

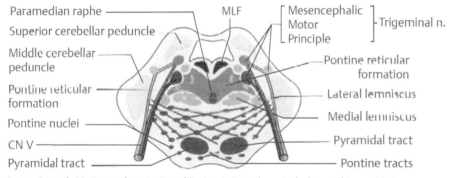

Source: Borsody M. Comprehensive Board Review in Neurology. 2nd Edition. Thieme; 2009.

Chapter 9
Midbrain

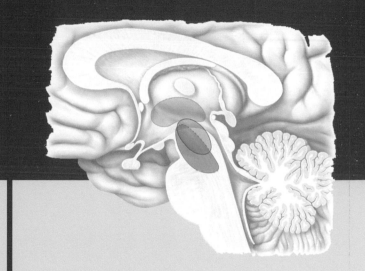

LEARNING OBJECTIVES

- ▶ Discuss the pathogenesis and clinical features of Parinaud's syndrome.
- ▶ Recognize the symptoms of peduncular hallucinosis and identify the region of the midbrain giving rise to the condition.
- ▶ Identify the symptoms and characteristic location of midbrain damage associated with Claude's syndrome.
- ▶ Identify the symptoms and characteristic location of midbrain damage associated with Benedikt's syndrome.
- ▶ Identify the symptoms and characteristic location of midbrain damage associated with Weber's syndrome.
- ▶ Describe the blood supply of the midbrain.
- ▶ Identify the colliculi in gross midbrain specimens. Describe their functions.
- ▶ Identify the trochlear nerve in CT scan and MRI. Describe its origin and functions.
- ▶ Locate the red nucleus within the midbrain.
- ▶ Identify in midbrain sections and recall the function of the crus cerebri.
- ▶ Know the role of the red nucleus in decorticate rigidity.
- ▶ Locate the hypothalamospinal sympathetic tract within the midbrain. Describe the etiopathogenesis and clinical features of Horner's syndrome.
- ▶ Identify the neurotransmitters associated with specialized neurons in the brainstem.
- ▶ Identify structures in a cross section of the brainstem at the level of the inferior colliculus. Describe the functions of the mesencephalic nucleus of trigeminal.

9.1 Questions

Easy	Medium	Hard

Consider the following case for questions 1 to 3:

Axial postgadolinium T1-weighted image at the level of the rostral midbrain of a 38-year-old male demonstrates a round, intensely enhancing mass (white arrow in the image below).

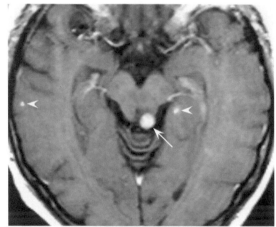

Source: Binder D, Sonne D, Fischbein N. Cranial Nerves: Anatomy, Pathology, Imaging. 1st Edition. Thieme; 2010.

1. Which of the following might be found in him?

A. Superior gaze palsy

B. Loss of pupillary light reflex

C. Hydrocephalus

D. A + C

E. A + B

F. A + B + C

2. Which of the following might be the principal feeder for the tumor?

A. Paramedian branches from bifurcation of basilar artery

B. Quadrigeminal branch of PCA

C. Thalamogeniculate branch of PCA

D. Thalamoperforating branches of PCA

E. Superior cerebellar artery

3. Which of the following might be an additional symptom for him?

A. Right hemiplegia

B. Left hemiplegia

C. Right-sided tremor

D. Left-sided tremor

E. Down and out right eye

F. Down and out left eye

Consider the following case for questions 4 and 5:

A 42-year-old right-handed female presents with a 2-week history of right-sided headache and a 3-day history of irritability, confusion, and visual hallucinations. History reveals general noncompliance with taking medication for hypertension and hyperlipidemia. Upon neurological exam, CN III palsy was present. During psychiatric exam, she described visions of animals and people that were sometimes shadows, and other times bright colors. These hallucinations, often of reduced size (lilliputian), were not frightening to the patient, and she was aware that they were not real. She had no past psychiatric history and reported no auditory hallucinations or delusions.

4. Which of the following is the diagnosis for her?

A. Weber's syndrome

B. Claude's syndrome

C. Benedikt's syndrome

D. von Monakow's syndrome

E. Peduncular hallucinosis

5. Which area of the brainstem is most likely affected in her?

A. Corticopontine tracts

B. Pyramidal tracts

C. Red nucleus

D. Substantia nigra, pars reticulata

E. Substantia nigra, pars compacta

Consider the following image for questions 6 to 9:

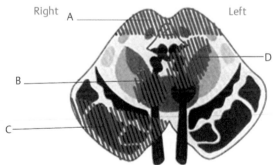

Source: Tsementzis S. Differential Diagnosis in Neurology and Neurosurgery. A Clinician's Pocket Guide. 1st Edition. Thieme; 1999.

6. A 68-year-old male farmer was admitted to the emergency department after reporting a sudden onset of dizziness and an inability to open his left eye. He had a history of uncontrolled hypertension and diabetes, with no prior history of stroke. Upon neurological examination, he was found to be alert and aware, and language was normal. Visual field and acuity were normal. Ptosis of the left eye was found, and there was no pupil response to light. In the primary position, the right eye was orthophoric and the left eye was exotropic. Left eye adduction, elevation, and depression were limited; however, abduction was normal. When examining the extremities, muscle power was grade 5 and the Babinski response was flexor. There was no presence of sensory disturbance. Dysmetria was present in the right limbs, as was an intention tremor. Further, the patient had a wide-based gait, swerving to the right when attempting to walk straight. Based on this information, what is the most likely location of midbrain damage?

A. Area A

B. Area B

C. Area C

D. Area D

7. A 75-year-old man was admitted to the emergency department following a collapse at his home. Diagnostic radiology was performed via a T2-weighted MRI, which showed increased signal within area B consistent with ischemic infarct. Which of the following might be a presenting symptom in him?

A. Left-sided ptosis

B. Left-sided mydriasis

C. Intention tremor of right upper limb

D. Astereognosis of right upper limb

E. Astereognosis of left upper limb

8. A 55-year-old male was taken to the emergency department after awaking at ~7:00 am with severe left-sided weakness. Neurological examination revealed a positive Babinski's response on the left. Diagnostic radiology was performed via a T2-weighted MRI, which showed increased signal within one of the areas A through D consistent with ischemic infarct. Which of the following might be an additional symptom in him?

A. Astereognosis of the left upper limb

B. Intention tremor of the left upper limb

C. Deviation of tongue to the left on attempted protrusion

D. Paralysis of the right buccinator muscle

E. Right eye deviated upward and inward

9. Which of the following vessels might have been involved for the patient in question 8?

A. P1 segment of the PCA

B. Thalamoperforating branches of PCA

C. Quadrigeminal branch of PCA

D. Medial posterior choroidal branch of PCA

E. Thalamogeniculate branch of PCA

Consider the following image for questions 10 to 12:

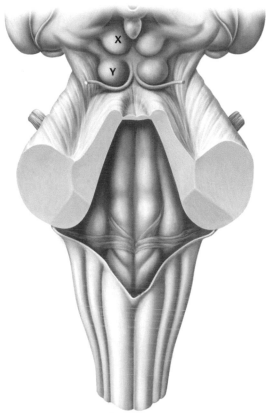

Source: Schünke M, Schulte E, Schumacher U et al. THIEME Atlas of Anatomy: Head, Neck, and Neuroanatomy. 2nd Edition, Thieme; 2016. Illustration by Karl Wesker/Markus Voll.

10. Which of the following areas are indicated by X and Y?

A. Mammillary bodies

B. Red nucleus

C. Tectum

D. Tegmentum

E. Basis pedunculi

11. Which of the following is a true statement regarding area X?

A. These receive input from ipsilateral lateral lemniscus.

B. These project to the medial geniculate nucleus of thalamus.

C. These project to the pulvinar nucleus of thalamus.

D. These overlie the internal genu of the facial nerve.

E. Lesions of these could cause contralateral ataxia.

77

12. Which of the following is a true statement regarding area Y?

A. These receive input exclusively from the ipsilateral cochlea.

B. These receive input from the ipsilateral lateral lemniscus.

C. These project to the lateral geniculate nucleus of thalamus.

D. These overlie the internal genu of the facial nerve.

E. Lesions of these could cause contralateral ataxia.

Consider the following image for questions 13 and 14:

A 27-year-old female presents with right-sided facial numbness. Coronal postcontrast T1-weighted image shows a homogeneously enhancing mass (asterisk) lateral to the pons (P) in the right cerebellopontine angle that represents a large CN V schwannoma. A second (smaller) enhancing mass (arrow) at the level of the left pontomesencephalic junction is also found, consistent with schwannoma involving another cranial nerve.

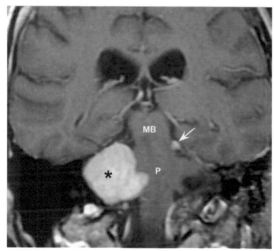

Source: Binder D, Sonne D, Fischbein N. Cranial Nerves: Anatomy, Pathology, Imaging. 1st Edition. Thieme; 2010.

13. Which of the following is the primary action of the muscle that might be compromised due to the second mass?

A. Abduction

B. Adduction

C. Elevation

D. Depression

E. Intorsion

F. Extorsion

14 Which of the following is the supply to the nucleus from which the nerve involved with the second mass arises?

A. Left quadrigeminal artery

B. P1 segment of left PCA

C. Left thalamogeniculate artery

D. Right quadrigeminal artery

E. P1 segment of right PCA

F. Right thalamogeniculate artery

Consider the following image for questions 15 to 18:

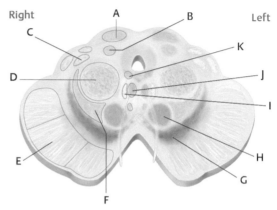

Source: Schünke M, Schulte E, Schumacher U et al. THIEME Atlas of Anatomy: Head, Neck, and Neuroanatomy. 2nd Edition. Thieme; 2016. Illustration by Karl Wesker/Markus Voll.

15. Following injury to the midbrain, a 51-year-old right-handed male presented with a slow tremor (~4 Hz) that responded well to levodopa. It was determined that this was a rubral tremor brought about from damage to the red nucleus. Which area in the presented image best corresponds to the region that was damaged?

A. Area D

B. Area F

C. Area H

D. Area I

E. Area J

16. A 60-year-old woman's tongue deviates to the left on protrusion and the angle of her mouth deviates to the right on an attempt to smile. Damage to which of the following areas in the presented image would most likely explain this woman's deficits?

A. Area A

B. Area B

C. Area C

D. Area D

E. Area E

17. A 78-year-old patient suffers from massive cerebral stroke, following which he develops decorticate posture. Which of the following areas in the presented image is primarily responsible for this phenomenon?

A. Area D

B. Area E

C. Area F

D. Area G

E. Area H

18. Following a brainstem infarction, a 56-year-old man presents with ptosis, miosis, enophthalmos, and anhidrosis at the face. Which of the following areas in the presented image might have been damaged for him?

A. Area C

B. Area F

C. Area I

D. Area J

E. Area K

19. A 26-year-old female was prescribed an antidepressant that acts by inhibiting selective serotonin reuptake by presynaptic neurons. Which of the following neurons might be influenced by the drug's action?

A. Substantia nigra, pars compacta

B. Substantia nigra, pars reticulata

C. Nucleus raphe magnus

D. Nucleus locus coeruleus

E. Nucleus Edinger–Westphal

F. Periaqueductal gray (PAG)

20. Following a pineal body tumor resection, an 83-year-old woman developed prominent speech perception impairment, despite only moderate sensorineural hearing loss. Postoperative MRI revealed damage to the inferior colliculi. If unilateral damage has occurred extensively to the brainstem at this level, which of the following might be an additional finding in her?

A. Loss of accommodation

B. Loss of upward gaze

C. Paralysis of orbicularis oculi

D. Loss of jaw jerk

E. Loss of eye adduction

9.2 Answers and Explanations

Easy	Medium	Hard

Consider the following explanation for answers 1 to 3:

The mass is centered on the left superior colliculi (observer's right is the patient's left and ventral aspect of brainstem is up on the image for axial CT scans and MRIs).

1. Correct: A + B + C (F)

A growing tumor pressing on the superior colliculi (lesion causes upward gaze palsy, **A**) will gradually involve the pretectal area (involved in pupillary light reflex, **B**), cerebral aqueduct (obstruction will cause hydrocephalus, **C**), and CN III nucleus. The combination of these defects is seen in Parinaud's syndrome.

2. Correct: Quadrigeminal branch of PCA (B)

Blood supply to the superior colliculi is provided by the quadrigeminal (P1) and posterior medial choroidal (P2) arteries.

Paramedian branches from the bifurcation of the basilar artery (**A**) supply the medial midbrain ventral to the cerebral aqueduct. The thalamogeniculate artery (**C**) supplies the posterior part of the thalamus including the medial and lateral geniculate bodies. Thalamoperforating arteries (**D**) supply the anterior nuclei of thalamus.

The superior cerebellar artery (**E**), along with the quadrigeminal artery, supplies the inferior colliculus, but has no significant contribution to blood supply at the level of the rostral midbrain.

3. Correct: Down and out left eye (F)

As noted earlier, the tumor will eventually involve the left CN III nucleus. This will lead to ptosis and loss of adduction, elevation, and extorsion of the eyeball—leading to a down and out left, not the right (**E**), eye.

Hemiplegia (**A** and **B**, lesion of corticospinal tract) or tremor (**C** and **D**, lesion of red nucleus or brachium conjunctivum) would result from structures further ventral than the scope of the tumor.

4. Correct: Peduncular hallucinosis (E)

Peduncular hallucinosis (**E**) is most consistent with the symptomology reported, with formation of hallucinations that are vivid, bizarre, and often cartoonish in nature being the defining characteristic. Importantly, these hallucinations are recognized by the patient as being unreal, and are purely visual in nature. Peduncular hallucinosis may also present with CN III palsy and disrupted sleep–wake cycles.

Weber's syndrome (**A**) would include contralateral hemiplegia, Claude's syndrome (**B**) would present with contralateral ataxia, Benedikt's syndrome (**C**) would include contralateral dyskinesia (such as parkinsonian tremor, chorea, and/or athetosis), and von Monakow's syndrome (**D**) would include contralateral hemisensory loss for vibratory and position sense, in addition to CN III palsy.

5. Correct: Substantia nigra, pars reticulata (D)

Specific lesions associated with peduncular hallucinosis have been localized to bilateral medial substantia nigra pars reticulata, with the symptoms possibly consequent to dysfunction of the mesencephalic reticular formation resulting in disinhibition of dream generation.

Lesions of the corticopontine tract (**A**) would most often result in deficits in the coordination of planned motor functions.

Lesions to the pyramidal tract (**B**) would result in upper motor neuron syndrome.

Lesions of the red nucleus (**C**) have an impact in locomotion, specifically controlling the muscles of the shoulder and upper arm (such as those utilized in swinging of the arms during bipedal movement). These may also result in resting tremor, abnormal muscle tone, and choreoathetosis, due to its projections to the cerebellum.

Dysfunction of the substantia nigra pars compacta (**E**), such as is seen in Parkinson's disease, results in resting tremor, rigidity, and slowness of movement and difficulty with walking.

Refer to the following image for answers 6 to 9:

6. Correct: Area D (D)

This patient is showing symptomology consistent with Claude's syndrome, specifically an ipsilateral CN III palsy with dilated pupil, and contralateral cerebellar signs and hemiataxia. Claude's syndrome is associated with damage to the red nucleus, brachium conjunctivum, and dorsal midbrain tegmentum, consistent with the lesion shown in area D.

Damage to the superior colliculi and medial longitudinal fasciculus (**A**) would present with upward gaze palsy along with CN III palsy, but would not manifest with cerebellar signs.

Damage to the red nucleus, brachium conjunctivum, and root fibers of CN III of the right side (**B**) would reverse the side of the deficits reported.

Damage to the corticospinal and corticopontine tracts, root fibers of CN III, and the substantia nigra (**C**) would cause accompanying hemiplegia and signs of parkinsonism. Cerebellar signs would not manifest.

7. Correct: Astereognosis of left upper limb (E)

Lesion for this patient is consistent with the diagnosis of Benedikt's syndrome—ipsilateral CN III palsy, contralateral involuntary movement of the limbs, and impaired contralateral vibratory and position sensation. Benedikt's syndrome involves damage to the midbrain tegmentum including the red nucleus, brachium conjunctivum, root fibers of CN III, and medial lemniscus. Consequently, the patient will demonstrate right oculomotor palsy (indicated by ptosis and mydriasis), not left (**A** and **B**); left-sided cerebellar signs (indicated by intention tremor), not right (**C**); and left-sided astereognosis, not right (**D**).

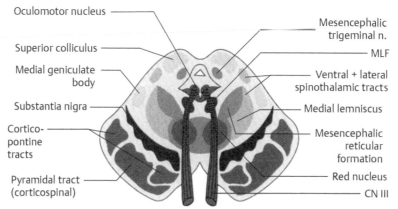

Source: Tsementzis S. Differential Diagnosis in Neurology and Neurosurgery. A Clinician's Pocket Guide. 1st Edition. Thieme; 1999.

8. Correct: Deviation of tongue to the left on attempted protrusion (C)

To have left-sided hemiparesis with a positive Babinski's sign, the lesion must contain the right corticospinal (pyramidal) tract. Hence, area C should describe the zone of infarction for the patient. The pyramidal tract also contains the corticobulbar fibers, lesion of which will lead to upper motor neuron paralysis for lower cranial nerves. Right-sided lesion of the corticobulbar fibers will result in left hypoglossal nerve palsy, leading to left genioglossus muscle palsy and deviation of the tongue to the left on attempted protrusion.

The patient should display signs of Weber's syndrome, specifically, CN III palsy, contralateral spastic hemiplegia, and contralateral weakness of the lower face and tongue.

This patient should display paralysis of the left, but not the right (**D**), buccinator muscle.

Astereognosis (**A**, lesion of medial lemniscus), intention tremor (**B**, lesion of red nucleus and/or brachium conjunctivum), or upward and inward deviation of eye (**E**, lesion of trochlear nerve) does not occur in lesions of ventral part of rostral midbrain (Weber's syndrome).

9. Correct: P1 segment of the PCA (A)

Structures damaged in the Weber's syndrome are supplied by the paramedian branches of the basilar bifurcation and P1 segment of the PCA.

Thalamoperforating arteries (**B**) supply the anterior nuclei of thalamus. Quadrigeminal (**C**) and medial posterior choroidal (**D**) arteries supply the tectal area of midbrain. Thalamogeniculate artery (**E**) supplies the posterior part of thalamus including the medial and lateral geniculate bodies.

Refer to the following image key for answers 10 to 12:

X, superior colliculus; Y, inferior colliculus

10. Correct: Tectum (C)

Superior and inferior colliculi represent dorsal mesencephalon—the tectum (refer to the accompanying image).

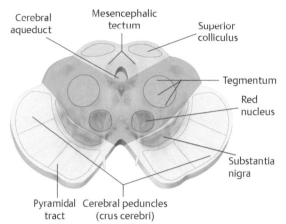

Source: Schünke M, Schulte E, Schumacher U et al. THIEME Atlas of Anatomy: Head, Neck, and Neuroanatomy. 2nd Edition. Thieme; 2016. Illustration by Karl Wesker/Markus Voll.

The mammillary bodies (**A**) are a pair of prominences on the ventromedial surface of the caudal hypothalamus. The red nucleus (**B**) is a part of the mesencephalic tegmentum (**D**), both being ventral to tectum. Basis pedunculi (**E**) comprises the crus cerebri and the substantia nigra, and is the ventral most part of midbrain.

11. Correct: These project to the pulvinar nucleus of thalamus (C)

The pulvinar nucleus of thalamus receives inputs primarily from the superior colliculus and visual cortex. It projects back to the visual cortices and mediates complex cognitive functions.

The inferior colliculus receives input from the ipsilateral lateral lemniscus (**A**) and projects to the medial geniculate nucleus of thalamus (**B**). The facial colliculus overlies the internal genu of the facial nerve (**D**). Superior collicular lesion produces paralysis of upward gaze and deficits in head turn to contralateral space due to its role in programming eye and head movements in visual grasp scenarios, and is not related to ataxia (**E**) or other cerebellar signs.

12. Correct: These receive input from the ipsilateral lateral lemniscus (B)

The inferior colliculus receives input from ipsilateral lateral lemniscus and projects to the medial, not the lateral (**C**), geniculate nucleus of thalamus.

Inputs for the inferior colliculus come from bilateral (though primarily contralateral) cochlea (**A**).

The facial colliculus overlies the internal genu of the facial nerve (**D**). Inferior collicular lesions produce defects in hearing and localizing sound, and are not related to ataxia (**E**) or other cerebellar signs.

Consider the following explanation for answers 13 and 14:

Since the second smaller mass is at the level of the caudal midbrain (pontomesencephalic junction), it is most likely a left CN IV schwannoma.

13. Correct: Intorsion (E)

CN IV supplies the superior oblique muscle, the primary action of which is intorsion of the eye. Actions of extraocular muscles on the eyeball can be summarized as:

Muscle	Primary action	Secondary action
Lateral rectus	Abduction	None
Medial rectus	Adduction	None
Superior rectus	Elevation	Adduction, intorsion
Inferior rectus	Depression	Adduction, extorsion
Superior oblique	Intorsion	Depression, abduction
Inferior oblique	Extorsion	Elevation, abduction

14. Correct: P1 segment of right PCA (E)

Left CN IV originates from the right trochlear nucleus, which is supplied by the right, not the left (**B**), P1 segment of the PCA.

The quadrigeminal artery (**A** and **D**) supplies the inferior colliculus at the level of the caudal midbrain. The thalamogeniculate artery (**C** and **F**) supplies the posterior part of thalamus including the medial and lateral geniculate bodies.

15. Correct: Area H (C)

The red nucleus can be identified as area H.

Areas D (**A**) can be identified as the reticular formation, F (**B**) as the medial lemniscus, I (**D**) as the medial longitudinal fasciculus, and J (**E**) as the oculomotor nucleus.

16. Correct: Area E (E)

Symptoms indicate that the patient has left lower face palsy and a left tongue weakness. Combination of these symptoms indicates injury to the right corticobulbar tract contained within the middle third of the crus cerebri, structure E in the image.

Superior colliculus (**A**), mesencephalic nucleus of CN V (**B**), lateral spinothalamic tract (**C**), and reticular formation (**D**) are not related to the corticobulbar fibers and, therefore, would not account for the pattern of deficits reported in this patient.

17. Correct: Area H (E)

Decorticate posture follows cerebral stroke. Activity of the red nucleus (area H), through the rubrospinal fibers, preferentially targets the flexor motor neurons of the contralateral cervical cord. The upper limbs, as a result, assume a flexed posture.

Reticular formation (area D [**A**]), crus cerebri (area E [**B**]), medial lemniscus (area F [**C**]), and substantia nigra (area G [**D**]) are not involved in decorticate rigidity.

Refer to the following image for answers 15 to 18:

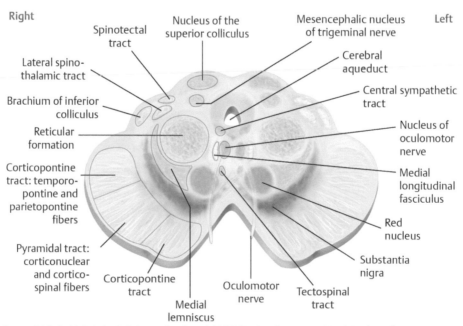

Source: Schünke M, Schulte E, Schumacher U et al. THIEME Atlas of Anatomy: Head, Neck, and Neuroanatomy. 2nd Edition. Thieme; 2016. Illustration by Karl Wesker/Markus Voll.

18. Correct: Area K (E)

The patient is suffering from Horner's syndrome, which is caused by lesions of the sympathetic fibers (area K) that descend from the hypothalamus to the intermediolateral cell column of the ipsilateral thoracolumbar cord.

Lesions of lateral spinothalamic tract (area C [**A**]), medial lemniscus (area F [**B**]), medial longitudinal fasciculus (area I [**C**]), and oculomotor nucleus (area J [**D**]) will not interrupt sympathetic fibers to cause Horner's syndrome.

19. Correct: Nucleus raphe magnus (C)

The drug should influence nucleus raphe magnus, which is a part of the midline raphe serotonergic neurons that project to extensive areas of the central nervous system.

Pars compacta (**A**) and pars reticulata (**B**) of substantia nigra contain dopaminergic neurons that project primarily to neostriatum and GABAergic neurons that project primarily to thalamus, respectively. These play crucial roles in functions of basal ganglia.

Nucleus locus coeruleus (**D**) contains adrenergic neurons that project to several areas of CNS and modulate sleep and wakefulness, and behavior.

Edinger–Westphal nucleus (**E**) is the preganglionic parasympathetic neuron for sphincter pupillae and ciliary muscles, and as a rule, is cholinergic.

Neurons in the PAG (**F**) are mostly enkephalinergic, and play important roles in autonomic and affective functions, and in pain modulation.

20. Correct: Loss of jaw jerk (D)

Among various structures located at the level of the inferior colliculus is the mesencephalic nucleus of trigeminal, which serves as the afferent neuron for the jaw jerk reflex (efferent being the motor nucleus of the trigeminal nerve). Lesion at this level, therefore, might interfere with this reflex.

Loss of accommodation (**A**) and eye adduction (**E**) occur with lesion of CN III. Both the nucleus and the emerging nerve lie at the level of the superior colliculus. Loss of upward gaze (**B**) is a classical finding with lesions of superior colliculus, which is at the level of rostral midbrain.

While corticobulbar fibers may be injured at the level of inferior colliculus, such injury will not involve the upper face (orbicularis oculi, **C**) but will paralyze the contralateral lower face.

Chapter 10
Cranial Nerves

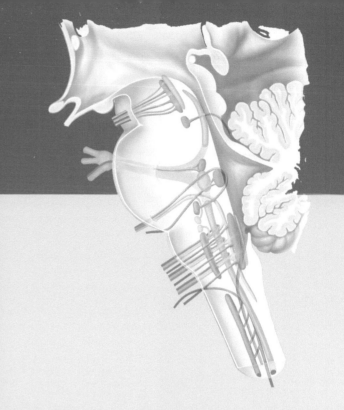

LEARNING OBJECTIVES

▶ Describe the contents of and the structures related to the cavernous sinus. Identify pathways and exit points for cranial nerves from skull base. Correlate functions of cranial nerves with the clinical features associated with their lesions.

▶ Trace the pathway for the corneal reflex. Analyze the clinical features of CN VII lesion.

▶ Trace the three orders of sensory neurons that constitute an afferent pathway.

▶ Analyze the clinical features of CN X palsy, LMN type.

▶ Analyze the clinical features of CN III lesion.

▶ Analyze the clinical features consequent to CN V3 palsy.

▶ Describe the innervation of tongue.

▶ Distinguish between UMN and LMN lesions of CN VII.

▶ Trace the pathways for taste sensation.

▶ Analyze clinical features of CN IV palsy.

▶ Analyze clinical features with lesions of the corticobulbar tract.

▶ Describe the adult derivatives of the embryonic brain vesicles. Describe the histogenesis of the developing neural tube.

▶ Trace the pathway of the secretomotor fibers for the parotid gland.

▶ Describe the pathway for lacrimation.

▶ Describe the trigeminothalamic tracts.

▶ Trace the pathway for carotid sinus baroreceptor reflex.

▶ Analyze the clinical features of CN XII palsy, LMN type.

10.1 Questions

Easy   Medium   Hard

1. A 26-year-old female presents with complete ophthalmoplegia of her right eye. Physical examination reveals anesthesia over the region of the forehead, orbit, and the upper jaw. Sensation over the lower jaw, however, is intact. Which of the following might be the likely location for a lesion in her?

A. Trigeminal ganglion

B. Foramen ovale

C. Foramen rotundum

D. Superior orbital fissure

E. Cavernous sinus

Consider the following case for questions 2 and 3:

When the left cornea of a 26-year-old female is touched with a wisp of cotton, her right eye, but not the left, blinks.

2. Which of the following might be an associated finding in her?

A. Loss of sensation over the left cheek

B. Loss of sensation over the right cheek

C. Absent jaw jerk

D. Deviation of angle of mouth to left on attempt to smile

E. Deviation of angle of mouth to right on attempt to smile

3. Which of the following is the location for the cell body of the primary afferent neuron involved in the reflex?

A. Principal sensory nucleus of trigeminal

B. Spinal nucleus of trigeminal

C. Mesencephalic nucleus of trigeminal

D. Trigeminal ganglion

E. Geniculate ganglion

4. A neurology resident is explaining the three orders of neurons that participate in a sensory pathway to her interns. Which of the following sensation is related to a first-order neuron, cell body for which lies within the CNS?

A. Discriminatory touch from skin overlying masseter muscle

B. Pain from skin overlying masseter muscle

C. Temperature from skin overlying masseter muscle

D. Conscious proprioception from skin overlying masseter muscle

E. Unconscious proprioception from masseter muscle

5. A 9-year-old boy has developed progressive difficulties swallowing and talking. Examination reveals symmetrical protrusion of his tongue and symmetrical smile, but slight drooping of his palate to the left and deviation of his uvula to the right when he says "ah." MRI reveals an intracranial growth. Which of the following is the most likely location of this tumor?

A. Middle third of right crus cerebri; midbrain

B. Middle third of left crus cerebri; midbrain

C. Vagal trigone; rhomboid fossa

D. Hypoglossal trigone; rhomboid fossa

E. Preolivary sulcus; medulla

F. Postolivary sulcus; medulla

6. A 54-year-old man presents with an aneurysm affecting the left posterior communicating artery. Which of the following might be an initial symptom for him?

A. Ptosis

B. Mydriasis

C. Inability to adduct eye

D. Inability to abduct eye

E. Vertical diplopia

7. A 58-year-old man's jaw deviates to the right side on attempted protrusion. Structures passing through which of the following areas might be lesioned in his case?

A. Crus cerebri of right midbrain

B. Crus cerebri of left midbrain

C. Foramen stylomastoid

D. Superior orbital fissure

E. Foramen ovale

F. Foramen rotundum

8. A 39-year-old female presents with a painful ulcer located at the base of her tongue. She is unable to differentiate sugar from salt when both were applied to the perilesional area. Which of the following structures might be defective in her case?

A. CN V

B. CN VII

C. CN IX

D. Chief sensory nucleus of trigeminal

E. Spinal nucleus of trigeminal

F. Nucleus of the solitary tract

9. A 60-year-old man presents with deviation of the angle of his mouth to the left on an attempt to smile. No asymmetry was noted when he was asked to raise his eyebrows. Which of the following might be a likely associated finding in him?

A. Unable to forcefully close his left eye against resistance

B. Unable to forcefully close his right eye against resistance

C. Paralyzed left buccinator muscle

D. Paralyzed right buccinator muscle

E. Absent lacrimation, left eye

F. Absent lacrimation, right eye

10. A 15-year-old girl could easily distinguish salt from sugar when each of these was separately applied to her epiglottis. Which of the following structures needs to be functional for being able to do so?

A. Trigeminal ganglion

B. Geniculate ganglion

C. Superior glossopharyngeal (jugular) ganglion

D. Inferior glossopharyngeal (petrous) ganglion

E. Superior vagal (jugular) ganglion

F. Inferior vagal (nodose) ganglion

11. A 58-year-old male presents with double vision. He states that he must tilt his head to the left during walking and finds it particularly difficult when going downstairs. Physical examination reveals vertical diplopia with his right eyeball deviated upward and slightly inward on forward gaze. Which of the following might be defective in him?

A. Right oculomotor nerve

B. Right oculomotor nucleus

C. Right trochlear nerve

D. Right trochlear nucleus

E. Right abducens nerve

F. Right abducens nucleus

12. A 72-year-old male presents with an infarction affecting the genu of his left internal capsule. Which of the following actions will most likely be unaffected in him?

A. Smiling

B. Whistling

C. Phonation

D. Shrugging of shoulder

E. Tongue movements

13. A male neonate presents with difficulty in suckling. Which of the following zones within the neural tube might have been affected in him?

A. Mesencephalon; basal plate

B. Mesencephalon; alar plate

C. Metencephalon; basal plate

D. Metencephalon; alar plate

E. Myelencephalon; basal plate

F. Myelencephalon; alar plate

14. A 39-year-old woman presents with an aneurysm affecting the internal carotid artery within the cavernous sinus. Which of the following might be the most likely presenting symptom for her?

A. Loss of adduction of eyeball

B. Loss of intorsion of eyeball

C. Loss of abduction of eyeball

D. Anesthesia over forehead

E. Anesthesia over upper jaw

15. An 18-year-old girl presents with a viral infection that affects the tympanic plexus within the middle ear. Which of the following locations represents the cell bodies of the postganglionic neurons which serve the dysfunctional gland in her case?

A. Within the pterygopalatine fossa

B. Within the infratemporal fossa

C. Within the orbit

D. On the hyoglossus muscle inferior to lingual nerve

E. Within the temporal bone

16. A 60-year-old man presents with deviation of the angle of his mouth to the left on an attempt to smile. During physical examination, he was unable to shrug his right shoulder. Which of the following might be a likely associated finding in him?

A. Unable to forcefully close his left eye against resistance

B. Unable to forcefully close his right eye against resistance

C. Deviation of tongue to the right side on attempted protrusion

D. Deviation of tongue to the left side on attempted protrusion

E. Complete paralysis of left masseter muscle

F. Complete paralysis of right masseter muscle

17. A foreign particle blown into the eye results in lacrimation. Which of the following represents the location of the cell bodies of the postganglionic neurons that form the efferent arc of this reflex?

A. Geniculate ganglion
B. Otic ganglion
C. Pterygopalatine ganglion
D. Superior salivatory nucleus
E. Inferior salivatory nucleus

18. A 68-year-old female presents with infarction of thalamus that involves his right VPM nucleus. Which of the following sensations might still be intact in her?

A. Pain sensation from left orbit
B. Discriminative touch sensation from left orbit
C. Pain sensation from left cheek
D. Discriminative touch sensation from left cheek
E. Pain sensation from left gum
F. Discriminative touch sensation from left gum

19. A 62-year-old male presents with unexplained frequent syncopal attacks and falls. In the clinic, he is diagnosed with carotid sinus hypersensitivity syndrome. Which of the following represents the primary location for the cell bodies of the preganglionic motor neurons that are responsible for his symptoms?

A. Solitary nucleus, rostral part
B. Solitary nucleus, caudal part
C. Nucleus ambiguus
D. Dorsal vagal nucleus
E. Spinal nucleus of trigeminal

20. The tongue of a 48-year-old female deviates to the right on attempted protrusion. Which of the following might be the most likely underlying lesion for her?

A. Infarction of right anterior spinal artery
B. Infarction of left anterior spinal artery
C. Infarction of right anterior inferior cerebellar artery
D. Infarction of left anterior inferior cerebellar artery
E. Infarction of right posterior inferior cerebellar artery
F. Infarction of left posterior inferior cerebellar artery

10.2 Answers and Explanations

Easy	Medium	Hard

1. Correct: Cavernous sinus (E)

GG – Gasserian ganglion
P – Pituitary gland
CC – Internal carotid artery
S – Sphenoid sinus

Coronal view through cavernous sinus

Source: Harnsberger HR. Handbook of Head and Neck Imaging. 2nd Edition. St. Louis, MO: Mosby, 1995. Reprinted with permission.

Complete ophthalmoplegia will result from involvement of CN III, IV, and VI. Anesthesia of the forehead and orbit (CN V1) and upper jaw (CN V2) indicates CN V involvement. Sparing of the lower jaw indicates that CN V3 is not involved in the lesion. All these facts together confirm the lesion to be within the cavernous sinus (CN III, IV, V1, and V2 related to the lateral wall and CN VI within the sinus adjacent to the cavernous portion of the internal carotid artery).

Lesion within the trigeminal ganglion (**A**) will not include CN III, IV, or VI, and will include CN V3.

Lesion within the foramen ovale (**B**) will include CN V3 but not CN III, IV, VI, V1, or V2.

Lesion within the foramen rotundum (**C**) will include CN V2 but not CN III, IV, VI, or V1.

Lesion within superior orbital fissure (**D**) will not include CN V2.

2. Correct: Deviation of angle of mouth to right on attempt to smile (E)

The corneal reflex is characterized by bilateral forced eye closure in response to stimulation of either cornea. Afferent limb of the reflex comprises CN V1 and chief sensory nucleus of CN V—a lesion of which causes loss of both direct and indirect reflexes. Efferent limb of the reflex comprises bilateral motor nuclei of CN VII and CN VII—a lesion of which causes unilateral loss of the reflex. Therefore, the left CN VII or its motor nucleus is dysfunctional in this patient. This causes deviation of angle of mouth to the strong, i.e., right, but not left (**D**), side on attempted smiling.

Loss of sensation over the cheek (**A** and **B**) would result from lesion of CN V, which, as explained before, is not the case here. Jaw jerk (**C**) also involves CN V for both the afferent and efferent arcs.

3. Correct: Trigeminal ganglion (D)

The trigeminal ganglion contains cell bodies of the primary (first-order) afferent neurons for all sensation carried by CN V, except for proprioception from muscles of mastication. For the corneal reflex, axon for the neuron is CN V1.

The principal sensory nucleus of CN V (**A**) contains cell bodies of the secondary (second-order) afferent neurons for the corneal reflex (for all discriminative touch sensation from face, for that matter).

Spinal nucleus of CN V (**B**) contains cell bodies of the secondary (second-order) afferent neurons for the pain and thermal sensation from the face.

The mesencephalic nucleus of CN V (**C**) contains cell bodies of the primary (first-order) afferent neurons for proprioception from muscles of mastication.

Lastly, the geniculate ganglion (**E**) contains cell bodies of the primary (first-order) afferent neurons for all sensation carried by CN VII.

4. Correct: Unconscious proprioception from masseter muscle (E)

Unconscious proprioception from the muscles of mastication is relayed to the mesencephalic nucleus of CN V. This nucleus is the only example of cell body of a first-order sensory neuron that is located within the CNS (a notable exception).

All other listed sensations (**A–D**) are carried by primary sensory neurons, cell bodies for which lie within the trigeminal ganglion. The trigeminal ganglion, as with any other ganglia containing cell bodies of primary (first-order) sensory neurons, is located outside the CNS.

5. Correct: Postolivary sulcus; medulla (F)

Clinical features indicate left vagal palsy of LMN type (ipsilateral palatal drooping and contralateral uvular deviation), either at the level of the nerve or the nucleus ambiguus. Since the nerve exits the brainstem through the postolivary sulcus, a tumor affecting the region is likely to cause the symptoms reported in this patient. UMN lesion (crus cerebri for example, **A** and **B**) is ruled out by symmetrical smile and a symmetrical protrusion of tongue (which also indicates multiple cranial nerves are not involved).

The vagal trigone (**C**) overlies the dorsal motor nucleus of vagus, which is not involved in motor supply of the palatal muscles.

Involvement of hypoglossal trigone (**D**, overlying hypoglossal nucleus) or medullary preolivary sulcus (**E**, attachment of hypoglossal nerve) would result in tongue deviation on attempted protrusion.

6. Correct: Mydriasis (B)

The course of CN III (between the posterior cerebral and superior cerebellar arteries, inferolateral to the posterior communicating artery) renders it vulnerable for damage consequent to aneurysm of the related vessels. Also, because of the peripheral location of the parasympathetic fibers within the nerve, these parasympathetic fibers are affected earlier than the somatomotor fibers in cases of compressive lesions, such as an aneurysm. Parasympathetic fibers carried within CN III acts on the sphincter pupillae to constrict the pupil (miosis), and on the ciliary muscle for lens accommodation. A lesion to such fibers, therefore, will cause mydriasis and loss of accommodation.

Loss of adduction (**C**, lesion of medial rectus muscle) and ptosis (**A**, lesion of levator palpebrae superioris) are consequent to damage of somatomotor fibers within CN III, and are not initial events during compression of the nerve.

Inability to abduct the eye (**D**, lesion of CN VI) or vertical diplopia (**E**, lesion of CN IV) does not occur in CN III palsy.

7. Correct: Foramen ovale (E)

The patient's jaw deviates to the paralyzed side (due to action of the intact contralateral lateral pterygoid muscle), consequent to a lesion of CN V3 (which exits skull through the foramen ovale).

Unilateral UMN lesions would not cause jaw deviation, since the motor nucleus of CN V has a bilateral UMN supply. A lesion of the corticobulbar tracts within the crus cerebri (**A** and **B**), therefore, is unlikely to cause jaw deviation.

Lesions of nerves passing through stylomastoid foramen (**C**, CN VII), superior orbital fissure (**D**, CN III, IV, V1, and VI), or foramen rotundum (**F**, CN V2) would not cause the jaw to deviate.

8. Correct: Nucleus of the solitary tract (F)

Both taste and pain sensation from the base (posterior third) of the tongue is conveyed by CN IX. Since sensation for pain is intact and that for taste is lost, the lesion lies at the nuclear level and not with the nerve (**C**). The rostral portion of the solitary nucleus is responsible for taste sensation.

CN V (**A**) and CN VII (**B**) convey general and taste sensation from the anterior two-thirds of tongue, respectively. Chief sensory (**D**) and spinal (**E**) nuclei of CN V are responsible for discriminatory touch, and pain and thermal sensation, from the face (including tongue), respectively.

9. Correct: Paralyzed right buccinator muscle (D)

Following facial paralysis, the angle of the mouth deviates to the strong side on an attempt to smile. Symmetrical elevation of eyebrows rules out upper face (and hence LMN) paralysis. Put together, the patient is suffering from a lower right facial paralysis consequent to a left UMN (corticobulbar) lesion. Therefore, his right buccinator muscle, and not the left (**C**), will be paralyzed.

Closing his eyes against resistance (**A** and **B**) requires functional orbicularis oculi, which are not involved in UMN lesions of CN VII (since upper face has bilateral UMN supply and is therefore spared in UMN lesions).

Lacrimation (**E** and **F**) requires a functional superior salivatory nucleus, which is also not involved in UMN lesions of CN VII.

10. Correct: Inferior vagal (nodose) ganglion (F)

Taste sensation from epiglottis and soft palate is carried by vagus nerve (contains peripheral process of the afferent neuron). Its cell body lies within the inferior vagal (nodose) ganglion, and its central process feeds into the rostral solitary nucleus.

The geniculate ganglion (**B**) contains cell bodies of the afferent neurons responsible for taste sensation from anterior two-thirds of tongue (via CN VII).

The inferior glossopharyngeal ganglion (**D**) contains cell bodies of the afferent neurons responsible for taste sensation from the posterior third of tongue (via CN IX).

Trigeminal (**A**), superior glossopharyngeal (**C**), or superior vagal (**E**) ganglia are not involved in pathways for taste sensation.

11. Correct: Right trochlear nerve (C)

The patient presents with classical signs of right trochlear nerve palsy, with upward (and slightly inward) deviation of the ipsilateral eyeball (due to a paralysis of the superior oblique muscle) and a contralateral tilting of the head to compensate for diplopia. The right trochlear nerve is fed by the left, not the right (**D**), trochlear nucleus, which is located at the level of the caudal midbrain. This is the only cranial nerve that crosses within the brainstem.

Clinical features seen in lesions of oculomotor nerve (**A**) or nucleus (**B**), and abducent nerve (**E**) or nucleus (**F**) are not consistent with the symptoms reported by this patient. Such lesions might cause horizontal diplopia with other characteristic features, but not vertical diplopia as reported in this case.

12. Correct: Phonation (C)

The genu of the internal capsule contains corticobulbar fibers. Muscles responsible for phonation are controlled by the nucleus ambiguus, which has a bilateral supply from the corticobulbar tract. Hence, unilateral lesions of these corticobulbar fibers will least affect phonation.

Corticobulbar fibers control the contralateral motor nucleus of CN VII that innervates lower facial muscles (smiling [**A**] and whistling [**B**]), the contralateral trapezius muscle (shrugging of shoulder [**D**]) via CN XI, and the contralateral motor nucleus of the hypoglossal nerve (tongue movements [**E**]). Each of these functions will be affected in unilateral lesion of the corticobulbar tract.

13. Correct: Metencephalon; basal plate (C)

Suckling requires coordinated activity between facial muscles, which are supplied by the motor nucleus of CN VII located in the caudal pons. Muscles of mastication, supplied by the motor nucleus of CN V located in the rostral pons, also play a secondary role in the act. Basal plates of the embryonic neural tube give rise to motor neurons, and the metencephalon develops into the pons and cerebellum.

Alar plates (**B**, **D**, and **F**) give rise to sensory neurons, and the mesencephalon (**A** and **B**) develops into the midbrain. The myelencephalon (**E** and **F**) develops into the medulla oblongata.

14. Correct: Loss of abduction of eyeball (C)

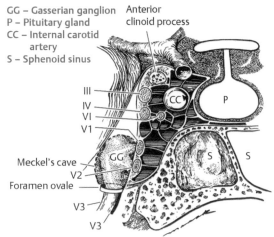

GG – Gasserian ganglion
P – Pituitary gland
CC – Internal carotid artery
S – Sphenoid sinus

Anterior clinoid process

Coronal view through cavernous sinus

Source: Harnsberger HR. Handbook of Head and Neck Imaging. 2nd Edition. St. Louis, MO: Mosby, 1995. Reprinted with permission.

CN III (**A**, supplying medial rectus, which is the primary adductor of eyeball), IV (**B**, supplying superior oblique, which primarily causes intorsion of eyeball), V1 (**D**, responsible for sensation of upper face), and V2 (**E**, responsible for sensation of midface) are related to the lateral wall of the cavernous sinus, while CN VI (supplies lateral rectus, which is the primary abductor of eyeball) lies within the sinus adjacent to the cavernous portion of the internal carotid artery. CN VI, therefore, is most likely to be involved by an aneurysm of the internal carotid artery.

15. Correct: Within the infratemporal fossa (B)

The tympanic plexus is formed by the glossopharyngeal nerve, which carries preganglionic parasympathetic fibers for the parotid gland. A lesion of the plexus will therefore impair salivary secretion from the parotid gland. Cell bodies of the postganglionic neurons that serve the parotid gland are within the otic ganglion, which itself is in the infratemporal fossa.

The pterygopalatine fossa (**A**, location of the pterygopalatine ganglion), orbit (**C**, location of ciliary ganglion), on the hyoglossus muscle inferior to lingual nerve (**D**, location of submandibular ganglion), or within the temporal bone (**E**, location of geniculate ganglion) are not anatomical regions where the otic ganglion is located.

16. Correct: Deviation of tongue to the right side on attempted protrusion (C)

Deviation of angle of the mouth to the left indicates a right facial palsy. Inability to shrug the right shoulder indicates right trapezius paralysis, which is supplied by the right CN XI. Involvement of multiple cranial nerves indicates involvement of the corticobulbar tract (UMN), the left one in this case. This would render paralysis of the right hypoglossal nucleus and nerve—the tongue would deviate to the right (the weak), and not left (**D**), side on attempted protrusion.

An inability to close eyes against resistance (**A** and **B**) would indicate upper facial (orbicularis oris) paralysis, which is not the case in corticobulbar tract (UMN) lesions.

The motor nucleus of CN V has bilateral UMN supply—therefore, unilateral lesions will not result in complete paralysis for muscles of mastication (including masseter, **E** and **F**).

17. Correct: Pterygopalatine ganglion (C)

Cell bodies for the pre- and postganglionic neurons for lacrimation are located in the superior salivatory (**D**) and the pterygopalatine ganglia, respectively.

The geniculate ganglion (**A**) contains cell bodies of the primary (first-order) afferent neurons for all sensation carried by CN VII.

Cell bodies for the pre- and postganglionic neurons for salivation from the parotid gland are located in the inferior salivatory (**E**) and the otic (**B**) ganglia, respectively.

18. Correct: Discriminative touch sensation from left gum (F)

Discriminative touch sensation from within the oral cavity reaches the ipsilateral VPM nucleus of thalamus via the dorsal trigeminothalamic tract.

All modalities of sensation from face (**A–D**), including pain and thermal sensation from within the oral cavity (**E**), reach the contralateral VPM nucleus of thalamus via the ventral trigeminothalamic tract (trigeminal lemniscus).

19. Correct: Dorsal vagal nucleus (D)

Carotid sinus hypersensitivity syndrome is an exaggerated response to carotid sinus baroreceptor stimulation. The hypersensitive receptors detect normal blood flow as excessive and trigger the reflex. It results in syncopal attacks from diminished cerebral perfusion consequent to vagal stimulation of the heart.

Normally, these stretch receptors can trigger impulses (on detection of raised blood pressure) that are carried via CN IX to the caudal part of the solitary nucleus (**B**). This comprises the afferent arc. Stimulation of the solitary nucleus activates neurons within the dorsal vagal nucleus, which contains cell bodies of the preganglionic parasympathetic neurons that supply the heart (and slows it down). This is the efferent component of the reflex arc.

The rostral part of the solitary nucleus (**A**) is involved with taste sensation. The nucleus ambiguus (**C**, motor supply to palate, pharynx, and larynx) or spinal nucleus of trigeminal (**E**, afferent for pain and thermal sensation from face) is not involved in parasympathetic stimulation of heart by vagus.

20. Correct: Infarction of right anterior spinal artery (A)

Deviation of the tongue can be consequent to hypoglossal nerve or nucleus, or corticobulbar tract palsy. All these structures are located within the ventromedial aspect of brainstem and the anterior spinal artery is the only vessel listed that supplies the ventromedial brainstem. Since, supply of the anterior spinal artery is limited to the medulla, the lesion has to be of the LMN, in which case it has to be the right (and not the left [**B**]) artery since the tongue deviates toward the weak side.

Anterior (**C** and **D**) and posterior (**E** and **F**) inferior cerebellar arteries primarily supply the dorsolateral medulla and pons.

Chapter 11

Ascending and Descending Tracts

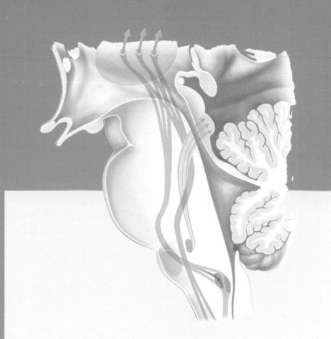

LEARNING OBJECTIVES

- ▶ Analyze the role of the vestibulospinal pathway in decerebrate posturing.
- ▶ Describe the location and function of the fasciculus cuneatus.
- ▶ Describe the symptoms associated with spinocerebellar ataxia, and relate those to damage within the spinocerebellar tract of the spinal cord.
- ▶ Describe the location and function of the fasciculus cuneatus.
- ▶ Describe the location and function of the spino-olivary tract.
- ▶ Describe the role and location of the rubrospinal tract.
- ▶ Describe the function and location of the sacral segments of the lateral spinothalamic tract.
- ▶ Describe the lateral corticospinal tract and its somatotopic organization.
- ▶ Describe the role of the posterior columns in discriminative touch and the somatotopy associated with the fasciculus gracilis and fasciculus cuneatus.
- ▶ Describe the role of the lateral funiculus as a descending autonomic tract within the spinal cord.
- ▶ Analyze the first-, second-, and third-order neurons of the spinothalamic tract.
- ▶ Describe the corticospinal tract, and relate lesion location to symptoms reported.
- ▶ Describe the location and function of the anterior corticospinal tract.

11.1 Questions

Easy	Medium	Hard

1. A 48-year-old woman arrives at the ER and is unconscious and unresponsive to sensory stimuli. A brain MRI reveals extensive damage to large areas of the midbrain. Upon examination, she demonstrates pronounced rigidity within all four limbs. Intact activity of which of the following brainstem pathways is likely responsible for the decerebrate posture observed?

A. Spinothalamic tract

B. Rubrospinal tract

C. Corticospinal tract

D. Lateral vestibulospinal tract

E. Medial vestibulospinal tract

Consider the following image for questions 2 to 6:

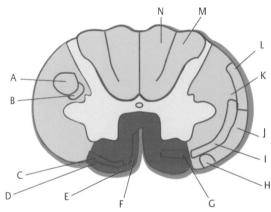

Source: Alberstone C, Benzel E, Najm I et al. Anatomic Basis of Neurologic Diagnosis. 1st Edition. Thieme; 2009.

2. A 21-year-old male receives a spinal injury to the dorsal funiculi at the level of T3. The patient displays a deficit in discriminative touch in the left arm. Which area in the image has most likely been damaged?

A. Area J

B. Area K

C. Area L

D. Area M

E. Area N

3. A 17-year-old right-handed girl presents with an imbalance in walking, with the tendency to reel and fall in an unpredictable direction. Although symptoms first appeared a year ago, they have been progressive in nature. The patient has no relevant past history and no recent exposure to alcohol, drugs, or toxins. Family history revealed similar symptoms in her mother and maternal uncle. Mental status and speech were normal, and there was no cranial nerve abnormality found upon neurological exam. Motor examination revealed normal bulk and power, normal tone, and preserved reflexes in all limbs. Cerebellar signs were present in both upper and lower limbs. Genetic testing revealed mutation of the ataxin 1 gene. In which area of the image would you most likely expect to see degeneration in this patient?

A. Area N

B. Area A

C. Area B

D. Area J

E. Area F

4. A 41-year-old right-handed male presents to the emergency department following a car accident in which substantial spinal trauma was observed. Although complete spinal cord lesion is not suspected, the patient is suffering from loss of pain and temperature sensation on the left side of his body, as well as upper motor neuron paralysis and loss of proprioception on the right side of his body. Which area on the image would be related to the loss of tactile discrimination, vibratory, and position sense observed?

A. Area A

B. Area C

C. Area E

D. Area H

E. Area M

5. A 22-year-old male is admitted to the emergency department following a gunshot wound. Physical examination revealed that the bullet had hit the ventral aspect of the spinal cord, with radiological testing revealing probable damage to the spino-olivary tract. Which area of the presented image best represents the suspected location of damage?

A. Area G

B. Area H

C. Area I

D. Area J

E. Area K

6. Which of the following areas represents the tract that originates within the red nucleus of the midbrain and terminates primarily within the cervical spinal cord, and has a role in upper, but less so in lower limb (primarily facilitates flexion) control?

A. Area A

B. Area B

C. Area C

D. Area D

E. Area E

Consider the following image for questions 7 to 10:

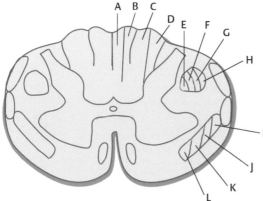

Source: Alberstone C, Benzel E, Najm I et al. Anatomic Basis of Neurologic Diagnosis. 1st Edition. Thieme; 2009.

7. A 72-year-old left-handed woman has noticed a progressive loss of light touch, vibration, and position sense in the right arm and upper trunk. A region of the spinal cord is found to be compressed by the presence of a tumor. Which area of the image is most likely affected?

A. Area A

B. Area B

C. Area C

D. Area D

E. Area E

8. A 29-year-old right-handed male presented to the emergency department following trauma from a pedestrian vs. car accident. Following the injury, a prominent hypalgesia in the posterior aspect of the ankle of his left leg was present. Diffusion tensor imaging would most likely reveal damage to which area identified in the presented image?

A. Area L

B. Area K

C. Area J

D. Area I

E. Area E

9. The area E in the presented image would be concerned with voluntary movement associated with which portion of the body?

A. Cervical segments

B. Thoracic segments

C. Lumbar segments

D. Sacral segments

E. Sacral and lumbar segments

10. A 28-year-old woman presents to her primary physician when she discovers she had difficulty in naming objects without looking at them. In the clinic, she is unable to identify common everyday objects placed on her hand with her eyes closed. Which area identified in the presented image would be required for this ability?

A. Area A

B. Area B

C. Area C

D. Area D

E. Area E

11. A junior intern in the neurology clinic is having difficulty localizing left versus the right side for a lesion. To her rescue, one of the residents hands her over a chart that has tracts listed as "crossed" and "uncrossed." Which of the following pathways all cross within the spinal cord?

A. Medial vestibulospinal tract, lateral spinothalamic tract, anterior spinothalamic tract

B. Anterior corticospinal tract, lateral spinothalamic tract, dorsal columns

C. Ventral spinocerebellar tract, dorsal spinocerebellar tract, lateral vestibulospinal tract

D. Anterior spinothalamic tract, lateral spinothalamic tract, anterior corticospinal tract

E. Medial vestibulospinal tract, lateral spinothalamic tract, anterior spinothalamic tract

12. A 57-year-old male patient presents to the emergency department displaying miosis, ptosis, anhidrosis, and enophthalmos. Upon diagnostic radiology, a lesion is found within the spinal cord. Where would you most likely expect this lesion to be?

A. Anterior funiculus

B. Posterior funiculus

C. Anterior horn

D. Intermediate zone gray matter

E. Lateral funiculus

Consider the following image for questions 13 and 14:

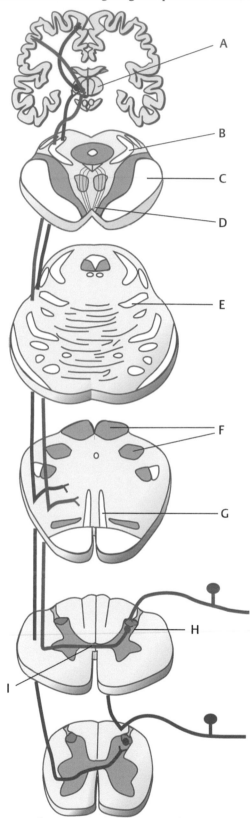

Source: Alberstone C, Benzel E, Najm I et al. Anatomic Basis of Neurologic Diagnosis. 1st Edition. Thieme; 2009.

13. Following a fall from her horse, a 17-year-old girl presented to the emergency department where diagnostic radiology was performed. A lesion in the tract in the presented image was identified. What type of deficit would you expect, if the damage were localized to L4?

A. Pain, temperature, and light touch of medial side of leg below the knee

B. Pain, temperature, and light touch of an oblique band below the inguinal ligament

C. Pain, temperature, and light touch of the umbilicus

D. Sense of position, vibration, and discriminatory touch of medial side of leg below the knee

E. Sense of position, vibration, and discriminatory touch of the umbilicus

14. Within the pathway presented, at which point does the ascending pathway transition from second-order to third-order neurons?

A. Area A

B. Area E

C. Area G

D. Area H

E. Area I

15. Within the medullary segment of the medial lemniscus, the body is represented in a(n):

A. Lying down position (arms medial, legs lateral)

B. Arms lateral, legs medial

C. Upright position (legs ventral, arms dorsal)

D. Inverted position (legs dorsal, arms ventral)

E. Non-specific organization

Consider the following image for questions 16 to 18:

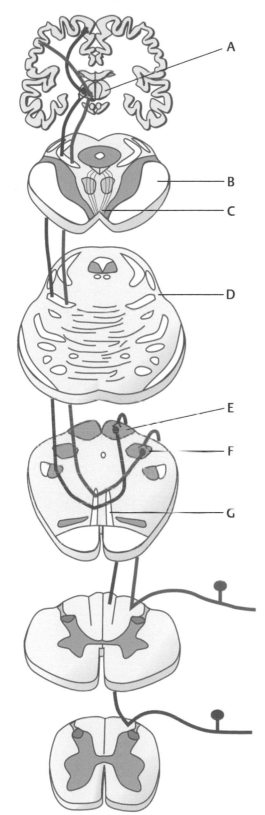

Source: Alberstone C, Benzel E, Najm I et al. Anatomic Basis of Neurologic Diagnosis. 1st Edition. Thieme; 2009.

16. A 66-year-old male is admitted to the emergency department under suspicion of stroke. Imaging reveals an occlusion to the paramedian branches of the basilar artery that has resulted in extensive damage to the pons. What type of deficits would be expected if the tract pictured above was damaged at area D?

A. Ipsilesional hypesthesia

B. Contralesional hypesthesia

C. Ipsilesional hemiparesis

D. Contralesional hemiparesis

E. Bilateral hemiplegia

17. In the pathway previously presented, the transition from second- to third-order neurons occurs within the:

A. Spinal ganglia

B. Fasciculus gracilis

C. Fasciculus cuneatus

D. Thalamus

E. Cerebral cortex

18. Damage to the area E would result in a hypesthesia in the:

A. Contralesional dermatomes above T6

B. Ipsilesional dermatomes above T6

C. Contralesional dermatomes below T6

D. Ipsilesional dermatomes below T6

Consider the following image for questions 19 to 21:

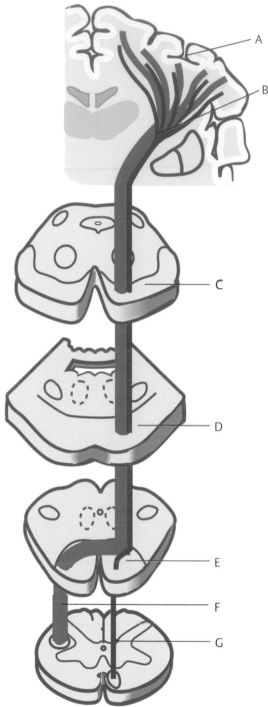

Source: Alberstone C, Benzel E, Najm I et al. Anatomic Basis of Neurologic Diagnosis. 1st Edition. Thieme; 2009.

19. A 52-year-old right-handed woman with a history of hypertension experiences an ischemic stroke to the M4 branch of the left middle cerebral artery, superior division, resulting in significant damage to the lateral surface of the brain, including the region identified in the area A. Based on this information, and the tract in the presented image, what type of clinical symptoms would this patient most likely present with?

A. Right face and arm spastic paresis

B. Left face and arm spastic paresis

C. Right face and arm flaccid paralysis

D. Right face and arm flaccid paralysis

E. Bilateral face and arm flaccid paralysis

20. A 22-year-old female is brought to emergency department following a bar fight in which she suffers blunt force trauma to her back. Diagnostic radiology revealed a bony fragment had penetrated the spinal cord and disrupted the tract denoted in area F, with the bone extending into the lateral portion of the identified tract. Which option best describes the damaged pathway and expected deficit?

A. Unilateral deficit in motor control of the right leg due to damage to the anterior corticospinal tract

B. Unilateral deficit in motor control of the right arm due to damage to the anterior corticospinal tract

C. Unilateral deficit in motor control of the right leg due to damage to the lateral corticospinal tract

D. Unilateral deficit in motor control of the right arm due to damage of the lateral corticospinal tract

E. Bilateral deficit in motor control of the legs due to damage to the lateral corticospinal tract

21. A 22-year-old female is brought to emergency department following a bar fight in which she suffers blunt force trauma to her back. Diagnostic radiology revealed a bony fragment had penetrated the spinal cord and disrupted the tract denoted in area F, with the bone extending into the lateral portion of the identified tract. The tract denoted in area G was preserved. What is the primary role of this preserved pathway?

A. Control of the left side axial muscles of the trunk

B. Bilateral control of axial muscles of the trunk

C. Control of the right side axial muscles of the trunk

D. Control of the left side upper extremity

E. Control of the right side upper extremity

11.2 Answers and Explanations

Easy	Medium	Hard

1. Correct: Lateral vestibulospinal tract (D)

Following damage to the midbrain, pathways from the cerebral cortex that normally suppress extensor tone would no longer be able to provide top-down inhibition to the lower motor neurons. In comparison, the lateral vestibulospinal tract will remain intact following such damage, as it does not receive input from cerebral cortex. As it facilitates extensor motor neurons and extensor reflexes, when the descending inhibitory pathways are no longer present, decerebrate rigidity is commonly observed.

The spinothalamic tract (**A**) carries nociceptive information from the periphery to the cerebral cortex. The rubrospinal tract (**B**) is involved in the mediation of voluntary movement, especially flexion of the upper extremities. Therefore, damage to the rubrospinal tract typically results in decorticate/flexor posture. The corticospinal tract (**C**) is similar to the rubrospinal tract, as it is the primary pathway involved in voluntary movement. Damage to this pathway will typically result in spastic paresis. The medial vestibulospinal tract (**E**) carries impulses from the vestibular system and mainly innervates muscles involved with the control of head and neck rotation and shoulder blades in response to changes in posture and balance.

Refer to the following image for answers 2 to 6:

2. Correct: Area M (D)

The dorsal funiculi consist of the fasciculus gracilis (area N) and the fasciculus cuneatus (area M). These tracts are both involved in the sensation of position, vibration, and discriminative touch. The fasciculus gracilis [area N (**E**)] transmits sensation from the legs, whereas the fasciculus cuneatus transmits sensation from the arms.

Areas J (**A**) and L (**C**) in the image correspond to the ventral and dorsal spinocerebellar tracts. These convey unconscious information (related to position, touch, and pressure sense) to the cerebellum, with damage resulting most often in ataxia. Area K (**B**) in the image is displaying the lateral spinothalamic tract, the main ascending nerve mediating pain and temperature sensation. Damage to this tract would often result in hypalgesia of the body.

3. Correct: Area J (D)

This patient is displaying symptomology consistent with spinocerebellar ataxia, which is confirmed via genetic testing revealing mutation of the ataxin 1 (SCA1) gene. This condition is hereditary, and often manifests with progressive cerebellar signs. Spinocerebellar ataxia results in atrophy of both the cerebellum and the spinal cord and brainstem pathways that send proprioceptive information to the cerebellum. Therefore, one would expect to see atrophy within area J, as this represents the anterior spinocerebellar tract.

The region identified in N (**A**) corresponds to the fasciculus gracilis, which contains proprioceptive, vibration, and tactile sensation information from the

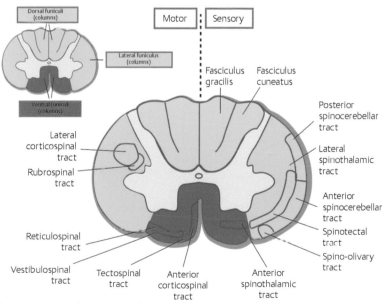

Source: Alberstone C, Benzel E, Najm I et al. Anatomic Basis of Neurologic Diagnosis. 1st Edition. Thieme; 2009.

legs. Area A (**B**) is denoting the lateral corticospinal tract, the primary descending pathway involved in voluntary movement. Area B (**C**) is pointing to the rubrospinal tract, which contributes to flexor muscle tone. Area F (**E**) is the anterior corticospinal tract, which consists of descending fibers involved in the control of axial and proximal limb muscles.

4. Correct: Area M (E)

The patient is displaying the classic signs associated with Brown-Séquard syndrome, a condition caused by damage to one half of the spinal cord, resulting in paralysis and loss of proprioception on the side of the body ipsilateral to the lesion and loss of pain and temperature sensation on the contralesional side. Area M, representing the fasciculus cuneatus, would carry information about position, vibration, and discriminative touch from the upper limbs.

The area labeled A (**A**) on the image is denoting the lateral corticospinal tract, the primary descending pathway involved in voluntary movement. Area C (**B**) is the reticulospinal tract, which is concerned primarily with motor control, especially automatic movements of locomotion and posture. Area E (**C**) is the descending tectospinal tract, which is concerned with reflexive postural movements of the head in response to visual and auditory stimuli. Area H (**D**) is the ascending spino-olivary tract, which conveys sensory information to the cerebellum.

5. Correct: Area H (B)

The spino-olivary tract (area H) lies just anterior to the spinocerebellar tract (area J [**D**]). Areas G (**A**), I (**C**), and K (**E**) represent the anterior spinothalamic, spinotectal tract, and the lateral spinothalamic tracts, respectively.

6. Correct: Area B (B)

The rubrospinal tract (area B) has been shown to play a much larger role in motor control in some nonhuman primates than it does in humans, and can assume much of the duties of the corticospinal tract (area A) when the latter is damaged.

Area C denotes the reticulospinal tract, which is also involved in motor control of the upper limbs. However, this tract originates from the reticular formation, and is largely involved in modulating the sensitivity of flexor responses to ensure that harmful stimuli do not elicit a withdrawal response when it would be harmful to do so.

Area D denotes the vestibulospinal tract, which is involved in the mediation of postural adjustments and head movements, while also helping to maintain balance by detecting and correcting small movements of the body via the vestibular system.

Area E in the presented image represents the tectospinal tract, a descending motor pathway that originates within the deep layers of the superior colliculus that is assumed to be involved in the reflexive turning of the head in response to abrupt visual stimuli.

Refer to the following image for answers 7 to 10:

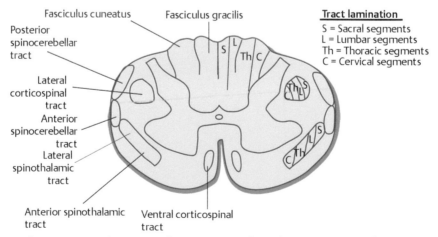

Source: Alberstone C, Benzel E, Najm I et al. Anatomic Basis of Neurologic Diagnosis. 1st Edition. Thieme; 2009.

7. Correct: Area D (D)

The area D represents the cervical segments of the fasciculus cuneatus, which when damaged would cause an absence in the sensation of light touch, vibration, and position sense in the right arm and upper trunk.

Areas A and B represent the sacral and lumbar segments of the fasciculus gracilis, which carry the same sensory information, but for regions below T6. The two fasciculi are separated by a septum.

Area C represents the thoracic portions of the fasciculus cuneatus, and therefore conveys similar senses for the thoracic segments of the body (not the arm).

Area E represents the cervical segments of the lateral corticospinal tract, damage of which would result in deficits in volitional movement.

8. Correct: Area I (D)

Areas I to L in the presented image represent the lateral spinothalamic tract, the pathway responsible for carrying pain and temperature information to the thalamus and ultimately to cortical and subcortical regions. It is somatotopically organized, with medial fibers concerned with sensation from the upper and lateral fibers concerned with sensation from the lower body. As the posterior ankle is represented by the S1 nerves, the correct answer would be area I, which represents the sacral segments.

Area J (C) contains the lumbar, area K (B) contains the thoracic, and area L (A) contains the cervical segments of the spinothalamic tract.

Area E (E) corresponds to the cervical segments of the lateral corticospinal tract, and is responsible for voluntary movement of the arm.

9. Correct: Cervical segments (A)

The lateral corticospinal tract conveys messages from primary motor cortex related to voluntary movement. This tract is somatotopically organized, with fibers that are associated with movement of the arms located medially, and those that are concerned with motor input to the legs being represented laterally. Therefore, area E would contain fibers related to movement of the cervical segments (A).

Thoracic (B), lumbar (C), and sacral (D) segments of the tract are represented by areas F, G and H, respectively.

Lastly, as the lateral corticospinal tract does not combine somatotopy from the upper and lower parts of the body as it ascends, there would be no single region responsible for both lumbar and sacral segments (E).

10. Correct: Area D (D)

The ability to recognize the form and texture of an unseen object, known as stereognosis, is dependent on the posterior column. Further, as the unknown objects were being placed on the hand of the patient, it would involve the cervical portion of the fasciculus cuneatus (area D) for stereognosis.

Fasciculus gracilis (areas A and B) also carry similar sorts of information from the lower body (below T6). Area C represents the thoracic segments of the fasciculus cuneatus, and therefore conveys position, vibratory, and discrimination senses for the thoracic segments of the body (not the hand). Area E corresponds to the cervical segments of the lateral corticospinal tract, and is responsible for voluntary movement of the arm.

11. Correct: Anterior spinothalamic tract, lateral spinothalamic tract, anterior corticospinal tract (D)

The lateral and anterior spinothalamic tracts cross to the contralateral white matter of the cord close to the cell bodies of origin before ascending to the thalamus. The anterior corticospinal tract, in contrast to the lateral corticospinal tract, does not decussate at the level of the medulla oblongata, but rather crosses over in the spinal level that it innervates.

The dorsal columns (B, fasciculus gracilis and cuneatus) do not cross over until they reach the cuneate nucleus at the level of the lower medullar oblongata.

Although the ventral spinocerebellar tract crosses within the spinal cord (and again to enter the cerebellum), the dorsal spinocerebellar tracts (C) do not decussate as they ascend the spinal cord. Neither the medial (A and E) nor the lateral vestibulospinal (C) tracts cross within the spinal cord.

12. Correct: Lateral funiculus (E)

The patient is displaying the classic signs related to Horner's syndrome, due to disruption of the hypothalamospinal tract. The hypothalamospinal tract connects the hypothalamus to the ciliospinal center of the intermediolateral cell column within the spinal cord (at the T1–T2 level). This tract is found in the posterior quadrant of the lateral funiculus.

The anterior funiculus (A) contains the spinothalamic, anterior corticospinal, medial longitudinal fasciculus, vestibulospinal, and reticulospinal tracts. The posterior funiculus (B) contains the cuneate and gracilis fasciculi. The anterior horn (C) contains Rexed's laminae VIII and IX, which consist primarily of interneurons associated with motor function. The intermediate zone gray matter (D), Rexed's lamina VII, contains Clark's column between T1 and L3 spinal cord levels and relays proprioceptive and tactile sensory inputs from spinal cord levels below T1 (trunk and lower limbs) to the cerebellum.

Refer to the following image for answers 13 and 14:

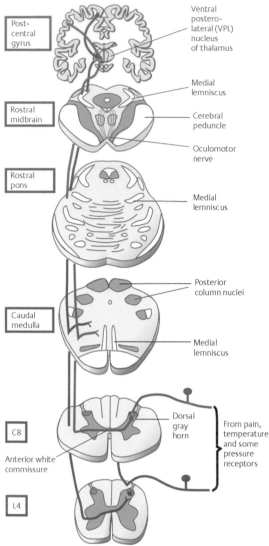

Source: Alberstone C, Benzel E, Najm I et al. Anatomic Basis of Neurologic Diagnosis. 1st Edition. Thieme; 2009.

13. Correct: Pain, temperature, and light touch of medial side of leg below the knee (A)

The presented image is displaying the spinothalamic tract, which is responsible for pain, temperature, and light touch sensation (**A, B,** and **C**). The dermatome ascribed to L4 consists of a small area of the medial side of the leg below the knee.

The dermatomes responsible for the oblique band below the inguinal ligament (**B**) and the umbilicus (**C**) are L1 and T10, respectively.

Sense of position, vibration, and discriminatory touch (**D** and **E**) are relayed to the brain via the dorsal column–medial lemniscus.

14. Correct: Area A (A)

The spinothalamic tract consists of first-order neurons with cell bodies within the dorsal root ganglion, which synapses within the nucleus proprius. The second-order neurons cross within the spinal cord, and ascend through the spinal cord, medulla, and pons to terminate within the ventral posterior lateral nucleus of thalamus. It is at this location, area A (**A**), that the third-order neurons within the ventral posterolateral nucleus of the thalamus send axons to the postcentral gyrus.

Areas E (**B**) and G (**C**) denote the medial lemniscus within the rostral midbrain and rostral pons, respectively. Area H (**D**) denotes the dorsal gray horn, where the pathway transition from first- to second-order neurons. Area I (**E**) denotes the anterior white commissure, where the second-order neurons that originate in the dorsal gray horn of the spinal cord cross the midline before projecting to the ventral posterolateral nucleus of the thalamus.

15. Correct: Upright position (legs ventral, arms dorsal) (C)

The dorsal column–medial lemniscus has the following somatotopy:

Within the dorsal columns (fasciculus gracilis and fasciculus cuneatus), caudal body parts are represented medially and rostral segments are represented laterally (**B**).

Within the medullary segment of the medial lemniscus, the body is represented in an upright position with the legs ventral and arms dorsal (**C**).

Within the pontine portion of the medial lemniscus, the somatotopy represents the body in a lying down position, with the arms medial and legs lateral (**A**).

Within the midbrain portion, the somatotopy is represented in an inverted position (**D**), with the legs dorsal and arms ventral.

The dorsal column-medial lemniscus, therefore, has a well-defined somatotopic organization (**E**) in each area of CNS that it traverses.

Refer to the following image for answers 16 to 18:

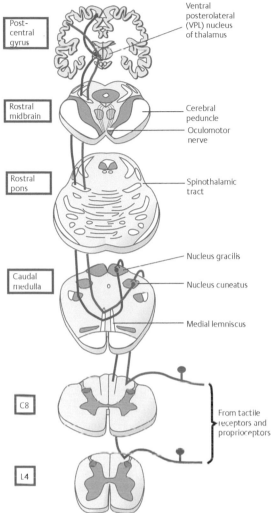

Post-central gyrus

Ventral posterolateral (VPL) nucleus of thalamus

Rostral midbrain

Cerebral peduncle

Oculomotor nerve

Rostral pons

Spinothalamic tract

Nucleus gracilis

Caudal medulla

Nucleus cuneatus

Medial lemniscus

C8

From tactile receptors and proprioceptors

L4

Source: Alberstone C, Benzel F, Najm I et al. Anatomic Basis of Neurologic Diagnosis. 1st Edition. Thieme; 2009.

16. Correct: Contralesional hypesthesia (B)

In the presented image of the tract, the dorsal column–medial lemniscus, mediates position sense and discriminative touch. Therefore, damage to this pathway would result in a hypesthesia. At area D (pons), decussation of the ascending tracts has occurred. Therefore, we would expect a contralesional hypesthesia.

An ipsilesional hypesthesia (**A**) would be expected if damage to the medial lemniscus was before the decussation at the level of the caudal medulla, or if damage was to the dorsal columns of the spinal cord.

A hemiparesis or hemiplegia (**C, D,** or **E**) would be expected if damage was to the primary descending tract responsible for volitional motor control, the lateral corticospinal tract.

17. Correct: Thalamus (D)

The transition from second- to third-order neurons occurs within the ventral posterolateral nucleus of the thalamus.

First-order neurons of the dorsal column–medial lemniscus are located within the spinal ganglia (**A**) at all levels of the spinal cord. Second-order neurons are located within the gracile and cuneate nuclei of the medulla (**B** and **C**). The ultimate destination for these fibers is the sensory areas of the cerebral cortex (**E**).

18. Correct: Ipsilesional dermatomes below T6 (D)

The medial lemniscus decussates at the level of the caudal medulla. Therefore, damage at or below this level, as indicated in area E, would result in an ipsilesional deficit (**B** or **D**) in position sense and discriminative touch. Further, the labeled region is indicating the nucleus gracilis, which is responsible for those dermatomes below T6, representing the lower extremities.

In order for a contralesional deficit to be present (**A** and **C**), the damage would have to be rostral to the decussation. In order for the damage to affect dermatomes above T6 (**A** and **B**), the nucleus cuneatus would need to be affected.

Refer to the following image for answers 19 to 21:

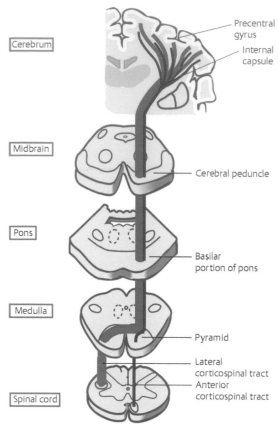

Cerebrum

Precentral gyrus

Internal capsule

Midbrain

Cerebral peduncle

Pons

Basilar portion of pons

Medulla

Pyramid

Lateral corticospinal tract

Anterior corticospinal tract

Spinal cord

Source: Alberstone C, Benzel E, Najm I et al. Anatomic Basis of Neurologic Diagnosis. 1st Edition. Thieme; 2009.

19. Correct: Right face and arm spastic paresis (A)

The pathway displayed in the image is the corticospinal tract, which is composed of projections primarily from the primary motor and supplementary motor cortices. Disruption of the corticospinal tract at the level of the cerebral cortex, as indicated in labeled area A, would result in an upper motor neuron disorder consisting of spastic paresis (**A** and **B**). Additionally, as the damaged region is denoted on the left side of cerebral cortex, and above the pyramidal decussation, so the deficit would involve the right (contralesional) face and arm (**A, C,** and **D**). Therefore, the correct answer would be a right-sided face and arm spastic paresis.

Flaccid paralysis (**C, D,** and **E**) would occur following damage to the lower motor neurons, caused by damage to the fibers travelling from the ventral horn of the spinal cord to the relevant muscle.

20. Correct: Unilateral deficit in motor control of the right leg due to damage to the lateral corticospinal tract (C)

The area F in the presented image corresponds to the lateral corticospinal tract (**C, D,** and **E**), which is composed of projections from the primary and supplementary motor cortices in addition to premotor cortex, and is responsible for conveying impulses concerned with voluntary movement. Since the damage is on the right side of the spinal cord following the pyramidal decussation, deficits would be ipsilesional. Lastly, since the lateral corticospinal tract is somatotopically organized with fibers for the arms represented medially and those for the legs represented laterally, the leg is most likely affected. Therefore, the correct answer would be a unilateral deficit in motor control of the right leg, but not the arm (**D**). A bilateral deficit (**E**) would require damaging both descending corticospinal tracts.

As evident by the symptoms reported, the anterior corticospinal tract (**A** and **B**) was not involved in the lesion.

21. Correct: Bilateral control of axial muscles of the trunk (B)

The indicated pathway is the anterior corticospinal tract—a descending pathway concerned with motor control primarily for the axial musculature (**A, B,** and **C**). Additionally, in comparison to the lateral corticospinal tract, most projections of the anterior corticospinal tract are bilateral, and not unilateral (**A** and **C**).

Control of the distal extremities (**D** and **E**), as previously noted, is handled by the lateral corticospinal tract.

Chapter 12
Thalamus

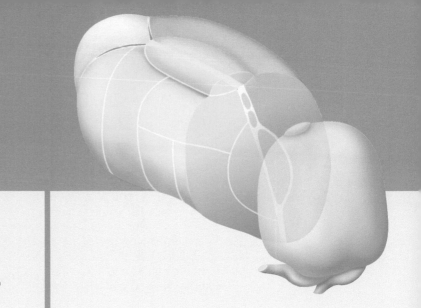

LEARNING OBJECTIVES

- ▶ Describe the connections and functions of thalamic nuclei. Describe the blood supply of thalamus.
- ▶ Trace the location of thalamic nuclei with relation to the ventricles.
- ▶ Identify the excitatory and inhibitory thalamic nuclei.
- ▶ Describe lesions of LGB. Describe the blood supply of thalamus.

12.1 Questions

Easy	Medium	Hard

Consider the following case for questions 1 and 2:

A 56-year-old woman was found unconscious on her kitchen floor. She was brought to the ER where she regained consciousness, but was admitted for resuscitation. Apart from slight slurring of speech, no other sensorimotor deficit was noted. A week after the incident, she can identify her family members and friends, but has no recollection of the incident that had led to her hospital admission.

1. Which of the following structures might have been affected by this patient's stroke?

A. VA nucleus of thalamus

B. VP nucleus of thalamus

C. DM nucleus of thalamus

D. Subthalamic nucleus

E. Genu of the internal capsule

2. Given the structure damaged, which of the following vessels is most likely to be involved in her case?

A. Thalamoperforating branch of posterior cerebral artery (P1)

B. Thalamogeniculate branch of the posterior cerebral artery (P2)

C. Medial posterior choroidal branch of the posterior cerebral artery (P2)

D. Lenticulostriate branch of middle cerebral artery

E. Medial striate branch of the anterior cerebral artery

Consider the following case for questions 3 to 5:

A 60-year-old woman presents with headache and blurred vision. MRI demonstrates moderate hydrocephalus with dilated left lateral ventricle, but normal-sized third ventricle, cerebral aqueduct, and fourth ventricle. A tumor mass, obstructing the ventricular system, was suggested as the probable cause for her symptoms.

3. Extension of the tumor might involve which of the following thalamic nuclei in her?

A. Pulvinar nucleus

B. LGB

C. MGB

D. Centromedian nucleus

E. Anterior nucleus

4. If the thalamic nucleus previously identified was involved, which of the following might be an associated finding in her?

A. Visual agnosia

B. Contralateral homonymous hemianopia

C. Contralateral deafness

D. Movement disorders

E. Amnesia

5. Which of the following is the primary supply for the thalamic nucleus that could potentially be involved in her case?

A. Thalamoperforating branch of posterior cerebral artery (P1)

B. Thalamogeniculate branch of the posterior cerebral artery (P2)

C. Medial posterior choroidal branch of the posterior cerebral artery (P2)

D. Lenticulostriate branch of middle cerebral artery

E. Medial striate branch of the anterior cerebral artery

Consider the following case for questions 6 and 7:

A 39-year-old woman presents with continuous pain and paresthesia affecting her extremities. She states that these are triggered by innocuous stimuli (a gentle breeze, for example), and is aggravated by emotional stimuli.

6. Which of the following thalamic nuclei might have been affected by a stroke in this patient?

A. VA

B. VL

C. VP

D. DM

E. Pulvinar

7. Which of the following is the primary supply for the involved thalamic nucleus in her case?

A. Thalamoperforating branch of posterior cerebral artery (P1)

B. Thalamogeniculate branch of the posterior cerebral artery (P2)

C. Medial posterior choroidal branch of the posterior cerebral artery (P2)

D. Lenticulostriate branch of middle cerebral artery

E. Medial striate branch of the anterior cerebral artery

8. Thalamic neurons prioritize and modulate sensory information on their way to the cerebral cortex. Which of the following is an inhibitory nucleus within the thalamus?

A. VA

B. VL

C. VPL

D. TRN

E. Pulvinar

Consider the following case for questions 9 to 11:

A 58-year-old man presents with deviation of the tongue to the right on attempted protrusion and paralysis of the right lower face. MRI demonstrates a tumor affecting the internal capsule.

9. In this patient, extension of the tumor might involve which of the following thalamic nuclei?

A. Pulvinar nucleus

B. Anterior nucleus

C. VP nucleus

D. VA nucleus

E. DM nucleus

10. If the previously identified thalamic nucleus was involved, which of the following might be an associated finding in this patient?

A. Visual agnosia

B. Contralateral homonymous hemianopia

C. Contralateral hemianesthesia

D. Movement disorders

E. Amnesia

11. Which of the following is the primary supply for the thalamic nucleus that could potentially be involved in his case?

A. Thalamoperforating branch of posterior cerebral artery (P1)

B. Thalamogeniculate branch of the posterior cerebral artery (P2)

C. Medial posterior choroidal branch of the posterior cerebral artery (P2)

D. Lenticulostriate branch of middle cerebral artery

E. Medial striate branch of the anterior cerebral artery

Consider the following case for questions 12 and 13:

A 36-year-old man presents with sudden-onset blindness affecting the left hemifield for both his right and left eyes.

12. In this patient, which of the following structures might be lesioned?

A. Left optic nerve

B. Right optic nerve

C. LGB of left thalamus

D. LGB of right thalamus

E. Optic chiasma

13. Given the structure damaged, which of the following vessels is most likely to be involved in his case?

A. Thalamoperforating branch of right posterior cerebral artery (P1)

B. Thalamoperforating branch of left posterior cerebral artery (P1)

C. Thalamogeniculate branch of the right posterior cerebral artery (P2)

D. Thalamogeniculate branch of the left posterior cerebral artery (P2)

E. Right ophthalmic artery

F. Left ophthalmic artery

Consider the following case for questions 14 and 15:

A 56-year-old man presents with tremor of his right fingers that worsens when he tries to grasp an object. He also has sinuous, rapid, and jerky movements that involve his right forearm.

14. Which of the following structures might be lesioned in this patient?

A. Posterior lobe of left cerebellar hemisphere

B. Posterior lobe of right cerebellar hemisphere

C. Left putamen

D. Right putamen

E. VL nucleus of left thalamus

F. VL nucleus of right thalamus

15. Given the structure damaged, which of the following vessels is most likely to be involved in his case?

A. Left posterior inferior cerebellar artery

B. Right posterior inferior cerebellar artery

C. Lenticulostriate branch of left middle cerebral artery

D. Lenticulostriate branch of right middle cerebral artery

E. Thalamoperforating branch of left posterior cerebral artery (P1)

F. Thalamoperforating branch of right posterior cerebral artery (P1)

Consider the following case for questions 16 to 18:

A 66-year-old woman presents with signs of increased intracranial pressure. MRI demonstrates moderate hydrocephalus with dilated lateral ventricles, but normal-sized cerebral aqueduct and fourth ventricle. A tumor affecting part of the ventricular system that develops from the diencephalon is identified as the probable cause for her symptoms.

16. Extension of the tumor might involve which of the following thalamic nuclei in her?

A. VPL nucleus

B. VPM nucleus

C. VL nucleus

D. VA nucleus

E. DM nucleus

17. If the previously identified thalamic nucleus was involved, which of the following might be an associated finding in this patient?

A. Visual agnosia

B. Contralateral homonymous hemianopia

C. Contralateral hemianesthesia

D. Movement disorders

E. Amnesia

18. Which of the following is the primary supply for the thalamic nucleus that could potentially be involved in her case?

A. Thalamoperforating branch of posterior cerebral artery (P1)

B. Thalamogeniculate branch of the posterior cerebral artery (P2)

C. Medial posterior choroidal branch of the posterior cerebral artery (P2)

D. Lenticulostriate branch of middle cerebral artery

E. Medial striate branch of the anterior cerebral artery

Consider the following case for questions 19 and 20:

A 46-year-old woman presents with lesion of the special visceral afferent (SVA) column of nuclei located in the pons.

19. Which of the following thalamic nuclei receives input from the involved nucleus?

A. VL

B. VPL

C. VPM

D. DM

E. Pulvinar

20. Which of the following is the primary supply for the thalamic nucleus in her case?

A. Thalamoperforating branch of posterior cerebral artery (P1)

B. Thalamogeniculate branch of the posterior cerebral artery (P2)

C. Medial posterior choroidal branch of the posterior cerebral artery (P2)

D. Lenticulostriate branch of middle cerebral artery

E. Medial striate branch of the anterior cerebral artery

12.2 Answers and Explanations

Easy	Medium	Hard

1. Correct: DM nucleus of thalamus (C)

The patient is suffering from anterograde amnesia, which is an inability to learn new information following the onset of amnesia. The DM nucleus of the thalamus receives extensive inputs from the limbic system and projects out to the cingulate, prefrontal, and orbitofrontal cortex. Via these connections, it forms part of an important circuit that is involved with consolidation of memories. Amnesia, both anterograde and retrograde, is observed with lesions of the nucleus.

The VA nucleus of thalamus (**A**) receives inputs primarily from the basal ganglia and is related to fine control of movements.

The VP nucleus of thalamus (**B**) receives inputs carried via the medial lemniscus, spinothalamic tracts, trigeminal lemniscus, trigeminothalamic tracts, etc., and is related to all modalities of sensation from the contralateral body and face. It projects out to the somatosensory cortex.

The subthalamic nucleus (**D**) participates in the indirect pathway of the basal ganglia circuit and, therefore, is related to fine control of movements.

Lastly, the genu of the internal capsule (**E**) contains the corticobulbar fibers. Lesion of the genu will not cause amnesia.

2. Correct: Medial posterior choroidal branch of the posterior cerebral artery (P2) (C)

DM nucleus of the thalamus is supplied by the medial posterior choroidal branch of the posterior cerebral artery (P2).

The thalamoperforating branch of posterior cerebral artery (**A**) supplies the anterior part of the thalamus, including the anterior, VA, and VL nucleus.

The thalamogeniculate branch of the posterior cerebral artery (**B**) supplies the posterior thalamus, including the LGB, MGB, pulvinar, VPL, and VPM nuclei.

The genu of the internal capsule is supplied by the lenticulostriate branch of middle cerebral artery (**D**).

The medial striate branch of the anterior cerebral artery (**E**) supplies the head of the caudate nucleus, anterior part of the lenticular nucleus, and the anterior limb of the internal capsule, among other structures, but provides no supply for thalamic nuclei.

3. Correct: Anterior nucleus (E)

Since the left lateral ventricle was dilated, and the third ventricle was of normal size, the tumor most likely is obstructing the left interventricular foramen (of Monro). This foramen lies between the column of fornix and the anterior nucleus of thalamus, which therefore will be the most likely affected by the tumor.

The pulvinar nucleus (**A**), LGB (**B**), and MGB (**C**) are located in the dorsal part of thalamus and are not related to the interventricular foramen. The centromedian nucleus (**D**) has an intralaminar midline location, and is also not related to the interventricular foramen.

4. Correct: Amnesia (E)

The anterior nucleus of thalamus receives extensive inputs from the mammillary bodies and fornix and projects out to the cingulate cortex. Via these limbic connections, it forms part of an important circuit that is involved with consolidation of memories. Amnesia, both anterograde and retrograde, is observed with lesions of the nucleus.

Visual agnosia (**A**, lesions of pulvinar nucleus), homonymous hemianopia (**B**, lesions of LGB), deafness (**C**, lesion of MGB), or movement disorders (**D**, lesion of VA/VL nuclei) would not occur from lesions of the anterior thalamic nucleus.

5. Correct: Thalamoperforating branch of posterior cerebral artery (P1) (A)

The thalamoperforating branch of the posterior cerebral artery supplies the anterior part of the thalamus, including the anterior, VA, and VL nucleus.

The thalamogeniculate branch of the posterior cerebral artery (**B**) supplies the posterior thalamus, including the LGB, MGB, pulvinar, VPL, and VPM nuclei.

The DM nucleus of the thalamus is supplied by the medial posterior choroidal branch of the posterior cerebral artery (**C**).

The genu and posterior limb of the internal capsule is supplied by the lenticulostriate branch of middle cerebral artery (**D**), but it provides no blood supply to the thalamus.

The medial striate branch of the anterior cerebral artery (**E**) supplies the head of caudate nucleus, anterior part of the lenticular nucleus, and the anterior limb of the internal capsule, among other structures, but has no blood supply to the thalamic nuclei.

6. Correct: VP (C)

The patient is suffering from thalamic pain syndrome (Dejerine–Roussy syndrome), which is often due to involvement of the VP nucleus. In this syndrome, pain and temperature sensations are diminished initially but over time return and become highly abnormal. Stimuli that would otherwise be considered as innocuous or even pleasant can be horribly painful (allodynia).

VA (**A**) and VL (**B**) nuclei of thalamus receive inputs primarily from the basal ganglia and cerebellum, and are related to prediction, coordination, and fine control of movements.

The DM nucleus of thalamus (**D**) receives extensive inputs from the limbic system and projects out to the cingulate, prefrontal, and orbitofrontal cortex. Via these connections, it forms part of an important circuit that is involved with consolidation of memories.

The pulvinar nucleus of the thalamus (**E**) receives inputs from the superior colliculus and projects out to the parietooccipital cortex. It serves as a relay station between subcortical visual centers and their respective association cortices.

7. Correct: Thalamogeniculate branch of the posterior cerebral artery (P2) (B)

The thalamogeniculate branch of the posterior cerebral artery supplies the posterior thalamus, including the pulvinar, LGB, MGB, VPL, and VPM nuclei.

The thalamoperforating branch of posterior cerebral artery (**A**) supplies the anterior part of the thalamus, including the anterior, VA, and VL nucleus.

The DM nucleus of the thalamus is supplied by the medial posterior choroidal branch of the posterior cerebral artery (**C**).

The middle cerebral artery (**D**) supplies the genu and posterior limb of the internal capsule but it has no supply for the thalamus.

The medial striate branch of the anterior cerebral artery (**E**) supplies the head of caudate nucleus, anterior part of the lenticular nucleus, and the anterior limb of the internal capsule, among other structures, but has no supply for thalamic nuclei.

8. Correct: TRN (D)

Among the nuclei listed, only the TRN is an inhibitory nucleus. Known as the "gatekeeper of the gatekeeper," the TRN receives (excitatory) feedback from the cerebral cortex about relayed information and accordingly inhibits other thalamic nuclei. Glutamate and aspartate (excitatory) are released from all thalamic nuclei except for TRN, which is GABAergic (inhibitory).

Consider the following explanation for answers 9 to 11:

Deviation of the tongue to the right on attempted protrusion and paralysis of right lower face indicates involvement of the left corticobulbar fibers (UMN) at the genu of the left internal capsule.

9.   Correct: VA nucleus (D)

The internal capsule passes lateral to the thalamus. The genu of the internal capsule is in the vicinity of the VA nucleus of the thalamus, separated only by the TRN. A tumor affecting the genu might, therefore, involve the nucleus.

The pulvinar (A) and VP nuclei (C) lie in the dorsal part of the thalamus and might be related to the posterior limb of the internal capsule. The anterior nucleus (B, related to the interventricular foramen) or DM nucleus (E, related to the third ventricle) are not related to the internal capsule.

10.   Correct: Movement disorders (D)

The VA nucleus of thalamus receives inputs primarily from the basal ganglia and is related to fine control of motor movements. Lesion to the nucleus will therefore cause movement disorders typical of basal ganglia lesions.

Visual agnosia (A, lesion of pulvinar), contralateral homonymous hemianopia (B, lesion of LGB), contralateral hemianesthesia (C, lesion of VP), or amnesia (E, lesion of anterior/DM nucleus) does not occur with lesions of the VA nucleus.

11.   Correct: Thalamoperforating branch of posterior cerebral artery (P1) (A)

The thalamoperforating branch of the posterior cerebral artery supplies the anterior part of the thalamus, including the anterior, VA, and VL nuclei.

The thalamogeniculate branch of the posterior cerebral artery (B) supplies the posterior thalamus, including the LGB, MGB, pulvinar, VPL, and VPM nuclei.

The DM nucleus of the thalamus is supplied by the medial posterior choroidal branch of the posterior cerebral artery (C).

The genu and posterior limb of the internal capsule is supplied by the lenticulostriate branch of middle cerebral artery (D), but provides no supply for the thalamus.

The medial striate branch of the anterior cerebral artery (E) supplies the head of the caudate nucleus, anterior part of the lenticular nucleus, and the anterior limb of the internal capsule, among other structures, but has no supply for thalamic nuclei.

12.   Correct: LGB of right thalamus (D)

The patient is suffering from a left homonymous hemianopia, which is caused by lesions of the right, but not the left (C), LGB.

Lesions of the optic nerves (A and B) would cause complete blindness in the respective eyes. Damage to the optic chiasma (E) would cause bitemporal hemianopia.

13.   Correct: Thalamogeniculate branch of the right posterior cerebral artery (P2) (C)

The right LGB is supplied by the thalamogeniculate branch of the right, and not the left (D), posterior cerebral artery.

The thalamoperforating branch of the posterior cerebral artery (A and B) supplies the anterior part of the thalamus, including the anterior, VA, and VL nucleus.

The ophthalmic artery (E and F) supplies the orbit and its contents (including the optic nerves).

Consider the following explanation for answers 14 and 15:

The patient has intention tremor (cerebellar sign) and choreoathetosis (basal ganglia sign)—this is possibly due to a lesion of the VL nucleus of thalamus. The nucleus is subdivided into two main parts: pars oralis (VLo) and pars caudalis (VLc). The internal segment of the pallidum projects to VLo, while the deep cerebellar nuclei project to VLc.

14.   Correct: VL nucleus of left thalamus (E)

Thalamic lesions produce contralateral movement disorders (since the VL nucleus relays to ipsilateral cortex that controls contralateral movements). Lesions of the left, and not the right (F), VL nucleus will, therefore, cause a right-sided intention tremor and choreoathetosis.

Cerebellar lesions (A and B) would not cause choreoathetosis, and putamen lesions (C and D) would not be expected to cause intention tremor.

15.   Correct: Thalamoperforating branch of left posterior cerebral artery (P1) (E)

The left VL nucleus is supplied by the thalamoperforating branch of the left, not right (F), posterior cerebral artery.

The posterior inferior cerebellar (A and B) and lenticulostriate branches of the middle cerebral (C and D) arteries do not supply thalamic nuclei.

16.   Correct: DM nucleus (E)

Since the lateral ventricles were dilated, and the cerebral aqueduct and fourth ventricle were of normal size, the tumor most likely is obstructing the third ventricle (develops from diencephalon). The DM nucleus of thalamus lies in the vicinity of the third ventricle, which therefore will be vulnerable from the tumor.

All other listed nuclei are located in the lateral aspect of thalamus and are not related to the third ventricle, which lies medial to thalamus.

17. Correct: Amnesia (E)

The DM nucleus of thalamus receives extensive inputs from the limbic system and projects to the cingulate, prefrontal, and orbitofrontal cortex. Via these connections, it forms part of an important circuit that is involved with consolidation of memories. Amnesia, both anterograde and retrograde, is observed with lesions of this nucleus.

Visual agnosia (**A**, lesion of pulvinar), contralateral homonymous hemianopia (**B**, lesion of LGB), contralateral hemianesthesia (**C**, lesion of VP), or movement disorders (**E**, lesion of VA/VL) do not commonly occur with lesions of the DM nucleus.

18. Correct: Medial posterior choroidal branch of the posterior cerebral artery (P2) (C)

The DM nucleus of the thalamus is supplied by the medial posterior choroidal branch of the posterior cerebral artery (P2).

The thalamoperforating branch of posterior cerebral artery (**A**) supplies the anterior part of the thalamus, including the anterior, VA, and VL nucleus.

The thalamogeniculate branch of the posterior cerebral artery (**B**) supplies the posterior thalamus, including the LGB, MGB, pulvinar, VPL, and VPM nuclei.

The lenticulostriate branch of middle cerebral artery (**D**) and the medial striate branch of the anterior cerebral artery (**E**) do not supply thalamic nuclei.

19. Correct: VPM (C)

The SVA column within the pons is represented by the rostral part of the nucleus of solitary tract, which is the second-order neuron in the pathway for taste sensation. The third-order neuron in the pathway, to which it relays, is the VPM nucleus of thalamus.

The VL nucleus of thalamus (**A**) receives inputs primarily from the basal ganglia and cerebellum, and is related to control of movements.

The VPL nucleus of thalamus (**B**) receives inputs carried via the medial lemniscus and spinothalamic tracts, and is related to all modalities of sensation from the contralateral body.

The DM nucleus of thalamus (**D**) receives extensive inputs from the limbic system.

The pulvinar nucleus of the thalamus (**E**) receives inputs primarily from the superior colliculus.

20. Correct: Thalamogeniculate branch of the posterior cerebral artery (P2) (B)

The thalamogeniculate branch of the posterior cerebral artery supplies the posterior thalamus, including the pulvinar, LGB, MGB, VPL, and VPM nuclei.

The thalamoperforating branch of the posterior cerebral artery (**A**) supplies the anterior part of the thalamus, including the anterior, VA, and VL nucleus.

The DM nucleus of the thalamus is supplied by the medial posterior choroidal branch of the posterior cerebral artery (**C**).

The lenticulostriate branch of middle cerebral artery (**D**) and the medial striate branch of the anterior cerebral artery (**E**) provide no blood supply for thalamic nuclei.

Chapter 13

Hypothalamus

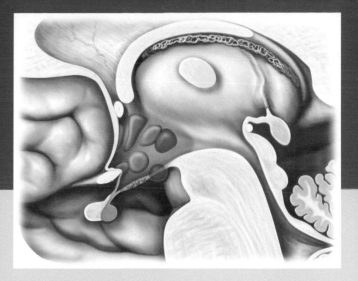

LEARNING OBJECTIVES

- ▶ Describe the role of hypothalamus in control of endocrine functions. Describe the blood supply of hypothalamus.
- ▶ Describe the morphological organization of hypothalamus.
- ▶ Describe the role of hypothalamus in temperature regulation.
- ▶ Describe the etiopathology and clinical features of Wernicke's encephalopathy and Korsakoff's psychosis.
- ▶ Describe the role of hypothalamus in regulation of feeding.
- ▶ Describe the primary connections of hypothalamus.
- ▶ Describe the role of hypothalamus in regulation of autonomic function.
- ▶ Describe the role of preoptic hypothalamic nucleus in sexual dimorphism.
- ▶ Describe the role of hypothalamus in regulation of sleep.

13.1 Questions

| Easy | Medium | Hard |

Consider the following case for questions 1 and 2:

A 26-year-old first-time pregnant woman presents with labor pain. However, progression of labor is not at the desired rate and she starts to fatigue. The attending decides to infuse a commonly used synthetic drug at a regulated dose to facilitate the delivery.

1. Which of the following hypothalamic neurons is the primary physiological source of the substance that was being infused in her?

A. Arcuate nucleus
B. Suprachiasmatic nucleus
C. Supraoptic nucleus
D. Paraventricular nucleus
E. Ventromedial nucleus

2. Which of the following blood vessels is primarily responsible to supply the related nucleus?

A. PCA
B. PCommA
C. ACA
D. MCA
E. Quadrigeminal artery

Consider the following case for questions 3 and 4:

A first-year medical student is confused with distribution of hypothalamic neurons. She just understands that the classification is based on a fiber bundle that runs through the hypothalamus and divides it into medial and lateral areas.

3. Which of the following hypothalamic neurons are the final targets for the fiber bundle?

A. Arcuate nucleus
B. Mammillary bodies
C. Supraoptic nucleus
D. Suprachiasmatic nucleus
E. Paraventricular nucleus

4. Which of the following thalamic neurons is the concerned fiber bundle connected to?

A. Lateral geniculate body
B. Medial geniculate body
C. Anterior nucleus
D. Ventral posterolateral nucleus
E. Ventral posteromedial nucleus

Consider the following case for questions 5 and 6:

A 46-year-old woman is hypertensive, diabetic, and obese. She presents with galactorrhea and secondary amenorrhea that she has had for the previous year. MRI with contrast reveals a microadenoma affecting her pituitary gland.

5. Which of the following hypothalamic neurons most likely controls the dysfunctional cells in her?

A. Arcuate nucleus
B. Suprachiasmatic nucleus
C. Supraoptic nucleus
D. Paraventricular nucleus
E. Ventromedial nucleus

6. Which of the following blood vessels is primarily responsible to supply the related nucleus?

A. PCA
B. PCommA
C. ACA
D. ACommA
E. Quadrigeminal artery

Consider the following case for questions 7 and 8:

A 66-year-old woman presents with mental retardation, seizures, stupor, and subnormal body temperature. Despite aggressive resuscitative measures, she suddenly collapses in the ER. Postmortem studies revealed hemorrhagic infarct involving the hypothalamus.

7. Involvement of which of the following hypothalamic neurons, most likely, is the cause of death for her?

A. Preoptic nucleus
B. Ventromedial nucleus
C. Dorsomedial nucleus
D. Anterior nuclear group
E. Posterior nuclear group

8. Which of the following blood vessels was, most likely, involved in the hemorrhagic infarct?

A. PCA
B. PCommA
C. ACA
D. ACommA
E. Quadrigeminal artery

Consider the following case for questions 9 and 10:

A 66-year-old man presents with confusion, unsteadiness, and headache. He had a history of frequent respiratory tract infections, which were successfully treated with antibiotics. Laboratory exams came back with severe hyponatremia, decreased serum, and increased urine osmolarity.

9. Which of the following is the most likely explanation of the symptoms for him?

A. Hyperactivity of the paraventricular nucleus

B. Hypoactivity of the paraventricular nucleus

C. Hyperactivity of the supraoptic nucleus

D. Hypoactivity of the supraoptic nucleus

E. Hyperactivity of the suprachiasmatic nucleus

F. Hypoactivity of the suprachiasmatic nucleus

10. Which of the following blood vessels is primarily responsible to supply the dysfunctional nucleus?

A. PCA

B. PCommA

C. ACA

D. MCA

E. Quadrigeminal artery

Consider the following case for questions 11 to 13:

A 48-year-old man presented to the ER following a fall from the staircase consequent to binge drinking at his house-warming party. The next morning, he was conscious, ataxic, and apathetic. When asked about the previous day's incident, he would not recall any drinking but had a spontaneous story of how he fell down while lifting weights. He also narrated how he had witnessed the death of his wife in a horrible accident 2 years ago, when, in reality, it was her who had brought him to the ER the previous day.

11. Which of the following might show significant atrophy in a brain MRI for the patient?

A. Ventromedial hypothalamic nucleus

B. Dorsomedial hypothalamic nucleus

C. Lateral geniculate bodies

D. Medial geniculate bodies

E. Mammillary bodies

12. Which of the following is the chief source of supply for the atrophied structure?

A. PCA

B. PCommA

C. ACA

D. ACommA

E. Quadrigeminal artery

13. Which of the following interventions, other than restriction of alcohol intake, might prove beneficial for him?

A. Administration of vitamin A

B. Administration of vitamin B1

C. Administration of vitamin B12

D. Administration of vitamin D

E. Administration of folic acid

14. A 12-year-old boy is brought to the clinic with the apprehension that he is not gaining weight. His mother reports that he has absolutely no appetite for any food, even for which used to be his favorites. She traces back this event to a head injury sustained due to fall from a bike, ~6 months before, following which he was transiently unconscious. No significant neurological deficit was noted at that time, and physical findings are within normal limits at the present time as well. Which of the following, most likely, would have a lesion on an MRI scan for him?

A. Anterior hypothalamic area

B. Posterior hypothalamic area

C. Medial hypothalamic area

D. Lateral hypothalamic area

E. Mammillary bodies

15. A 26-year-old man presents with marked changes in emotional behavior, irritability, impulsivity, and rage. This has occurred a day after he has regained consciousness following brain surgery for tumor resection. Which of the following structures, connecting medial amygdala to the medial hypothalamus, might have suffered from iatrogenic injury?

A. Stria terminalis

B. Stria medullaris

C. Fornix

D. Ventral amygdalofugal fibers

E. Medial forebrain bundle

16. A 38-year-old man presents with hydrocephalus with a hugely dilated third ventricle. On the second postoperative day following a ventriculoperitoneal shunt insertion, the surgeon notices slight drooping of the patient's eyelids with constricted pupils on the left side. The patient also stated that there is dryness over the left half of face, which he noticed when he was sweating earlier in the day. Which of the following, most likely, would have a lesion on an MRI scan for him?

A. Anterior hypothalamic area

B. Posterior hypothalamic area

C. Medial hypothalamic area

D. Lateral hypothalamic area

E. Mammillary bodies

Consider the following options for questions 17 to 20:

A. Suprachiasmatic nucleus

B. Ventromedial nucleus

C. Preoptic nucleus

D. Posterolateral hypothalamic area

E. Anterior hypothalamic area

17. Functioning of the hypothalamic nuclei has been related to greater arousal in men, with lesions of these having deleterious effects on copulation for males. Which of the presented structures is sexually dimorphic and is larger in males?

18. During the annual parent–teacher meeting, parents of a 13-year-old girl received complaints about their daughter falling asleep during several sessions. They were surprised to hear this, since the girl slept well at night. Neurological consultation might find out defective functioning of neurons within which of the presented structures?

19. A 56-year-old woman presents to the clinic with emotional distress. She says she has no tears despite the fact that she is sad and is "crying her lungs out." Which of the presented structures might have a lesion in her?

20. Following neurosurgery, a 42-year-old woman cannot stop eating. She seems to be hungry all the time and her appetite is not satisfied regardless of the size of her meals. Which of the presented structures might have suffered from an iatrogenic injury?

13.2 Answers and Explanations

Easy	Medium	Hard

Consider the following explanation for answers 1 and 2:

Intravenous administration of oxytocin is the most effective medical means of inducing labor. It exaggerates the inherent rhythmic pattern of uterine motility and facilitates the progression of labor.

1. Correct: Paraventricular nucleus (D)

The paraventricular nucleus of hypothalamus is the primary physiological source of oxytocin.

The arcuate nucleus (**A**) is involved with the production of regulatory hormones for the adenohypophysis. Cyclical activity of the suprachiasmatic nucleus (**B**) is responsible for the entrainment of the circadian rhythm. Although the supraoptic nucleus (**C**) can produce oxytocin, it is the chief producer of vasopressin/ADH. The ventromedial nucleus (**E**) acts as the satiety center within the tuberal region of the medial hypothalamus and is not related to synthesis of oxytocin.

2. Correct: ACA (C)

The paraventricular nucleus is located within the anterior area of medial hypothalamus and is supplied primarily by branches of ACA and ACommA

The PCA (**A**) is the primary supply to the posterior hypothalamic nuclei including the mammillary bodies.

The PCommA (**B**) is the primary supply to the middle or tuberal region of hypothalamus including the arcuate, dorsomedial, and ventromedial nuclei.

The MCA (**D**) supplies major areas of lateral surfaces of the cerebral hemispheres and parts of the internal capsule and the basal ganglia. It does not supply the hypothalamus.

The quadrigeminal artery (**E**), branch of P1, supplies the superior and inferior colliculi (corpora quadrigemina) of the midbrain. It is also not responsible for supply to the hypothalamus.

Consider the following explanation for answers 3 and 4:

The column of fornix is the major outflow pathway of the hippocampal formation. The fibers of fornix pass through the hypothalamus on the way to the mammillary body, dividing the hypothalamus into medial and lateral areas. This component of the fornix, referred to as the postcommissural fornix, also projects to the anterior thalamic nucleus. The other component, precommissural fornix, is distributed to the septal area. The hippocampal formation and septal area are involved in central regulation of emotional behavior, memory, etc.

3. Correct: Mammillary bodies (B)

4. Correct: Anterior nucleus (C)

Consider the following explanation for answers 5 and 6:

The patient is suffering from prolactinoma, possibly due to a tumor arising from the lactotrophs in the anterior pituitary gland. Increased secretion of prolactin by a functioning pituitary microadenoma suppresses FSH and LH secretion and produces lactation. Women present with galactorrhea and amenorrhea.

5. Correct: Arcuate nucleus (A)

The arcuate nucleus, as well as several other nuclei of the hypothalamic tuberal region, is involved with the production of regulatory hormones for the adenohypophysis.

Cyclical activity of the suprachiasmatic nucleus (**B**) is responsible for entrainment of the circadian rhythm. The supraoptic nucleus (**C**) is the chief producer of vasopressin/ADH. The paraventricular nucleus (**D**) of hypothalamus is the primary physiological source of oxytocin. Lastly, the ventromedial nucleus (**E**) acts as the satiety center within the tuberal region of the medial hypothalamus and is not related to synthesis of oxytocin.

6. Correct: PCommA (B)

The PCommA is the primary supply to the middle or tuberal region of the hypothalamus including the arcuate, dorsomedial, and ventromedial nuclei.

PCA (**A**) is the primary supply to the posterior hypothalamic nuclei including the mammillary bodies.

The preoptic and the anterior area of hypothalamus are supplied primarily by branches of ACA (**C**) and ACommA (**D**).

Quadrigeminal artery (**E**), branch of P1, supplies the superior and inferior colliculi (corpora quadrigemina) of midbrain. It does not supply hypothalamus.

Consider the following explanation for answers 7 and 8:

The cause of death for this patient is undoubtedly hypothermia. Other presenting symptoms are not usual causes of death during such an early course of the disease.

7. Correct: Posterior nuclear group (E)

The posterior hypothalamic neurons are involved in heat conservation. When body temperature falls, these neurons discharge to activate autonomic centers within the brainstem and the spinal cord and cause vasoconstriction, shivering, increased basal metabolic rate, and other heat-gaining mechanisms. Lesion of the posterior neurons, therefore, causes hypothermia.

The preoptic nucleus (**A**) is dimorphic, is larger in males, and possibly produces gonadotrophic-releasing hormones.

The ventromedial nucleus (**B**) of the hypothalamus is considered as the satiety center, with lesion producing central obesity.

The dorsomedial nucleus (**C**) functions in behavioral expressions (such as placidity and tameness), with lesion producing expressions of rage.

The anterior hypothalamic neurons (**D**) are heat sensitive and function as a heat-loss center. Lesion to these neurons produces hyperthermia.

8. Correct: PCA (A)

Branches from the P1 segment of the PCA are the primary supply to the posterior hypothalamic nuclei.

PCommA (**B**) is the primary supply to the middle or tuberal region of hypothalamus including the arcuate, dorsomedial, and ventromedial nuclei.

The preoptic and the anterior area of hypothalamus are supplied primarily by branches of ACA (**C**) and ACommA (**D**).

Quadrigeminal artery (**E**), branch of P1, supplies the superior and inferior colliculi (corpora quadrigemina) of midbrain. It does not supply hypothalamus.

Consider the following explanation for answers 9 and 10:

The patient is suffering from syndrome of inappropriate antidiuretic hormone with increased levels of ADH. This is commonly caused by diseases of the lungs (tuberculosis, bronchiectasis, pneumonia, etc.) and presents with headache, confusion, and vomiting in milder, and seizures and coma in more severe cases. Laboratory findings are significant for hyponatremia, increased serum osmolarity, and hyperconcentrated urine.

9. Correct: Hyperactivity of the supraoptic nucleus (C)

The supraoptic nucleus is the chief producer of the hormone ADH. Its hyperactivity will likely be responsible for SIADH.

The paraventricular nucleus (**A** and **B**) of the hypothalamus is the primary physiological source of oxytocin. Lesion is not likely to cause alteration of serum or urine osmolarity.

Hypoactivity of supraoptic nucleus (**D**) will cause diabetes insipidus, with increased serum and decreased urine osmolarity.

Cyclical activity of the suprachiasmatic nucleus (**E** and **F**) is responsible to set up a circadian rhythm. Again, lesion is not likely to cause alteration of serum or urine osmolarity.

10. Correct: ACA (C)

The supraoptic nucleus is located within the anterior area of medial hypothalamus and is supplied primarily by branches of anterior and anterior communicating arteries.

The PCA (**A**) is the primary supply to the posterior hypothalamic nuclei including the mammillary bodies.

The PCommA (**B**) is the primary supply to the middle or tuberal region of hypothalamus including the arcuate, dorsomedial, and ventromedial nuclei.

The MCA (**D**) supplies major areas of lateral surfaces of the cerebral hemispheres and parts of the internal capsule and the basal ganglia. It does not supply the hypothalamus.

The quadrigeminal artery (**E**), branch of P1, supplies the superior and inferior colliculi (corpora quadrigemina) of midbrain. It does not supply hypothalamus either.

Consider the following explanation for answers 11 to 13:

The patient is suffering from Korsakoff's psychosis, with classical features of amnesia and confabulation consequent to thiamine deficiency as a result of chronic alcoholism. This almost always follows Wernicke's encephalopathy, which causes lesions localized to periventricular structures at the level of third and fourth ventricles.

11. Correct: Mammillary bodies (E)

The mammillary bodies are primarily atrophied in Wernicke's encephalopathy and their lesion is related to endothelial swelling and tissue edema. The dorsomedial and anterior nuclei of thalamus are also severely atrophied.

None of the other listed structures (**A, B, C,** and **D**) are as significantly involved.

12. Correct: PCA (A)

Branches from the P1 segment of PCA are the primary supply to the mammillary bodies.

The PCommA (**B**) is the primary supply to the middle or tuberal region of hypothalamus including the arcuate, dorsomedial, and ventromedial nuclei.

The preoptic and the anterior area of hypothalamus are supplied primarily by branches of ACA (**C**) and ACommA (**D**).

The quadrigeminal artery (**E**), branch of P1, supplies the superior and inferior colliculi (corpora quadrigemina) of midbrain. It does not supply hypothalamus.

13. Correct: Administration of vitamin B1 (B)

Thiamine (vitamin B1) is an effective treatment for Wernicke's encephalopathy. The other listed substances (**A, C, D,** and **E**) have not been reported for treatment of the disease.

14. Correct: Lateral hypothalamic area (D)

The lateral hypothalamic area contains neurons that function as the "feeding" or "hunger" center. Lesion to this area causes anorexia, which is the likely cause for this boy, and results in age-inappropriate growth.

Anterior hypothalamic area (**A**) contains temperature-regulatory, heat-sensitive, and parasympathetic-regulatory neurons.

Posterior hypothalamic area (**B**) contains temperature-regulatory, cold-sensitive, and sympathetic-regulatory neurons.

Ventromedial hypothalamic area (**C**) contains neurons that function as the "satiety" center—lesion causes obesity.

Mammillary bodies (**E**) connect to the hippocampal formation via fornix—lesion causes memory deficits.

15. Correct: Stria terminalis (A)

Modulation of rage, aggression, emotional behavior, etc., is achieved by virtue of inputs from amygdala to the hypothalamus and the periaqueductal gray (PAG). Stria terminalis is the primary pathway that connects the medial amygdala to medial hypothalamus.

Stria medullaris (**B**) connects the habenular nuclei to the rostral forebrain, but is not connected to either amygdala or hypothalamus.

Fornix (**C**) connects the hippocampal formation to the mammillary bodies and the anterior thalamic nuclei.

Ventral amygdalofugal fibers (**D**) connect the lateral amygdala to the lateral hypothalamus.

Medial forebrain bundle (**E**) connects the septal and several brainstem areas to wide areas of the hypothalamus and the limbic cortex.

16. Correct: Posterior hypothalamic area (B)

The patient has Horner's syndrome with classical features such as ptosis, miosis, and anhidrosis. This can occur with a lesion affecting any part of the sympathetic pathway from the hypothalamus to the intermediolateral cell column of the spinal cord. Also, the posterior hypothalamus contains neurons that activate the sympathetic system. Lesion of this area, therefore, is likely to cause Horner's syndrome.

The anterior hypothalamic area (**A**) contains temperature-regulatory, heat-sensitive, and parasympathetic-regulatory neurons.

The ventromedial hypothalamic area (**C**) contains neurons that function as the "satiety" center—lesion to this area causes obesity.

The lateral hypothalamic area (**D**) contains neurons that function as the "feeding" or "hunger" center. Lesion to this area causes anorexia.

The mammillary bodies (**E**) connect to the hippocampal formation via fornix. Lesion to these structures causes memory deficits.

17. Correct: Preoptic nucleus (C)

Preoptic (Onuf's) nucleus (**C**) is sexually dimorphic (larger in males), and might be related to production of gonadotrophic-releasing hormone.

18. Correct: Posterolateral hypothalamic area (D)

Excessive daytime sleepiness or narcolepsy is due to loss of orexin-containing neurons in the posterolateral areas of hypothalamus (**D**). The ventral lateral preoptic nucleus (VLPO) is related to regulation of sleep and lesion causes insomnia.

19. Correct: Anterior hypothalamic area (E)

Lacrimation is a parasympathetic reflex. Cell bodies for the preganglionic neurons are located in the superior salivatory nucleus of the facial nerve and those for the postganglionic neurons are located in the pterygopalatine ganglion. These structures are regulated by neurons located within the anterior hypothalamic areas (**E**) that activate the parasympathetic system.

20. Correct: Ventromedial nucleus (B)

Ventromedial hypothalamic area (**B**) contains neurons that function as the "satiety" center. Lesion causes hyperphagia and obesity.

Cyclical activity of the suprachiasmatic nucleus (**A**) is responsible to set up a circadian rhythm that governs endocrine function and set up a sleep–wake cycle.

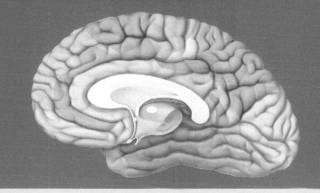

Chapter 14

Cerebral Cortex

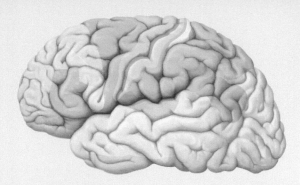

LEARNING OBJECTIVES

▶ Correlate functional areas of the cerebral cortex with clinical features related to their lesions.

▶ Describe the components and functions of the different parts of the internal capsule; correlate the clinical features with lesions of these.

▶ Describe the speech function of human brain. Define types of aphasias and correlate the symptoms with damage of structure and function. Describe the blood supply to cortical areas related to language; correlate aphasic symptoms with lesions of these.

▶ Correlate the pathogenesis with clinical features of prosopagnosia.

▶ Identify the internal capsule in CT scans and MRIs.

▶ Describe the arterial supply to the functional areas of the cortex. Correlate clinical features with stroke affecting these arteries.

▶ Correlate the pathogenesis with the clinical features of Gerstmann's syndrome.

▶ Illustrate the histological layers of the neocortex; correlate structure of cortical tissue with distribution and functions.

14.1 Questions

Easy	Medium	Hard

1. A 38-year-old right-handed male presents with right-sided weakness and loss of pain sensation and discriminative touch on his right upper and lower extremities. Which of the following is the most likely location of lesion?

A. Left precentral gyrus

B. Left postcentral gyrus

C. Left paracentral lobule

D. VPL nucleus of left thalamus

E. Posterior limb of left internal capsule

Consider the following case for questions 2 and 3:

A 39-year-old woman presents with aphasia. She is unable to construct sentences, but can repeat words after they are spoken by the examiner. She is fully aware of her situation and understands what she is being asked.

2. Which of the following is the likely diagnosis?

A. Global aphasia

B. Broca's aphasia

C. Wernicke's aphasia

D. Conduction aphasia

E. Transcortical motor aphasia

F. Transcortical sensory aphasia

3. Which of the following blood vessels or vascular zones might have been affected?

A. Stem of the MCA in lateral sulcus

B. Superior division of MCA

C. Inferior division of MCA

D. Watershed territory between MCA and ACA

E. Watershed territory between MCA and PCA

4. A 78-year-old man presents with right hemiplegia. Examination reveals paralysis of his facial and upper and lower limb muscles, all on the right side. Which of the following is the likely location of lesion for him?

A. Left paracentral lobule

B. Left precentral gyrus

C. Left internal capsule

D. Left caudal pons

E. Left caudal medulla oblongata

5. A 58-year-old-man presents with difficulty in performing activities of daily living such as dressing himself, brushing his teeth, shaving, and combing. His strength in the upper limbs is slightly reduced compared with what would be normal for his age. He is otherwise completely oriented to place and time, and his speech is well articulated. Which of the following is the likely location of lesion for him?

A. Primary motor cortex

B. Premotor cortex

C. Inferior frontal gyrus

D. Superior parietal lobule

E. Inferior parietal lobule

6. A 60-year-old man presents with a localized lesion affecting the inferior part of the cuneus and the adjacent lingual gyrus. Which of the following might be a likely symptom in him?

A. Motor aphasia

B. Astereognosis

C. Sensory aphasia

D. Prosopagnosia

E. Visual agnosia

7. A 56-year-old woman presents with slurring of speech and deviation of the angle of her mouth to the left on attempt to smile. She can tightly close both of her eyes against resistance, but her tongue deviates to the right on attempted protrusion. Which of the following represents the most likely location of a lesion for her?

A. Right internal capsule

B. Left internal capsule

C. Right caudal pons

D. Left caudal pons

E. Right rostral medulla

F. Left rostral medulla

Consider the following case for questions 8 and 9:

A 56-year-old man presents with confusion and reports that his house has been invaded by strange people. While he admits that they are kind to him and have the "same voices" and "wear the same clothes" as his wife and children, he claims that he has never seen them before.

8. Which of the following areas might have been affected by a stroke?

A. Superior parietal lobule

B. Inferior parietal lobule

C. Superior temporal gyrus

D. Inferior frontal gyrus

E. Inferior occipitotemporal gyrus

9. Which of the following blood vessels might have been involved in the stroke?

A. ACA

B. PCA

C. Stem of the MCA

D. Superior division of the MCA

E. Inferior division of the MCA

10. A 56-year-old male presents with aphasia. His speech is nonfluent and he has trouble repeating phrases spoken by the examiner. However, he is able to comprehend what is being asked. Which of the following cortical areas or structures, within the dominant hemisphere, might have been affected in him?

A. Superior frontal gyrus

B. Inferior frontal gyrus

C. Superior temporal gyrus

D. Inferior temporal gyrus

E. Arcuate fasciculus

11. A 48-year-old female attends a neurology clinic 2 weeks after she had suffered from a stroke. During physical examination, the only notable neurodeficit was her inability to identify objects placed on her hand with her eyes closed. Which of the following regions in her brain has been affected?

A. Prefrontal cortex

B. Striate cortex

C. Superior parietal lobule

D. Posterior paracentral lobule

E. Postcentral gyrus

Consider the following case for questions 12 and 13:

A 68-year-old male presents with a tumor affecting the region indicated by the arrow in the following CT scan.

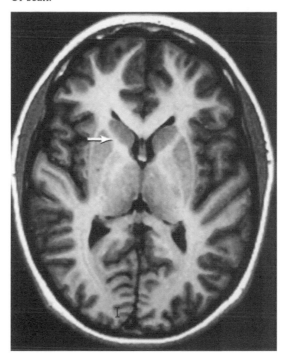

12. Which of the following fiber bundles is found within the structure indicated by the arrow?

A. Corticospinal

B. Corticobulbar

C. Frontopontine

D. Acoustic radiation

E. Optic radiation

13. Which of the following might be a presenting symptom in this patient?

A. Loss of pain sensation from upper limb

B. Deviation of tongue on attempted protrusion

C. Hemiplegia

D. Memory deficit

E. Resting tremor

14. A 48-year-old man presents with a stroke affecting the inferior division of his right MCA. Which of the following might be a clinical finding for him?

A. Inability to articulate, to construct sentences, to understand what is being asked, or to repeat after the examiner

B. Inability to understand what is being asked or to repeat; fluent meaningless speech

C. Inability to articulate, to construct sentences, or to repeat; completely understands what is being asked

D. Inability to attend to food on the left side of his plate

E. Inability to recognize faces

15. A 72-year-old-man presents with severe weakness of his right lower limb, but has age-appropriate strength in both of his upper limbs. Which of the following might be the location of a lesion in him?

A. Anterior paracentral lobule

B. Posterior paracentral lobule

C. Precentral gyrus

D. Postcentral gyrus

E. Posterior limb, internal capsule

16. A week following brain surgery, a 78-year-old man is reported to demonstrate social aggressiveness. He is completely conscious, oriented, and not in pain. His social behavior has become awkward, and his interaction with friends and family has called for concern. Which of the following cortical areas might have suffered from iatrogenic injury?

A. Superior parietal lobule

B. Inferior parietal lobule

C. Prefrontal cortex

D. Precentral gyrus

E. Fusiform gyrus

17. A 70-year-old man presents with an inability to write and do simple arithmetic calculations while shopping at the local grocery store. When asked to raise his left hand, he raises his right. When asked to show his thumb, he presents his ring finger. Which of the following might be damaged in him?

A. Left angular gyrus

B. Right angular gyrus

C. Right transverse temporal gyrus

D. Left transverse temporal gyrus

E. Right superior frontal gyrus

F. Left superior frontal gyrus

18. A 62-year-old man presents with a stroke affecting the cortical area (bilaterally) colored blue in the following image. Which of the following, consequently, might he be suffering from?

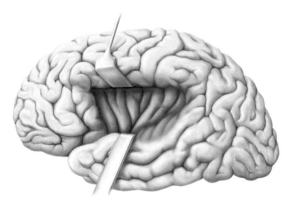

Source: Schünke M, Schulte E, Schumacher U et al. THIEME Atlas of Anatomy: Head, Neck, and Neuroanatomy. 2nd Edition. Thieme; 2016. Illustration by Karl Wesker/Markus Voll.

A. Anesthesia

B. Visual agnosia

C. Astereognosis

D. Prosopagnosia

E. Deafness

Consider the following image for questions 19 and 20:

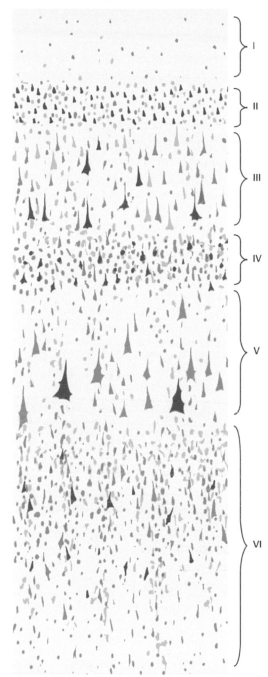

Source: Schünke M, Schulte E, Schumacher U et al. THIEME Atlas of Anatomy: Head, Neck, and Neuroanatomy. 2nd Edition. Thieme; 2016. Illustration by Karl Wesker/Markus Voll.

19. Which of the following layers will be expanded if the section was from the inferior parietal lobule?

A. Layers II and III

B. Layers II and IV

C. Layers III and IV

D. Layers III and V

E. Layers IV and V

20. Which of the following layers will be expanded if the section was from the striate cortex?

A. Layers II and III

B. Layers II and IV

C. Layers III and IV

D. Layers III and V

E. Layers IV and V

14.2 Answers and Explanations

Easy	Medium	Hard

1. Correct: Posterior limb of left internal capsule (E)

A lesion of the posterior limb of the internal capsule will result in contralateral hemiplegia (due to damage to corticospinal fibers) and contralateral hemianesthesia (arising from damage to thalamocortical fibers from the VPL nucleus of thalamus).

A lesion in the precentral gyrus (**A**) will cause paralysis of contralateral upper but not lower limbs (as lower limbs are controlled by the paracentral lobule). Additionally, such damage would be unlikely to cause hemianesthesia.

A lesion in the postcentral gyrus (**B**) will cause contralateral hemianesthesia but not hemiplegia.

A lesion in the paracentral lobule (**C**) might cause hemiplegia and hemianesthesia of contralateral lower limbs, but should not affect the upper limbs.

Lesion of VPL nucleus (**D**) will cause contralateral hemianesthesia but not hemiplegia.

2. Correct: Transcortical motor aphasia (E)

The patient is suffering from transcortical motor aphasia, in which connections from other cortical areas (related to language) within the frontal lobe to Broca's area are destroyed. The hallmark for diagnosis of transcortical aphasia is that repetition is spared (since the perisylvian arcuate fasciculus is intact).

Clinical features for different types of aphasias are as follows:

Global aphasia (**A**)—nonfluent speech, absent repetition, and inability to comprehend.

Broca's aphasia (**B**)—nonfluent speech, absent repetition, and intact comprehension.

Wernicke's aphasia (**C**)—fluent speech, absent repetition, and inability to comprehend.

Conduction aphasia (**D**)—fluent speech, absent repetition, and intact comprehension.

Transcortical sensory aphasia (**F**)—fluent speech, intact repetition, and inability to comprehend.

3. Correct: Watershed territory between MCA and ACA (D)

Transcortical motor aphasia is commonly caused by MCA–ACA watershed infarct.

Blood vessels/vascular zones involved in different types of aphasia are as follows:

Stem of the left MCA (**A**)—global aphasia.

Superior division of the left MCA (**B**)—Broca's aphasia.

Inferior division of the left MCA (**C**)—Wernicke's aphasia.

Watershed territory between left MCA and PCA (**E**)—transcortical sensory aphasia.

4. Correct: Left internal capsule (C)

A lesion within the internal capsule will cause contralateral hemiplegia affecting both facial (damage to corticobulbar fibers in the genu) and limb (damage to corticospinal fibers in the posterior limb) muscles.

A lesion within the left paracentral lobule (**A**) could paralyze right lower limb muscles but not facial and upper limb muscles.

A lesion within the left precentral gyrus (**B**) could paralyze right upper but not lower limb muscles (as lower limbs are represented in the paracentral lobule).

A lesion of the left caudal pons (**D**) could paralyze left facial (lower motor neuron type due to damage of facial motor nucleus) and right limb muscle (upper motor neuron type due to damage of corticospinal fibers) paralysis.

Lesion of the left caudal medulla (**E**) could cause limb (damage to corticospinal fibers) but not facial paralysis.

5. Correct: Premotor cortex (B)

The patient is suffering from apraxia, which is defined as a deficit in learned, skilled motor activity in the absence of paralysis. It is due to lesion of the premotor or supplementary motor (unimodal association) cortex located rostrally adjacent to precentral gyrus.

Precentral gyrus is the primary motor cortex (**A**) for upper limbs, face, and trunk. Lesions in this area cause contralateral hemiplegia.

The inferior frontal gyrus (**C**) contains the motor speech area (in the dominant hemisphere)—therefore, a lesion in this area would cause nonfluent speech.

The superior parietal lobule (**D**) is a unimodal sensory association area—a lesion to this region would cause astereognosis.

The inferior parietal lobule (**E**) is a heteromodal sensory association area—a lesion to this area is likely to cause agraphia, acalculia, visual agnosia, etc.

6. Correct: Visual agnosia (E)

The cuneus and lingual gyrus contain the striate (primary visual) and extrastriate (secondary visual) cortices. These brain regions are associated with processing visual stimuli and the perception of color, motion, and depth of vision. Therefore, lesion to these areas could result in visual agnosia.

Motor aphasia (**A**) could result from lesion in inferior frontal gyrus of the dominant hemisphere (Broca's area).

Astereognosis (**B**) could result from lesion in the superior parietal lobule.

Sensory aphasia (**C**) could result from lesion in the superior temporal gyrus of the dominant hemisphere (Wernicke's area).

Prosopagnosia (**D**) could result from lesion in the inferior occipitotemporal or fusiform gyrus.

7. Correct: Left internal capsule (B)

It is evident from the symptoms that the patient has lower facial palsy of the right side (angle of mouth deviates to the strong side) and paralyzed right genioglossus muscle (tongue deviates toward the paralyzed side). A lesion in the left, but not right (**A**), internal capsule (damage to corticobulbar fibers within the genu) is a possible explanation for such clinical features.

A lesion in the caudal pons (**C** and **D**) would cause ipsilateral complete facial palsy (lower motor neuron type, due to damage to facial motor nucleus) and contralateral genioglossus palsy (upper motor neuron type due to damage to corticobulbar fibers).

Rostral medullary lesions (**E** and **F**) would not cause facial palsy—it would cause ipsilateral genioglossus palsy (lower motor neuron type due to damage to hypoglossal nucleus).

Consider the following explanation for answers 8 and 9:

The patient is suffering from acquired prosopagnosia, which is inability to recognize faces. As reported, the patient can recognize the voices and clothes of the individual, just not the face.

8. Correct: Inferior occipitotemporal gyrus (E)

Acquired prosopagnosia is caused by lesions of the inferior occipitotemporal (fusiform) gyrus.

The superior parietal lobule (**A**) is a unimodal sensory association area—a lesion would cause astereognosis.

The inferior parietal lobule (**B**) is a heteromodal sensory association area—a lesion would cause agraphia, acalculia, visual agnosia, etc.

The superior temporal gyrus (**C**) is related to auditory areas and the sensory speech area (in the dominant hemisphere)—a lesion to this region may cause auditory deficits and Wernicke's aphasia (dominant hemisphere lesion).

The inferior frontal gyrus (**D**) includes the motor speech area (in the dominant hemisphere)—a lesion in this area may cause nonfluent speech.

9. Correct: PCA (B)

The fusiform gyrus is supplied by the PCA—a stroke involving this artery is a common cause for acquired prosopagnosia.

10. Correct: Inferior frontal gyrus (B)

The patient is suffering from Broca's aphasia, which is most commonly a result of damage to the motor speech area contained within the pars triangularis and pars opercularis of the inferior frontal gyrus of the dominant hemisphere.

A lesion of the superior temporal gyrus (**C**) might cause Wernicke's aphasia—in such conditions, a patient would not be able to comprehend but would retain fluency of speech.

A lesion of the arcuate fasciculus (**E**) could cause conduction aphasia—a condition in which both motor and sensory elements of speech would be retained; however, repetition would be lost.

Lesions of the superior frontal (**A**) or inferior temporal (**D**) gyri are not related to specific types of aphasias.

11. Correct: Superior parietal lobule (C)

The superior parietal lobule is a unimodal sensory association cortex which supports the ability to combine touch, pressure, and proprioceptive input to interpret the significance of sensory information. The patient is suffering from astereognosis, which commonly results from a lesion in this area.

The prefrontal cortex (**A**) is a multimodal association cortex involved in thought, cognition, behavior, working memory, etc. Lesions in this area are related to abrupt changes in behavior and personality.

The striate cortex (**B**) is the primary visual cortex—unilateral lesions in this area would cause contralateral homonymous hemianopia.

The posterior paracentral lobule (**D**) is the primary sensory area for lower limbs and genitalia—lesion would cause contralateral hemianesthesia for these areas.

The postcentral gyrus (**E**) is the primary motor area for upper limbs, trunk, and face—lesion will cause contralateral weakness for these areas.

Refer to the following image for answers 12 and 13:

As evident from the following image, the arrow indicates the anterior limb of the internal capsule.

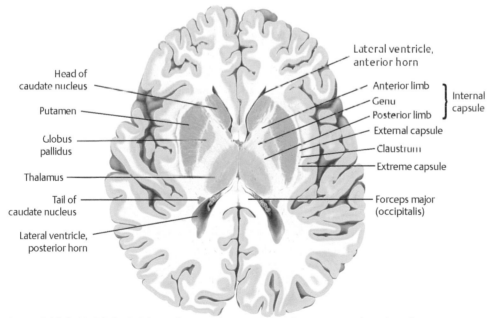

Source: Schünke M, Schulte E, Schumacher U et al. THIEME Atlas of Anatomy: Head, Neck, and Neuroanatomy. 2nd Edition. Thieme; 2016. Illustration by Karl Wesker/Markus Voll.

12. Correct: Frontopontine (C)

Fibers that traverse the anterior limb are the corticopontine and thalamocortical (anterior thalamic radiation from anterior and dorsomedial thalamic nuclei) pathways.

Corticospinal (**A**) and corticobulbar (**B**) fibers are carried in the posterior limb and the genu of the internal capsule, respectively.

The acoustic (**D**) and optic (**E**) radiations are carried in the sublentiform and retrolentiform part of the internal capsule, respectively.

13. Correct: Memory deficit (D)

Thalamocortical fibers that traverse the anterior limb of the internal capsule originate from the anterior and dorsomedial thalamic nuclei. These nuclei receive inputs from different components of the limbic system (mammillary body, fornix, etc.) and send outputs to the cingulate, prefrontal, and orbitofrontal cortex. This circuit is related to functions such as consolidation of memories, directing attention, motivation, and planning appropriate behavior. Amnesia is a frequent symptom due to lesion of this circuit.

A loss of pain sensation from the upper limb (**A**) can result from damage of thalamocortical fibers from the VPL nucleus of thalamus, which are carried in the posterior limb of the internal capsule.

A deviation of the tongue to the right (**B**) can result from damage to corticobulbar fibers, which are carried in the genu of the internal capsule.

Hemiplegia (**C**) can result from damage to corticospinal fibers that are carried in the posterior limb of the internal capsule.

Resting tremor (**E**) can result from damage to thalamocortical fibers from the VA and VL nuclei of thalamus (since they form part of the circuit connecting basal ganglia and cortex), which are carried in the posterior limb of the internal capsule.

14. Correct: Inability to attend to food on the left side of his plate (D)

The inferior division of the right MCA supplies the multimodal association areas of the posterior parietal cortex (at the junction of the parietal, temporal, and occipital lobes on the superolateral surface). This area, in the nondominant (i.e., right unless otherwise specified) hemisphere, is involved in spatial attention—a lesion most commonly causes a severe left hemineglect.

Global (**A**), Wernicke's (**B**), and Broca's (**C**) aphasia are related to the dominant hemisphere—these would result from lesions in the stem, inferior division, or superior division, respectively, of the left MCA.

Prosopagnosia (**E**) is related to lesion of the fusiform (inferior occipitotemporal) gyrus, which is supplied by the PCA.

15. Correct: Anterior paracentral lobule (A)

Anterior part of the paracentral lobule is the primary motor area for the lower limbs.

The posterior part of the paracentral lobule (**B**) is the primary sensory area for the lower limbs and genitalia. A lesion of this area of cortex will cause contralateral hemianesthesia for these areas.

The precentral (**C**) and postcentral (**D**) gyri are primary motor and sensory areas, respectively, for the upper limbs, face, and trunk. Lesions will cause contralateral hemiplegia and contralateral hemianesthesia, respectively, for these areas.

The posterior limb of the internal capsule (**E**) carries corticospinal fibers—a lesion in this region would cause contralateral hemiplegia and will not spare the upper limbs.

16. Correct: Prefrontal cortex (C)

Important functions of the prefrontal cortex are related to thought, cognition, behavior, planning, working memory, etc. Lesions in this area may cause abrupt change in behavior and personality, which can be expressed as social aggressiveness and explosive emotional lability.

Lesions of the superior parietal lobule (**A**), inferior parietal lobule (**B**), precentral gyrus (**D**), and fusiform gyrus (**E**) might cause astereognosis, language disorders (agraphia, acalculia, etc.), hemiplegia, and prosopagnosia, respectively—none of these are related to abrupt changes in behavior.

17. Correct: Left angular gyrus (A)

Agraphia, acalculia, right–left disorientation, and finger agnosia are the classic tetrad of symptoms for Gerstmann's syndrome—caused by a lesion localized to the dominant inferior parietal lobule (angular and supramarginal gyri). The location of the language areas defines the dominant hemisphere. In almost all right-handed people (~98%) and most left-handed people (~70%), the main centers for language are in the left hemisphere. Therefore, the left, and not the right (**B**), angular gyrus is the probable location of lesion in this patient.

The transverse temporal gyri (**C** and **D**) contain primary auditory areas—damage will primarily lead to auditory deficits.

The superior frontal gyri (**E** and **F**) are related to thought, cognition, behavior, planning, working memory, etc. Lesions in these areas are related to abrupt changes in behavior and personality.

18. Correct: Deafness (E)

The blue colored cortical area represents the transverse temporal (Heschl's) gyrus (area 41), which lodges the primary auditory area. Bilateral lesions involving the area would result in cortical deafness.

Anesthesia (**A**, lesion of primary somatosensory cortex [areas 3, 1, and 2]), visual agnosia (**B**, lesion of visual association cortex [areas 18, 19]), astereognosis (**C**, lesion of superior parietal lobule [areas 5, 7]), and prosopagnosia (**D**, lesion of inferior occipitotemporal or fusiform gyrus [area 37, 20]) are not related to lesions of the transverse temporal gyrus.

Refer to the following table for answers 19 and 20:

Histological organization of the neocortex is summarized in the table below:

Cell Layers of the Neocortex			
Layer	Name	Description	Major connections
I	Molecular layer	Cell sparse	Dendrites and axons from other layers
II	External granular layer	Scattered granular cells	Intra and inter cortical connections
III	External pyramidal layer	Scattered pyramidal cells	Intra and inter cortical connections
IV	Internal granular layer	Densely packed Granular cells	Receives inputs from thalamus
V	Internal pyramidal layer	Densely packed pyramidal cells	Send outputs to subcortical structures
VI	Multiform layer	Polymorphic layer	Sends output to thalamus

19. Correct: Areas II and III (A)

Layers II and III comprise smaller granular and pyramidal neurons which largely populate areas of association cortex. The inferior parietal lobule is heteromodal association cortex and therefore will have a relatively larger representation of these neurons.

Layers II and IV (**B**) represent granular neurons which largely populate sensory areas of the cortex.

Layers III and V (**D**) represent pyramidal neurons which largely populate motor areas of the cortex.

Expanded layers III and IV (**C**) or IV and V (**E**), in these combinations, would rarely be found in any functional areas.

20. Correct: Areas II and IV (B)

Layers II and IV represent granular neurons, which largely populate sensory areas of the cortex. Striate cortex is the primary visual cortex, and therefore will have larger representation of these neurons.

Layers II and III (**A**) comprise smaller granular and pyramidal neurons, which largely populate association areas of the cortex.

Layers III and V (**D**) represent pyramidal neurons which largely populate motor areas of the cortex.

Expanded layers III and IV (**C**) or IV and V (**E**), in these combinations, would rarely be found in any functional areas.

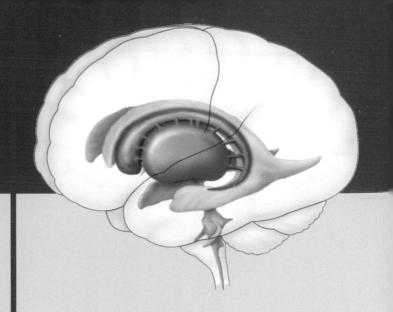

Chapter 15

Basal Ganglia

LEARNING OBJECTIVES

- ▶ Analyze the etiopathogenesis, clinical features, diagnosis, complications, and prognosis for parkinsonism.

- ▶ Analyze the etiopathogenesis, clinical features, diagnosis, complications, and prognosis for Wilson's disease.

- ▶ Identify components of basal ganglia in CT scan and MRI. Describe the blood supply for the basal ganglia.

- ▶ Define the role of excitatory and inhibitory neurons in the circuit that connects basal ganglia to cerebral cortex.

- ▶ Define the spatial relationship of the components of the basal ganglia.

- ▶ Analyze the etiopathogenesis, clinical features, diagnosis, complications, and prognosis for hemiballism.

15.1 Questions

Easy	Medium	Hard

Consider the following case for questions 1 to 4:

A 66-year-old man presents with reduced facial expression, slowness of movements, and resting tremor. Physical examination reveals rigidity and resistance to passive movement.

1. Which of the following is the likely diagnosis?

A. Chorea
B. Hemiballism
C. Athetosis
D. Dystonia
E. Parkinsonism

2. Which of the following is the most likely seat for his lesion?

A. Caudate nucleus
B. Putamen
C. Globus pallidus, internal segment
D. Globus pallidus, external segment
E. Subthalamic nucleus (STN)
F. Substantia nigra

3. Which of the following provides blood supply to the structure lesioned in him?

A. Anterior choroidal artery
B. Medial striate artery
C. Lateral striate artery
D. Posterior cerebral artery
E. Anterior cerebral artery

4. Which of the following might be the underlying pathophysiology for his symptoms?

A. Loss of excitatory input to neostriatum from cerebral cortex
B. Loss of inhibitory input to thalamus from basal ganglia
C. Loss of inhibitory input to internal segment of globus pallidus
D. Loss of excitatory input to STN
E. Loss of inhibitory input to globus pallidus, external

Consider the following case for questions 5 to 9:

A 20-year-old male presents with jaundice. History reveals that he had jaundice ~9 months ago that was treated conservatively. Physical examination reveals resting tremor involving all extremities. The tremor started 3 months before with his right upper limb and has gradually progressed to involve all limbs. His friends have reported severe mood changes for him recently.

5. Which of the following is the most likely diagnosis?

A. Huntington's disease
B. Parkinson's disease
C. Wilson's disease
D. Progressive supranuclear palsy
E. Friedreich's ataxia

6. Which of the following might be the underlying cause for his defects?

A. Mutations of ATM gene on chromosome 11
B. Mutations of ATP7B gene on chromosome 13
C. Mutations of SNCA gene on chromosome 4
D. Numerous CAG repeats on chromosome 4
E. Expansion of GAA repeat on chromosome 9

7. Which of the following areas is most likely to have undergone atrophy in him?

A. Putamen
B. Caudate nucleus
C. Inferior olive
D. Dentate nucleus
E. Substantia nigra, pars compacta

8. Which of the following might be the most likely additional finding in him?

A. Truncal ataxia
B. Sensory loss over limbs
C. Profound motor impairment for the limbs
D. Pigmented cornea
E. Cardiomyopathy

9. Which of the following is a true statement that the attending would want for his family to know?

A. This etiology for the disease is unknown and it cannot be inherited.

B. This is an unusual presentation for the disease since it primarily affects the elderly.

C. The disease is always fatal, regardless of the treatment modality.

D. The disease might not be fatal but will progress with further neurological disabilities, regardless of the treatment modality.

E. Prognosis for the disease is excellent based on the stage and the treatment instituted.

10. A 56-year-old woman presents with a stroke involving the medial striate artery (of Heubner). Which of the following areas are likely to be affected?

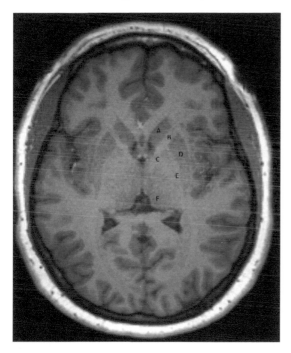

A. Areas A and B

B. Areas B and C

C. Areas C and D

D. Areas D and E

E. Areas E and F

11. An intern in the neurology clinic is reviewing the direct and indirect pathways of the circuit involving the basal ganglia and the cerebral cortex. To understand the pathophysiology of movement disorders, she is trying to analyze the excitatory and inhibitory neurons within the circuit. Which of the following is an excitatory pathway in the circuit?

A. Dopaminergic neurons originating from substantia nigra and acting on D1 receptors in neostriatum

B. Dopaminergic neurons originating from substantia nigra and acting on D2 receptors in neostriatum

C. Neurons projecting from the neocortex to the external segment of globus pallidus

D. Neurons projecting from the neocortex to the internal segment of globus pallidus

E. Neurons projecting from the globus pallidus to thalamus

12. A 36-year-old woman presents with a tumor affecting the lateral wall of the anterior horn of the lateral ventricle. Which of the following structures might be affected?

A. Caudate nucleus, head

B. Caudate nucleus, tail

C. Putamen

D. Globus pallidus

E. Dorsomedial nucleus of thalamus

Consider the following case for questions 13 to 16:

A 52-year-old male patient presents with violent and flinging movements of his right upper limb. The abnormal movements have started about a week ago and seem to primarily affect his proximal limb muscles.

13. Which of the following is the likely diagnosis?

A. Hemiballism

B. Chorea

C. Athetosis

D. Dystonia

E. Parkinsonism

14. Which of the following is the most likely seat for his lesion?

A. Caudate nucleus

B. Putamen

C. Globus pallidus, internal segment

D. Globus pallidus, external segment

E. STN

F. Substantia nigra

15. Which of the following provides blood supply to the lesioned structure?

A. Anterior choroidal artery

B. Medial striate artery

C. Lateral striate artery

D. Posterior cerebral artery

E. Anterior cerebral artery

16. Which of the following might be the underlying pathophysiology for his symptoms?

A. Loss of excitatory input to neostriatum

B. Loss of inhibitory input to neostriatum

C. Loss of excitatory input to globus pallidus, internal

D. Loss of inhibitory input to globus pallidus, internal

E. Loss of excitatory input to globus pallidus, external

F. Loss of inhibitory input to globus pallidus, external

Consider the following case for questions 17 to 20:

A 10-year-old boy presented with generalized edema, ascites, and proteinuria. Over the next 3 weeks, he developed conjugated hyperbilirubinemia, severe coagulopathy, rigidity, tremors at rest, shuffling gait, slurred speech, and emotional lability. Slit-lamp examination of his eyes revealed a pigmented corneal ring.

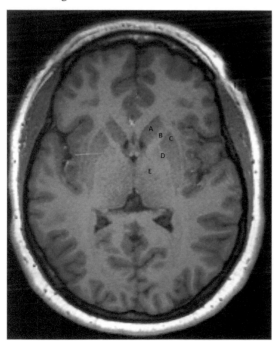

17. Which of the following might be the most affected area for the patient?

A. Area A

B. Area B

C. Area C

D. Area D

E. Area E

18. Which of the following might be an underlying pathophysiology for his case?

A. Impaired copper excretion in bile

B. Impaired copper excretion in urine

C. Impaired copper deposition in liver

D. Impaired copper deposition in brain

E. Impaired copper deposition in eye

19. Which of the following might be an important diagnostic finding for this patient?

A. Increased serum ceruloplasmin

B. Decreased serum ceruloplasmin

C. Increased serum copper

D. Decreased serum copper

E. Decreased urine copper

20. Which of the following might be an additional finding in this case?

A. Scoliosis

B. Cardiomyopathy

C. Pes cavus

D. Hemolytic anemia

E. Peptic ulcer

15.2 Answers and Explanations

Easy	Medium	Hard

1. Correct: Parkinsonism (E)

The abnormal movement described is classical for parkinsonism, which is characterized by the clinical triad of hypokinesia, rigidity, and resting tremor.

Chorea (**B**) is characterized by involuntary, arrhythmic, rapid, and jerky movements that typically involve distal parts of limbs early. Hemiballism (**A**), classified as a type of chorea, is characterized by unwanted flailing, flinging, ballistic movements that are often unilateral and initially affect proximal muscles of limbs. Athetosis (**C**) is characterized by slow, sinuous, and purposeless movements that often affect all limbs, neck, face, and tongue. Dystonia (**D**) is characterized by slow, sustained, and involuntary movements or postures that often involve larger trunk or limb girdle muscles.

2. Correct: Substantia nigra (F)

Lesions of substantia nigra result in parkinsonism.

Unilateral lesions of the caudate nucleus (**A**) can cause contralateral choreoathetosis, abulia, and behavioral disinhibition. Unilateral lesions of the putamen (**B**) can cause contralateral hemidystonia, hypophonic dysarthria, and impairment of short-term memory. Unilateral lesions of the globus pallidus (**C** and **D**) can cause contralateral hemidystonia, abulia, and short-term memory loss. Bilateral lesions may also cause akinetic mutism. Hemiballism is known to occur due to lesion in the contralateral STN (**E**).

3. Correct: Posterior cerebral artery (D)

The substantia nigra is supplied by the posterior cerebral and posterior communicating arteries.

Among structures related to basal ganglia, the anterior choroidal artery (**A**, branch of internal carotid) supplies the posterior part of putamen and globus pallidus. The medial striate artery of Heubner (**B**, branch of anterior cerebral/anterior communicating arteries) and anterior cerebral artery (**E**, branch of internal carotid artery) supply the head of the caudate nucleus, and the lateral striate arteries (**C**, branch of middle cerebral artery) supply most of the putamen and globus pallidus.

4. Correct: Loss of inhibitory input to internal segment of globus pallidus (C)

Loss of dopaminergic neurons in the substantia nigra, as is explained in the following flowchart, leads to loss of inhibitory input (via a direct pathway) and enhancement of excitatory input (via an indirect pathway) for the internal segment of the globus pallidus. This leads to enhancement of its inhibitory outputs on the thalamic projection nuclei and their target regions in the motor cortex, causing the hypokinesia.

As evident from the flow chart, none of the other listed options can explain the pathogenesis of parkinsonism.

Consider the following explanation for answers 5 to 9:

The presenting symptoms of recurrent hepatic dysfunction, bilateral resting tremor, and behavior changes hint toward Wilson's disease. The age for the patient also strongly suggests Wilson's disease, given the most common onset for the disease is during the second decade of life.

5. Correct: Wilson's disease (C)

Huntington's disease (**A**) presents, most commonly, during the fourth or fifth decade of life. Clinical features involve choreiform movements affecting all parts of the body and cognitive dysfunction, but jaundice (liver involvement) is not a known association.

Parkinson's disease (**B**), in its common sporadic form, presents commonly in the sixth decade of life. Although rare inherited forms can have an early onset, hepatic involvement is unlikely.

Progressive supranuclear palsy (**D**) presents commonly in the fourth decade of life with rigidity, frequent backward falls due to an abnormal gait, and dementia. Hepatic involvement is unknown.

Friedreich's ataxia (**E**) commonly presents in infancy. Gait and limb ataxia, nystagmus, dysarthria, sensory neuropathy, and cardiomyopathy are common clinical features. Hepatic involvement is unknown.

6. Correct: Mutations of ATP7B gene on chromosome 13 (B)

Wilson's disease is caused by mutations of the ATP7B gene on chromosome 13, which codes for a membrane-bound copper-transporting ATPase that secretes copper into bile. Deficiency of the protein causes impairment of copper incorporation into ceruloplasmin and inhibits ceruloplasmin secretion into blood.

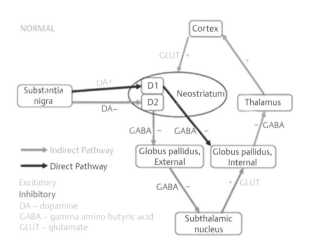

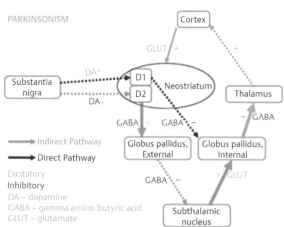

135

Mutations of ATM gene (**A**) on chromosome 11 (ataxia-telangiectasia), mutations of SNCA gene (**C**) on chromosome 4 (early-onset parkinsonism), numerous CAG (**D**) repeats on chromosome 4 (Huntington's disease), and expansion of GAA repeat (**E**) on chromosome 9 (Friedreich's ataxia) are not the underlying defects for Wilson's disease.

7. Correct: Putamen (A)

Accumulation of copper causes degeneration of the basal ganglia. The putamen is particularly affected by atrophy and even cavitation. None of the other listed structures are primarily affected in Wilson's disease.

8. Correct: Pigmented cornea (D)

Almost all patients diagnosed with Wilson's disease with neurological involvement present with copper deposition on their corneas (green/brown Kayser–Fleischer rings), which is usually asymptomatic.

Neurological deficits in these patients primarily present as movement disorders. Sensory (**B**) or motor (**C**) losses are usually not found in these patients. Truncal ataxia (**A**) and cardiomyopathy (**E**), as seen with Friedreich's ataxia, for example, are not common findings either.

9. Correct: Prognosis for the disease is excellent based on the stage and the treatment instituted (E)

Early diagnosis and treatment (with copper chelating agents, for example) have significantly improved the prognosis for Wilson's disease. Neuropsychiatric components for the disease improve in more than half of the patients and at least remain stable for another significant proportion (ruling out **C** and **D**).

Wilson's disease is caused by mutations of the ATP7B gene on chromosome 13 and can be inherited by autosomal recessive pattern (**A**). Onset of the disease can be variable (10–40 years of age) with most common presentation during the second decade of life (**B**).

10. Correct: Areas A and B (A)

Image key: A, head of caudate nucleus; B and E, anterior and posterior limbs of internal capsule; C and F, anterior and posterior parts of thalamus; D, putamen and globus pallidus.

Blood supplies for each of these structures are as follows:

Head of caudate nucleus—medial striate artery (of Heubner), branch of anterior cerebral/anterior communicating arteries.

Anterior limb of internal capsule—overlap between medial striate branch of anterior cerebral/anterior communicating and lateral striate (lenticulostriate) branch of middle cerebral arteries.

Anterior thalamus—thalamoperforating branch of posterior cerebral artery.

Putamen and globus pallidus—lateral striate branch of middle cerebral artery.

Posterior limb of internal capsule—lateral striate branch of middle cerebral and anterior choroidal branch of internal carotid arteries.

Posterior thalamus—thalamogeniculate branch of posterior cerebral artery.

11. Correct: Dopaminergic neurons originating from substantia nigra and acting on D1 receptors in neostriatum (A)

Excitatory and inhibitory neurons of the basal ganglia circuit can be easily understood from the following flowchart:

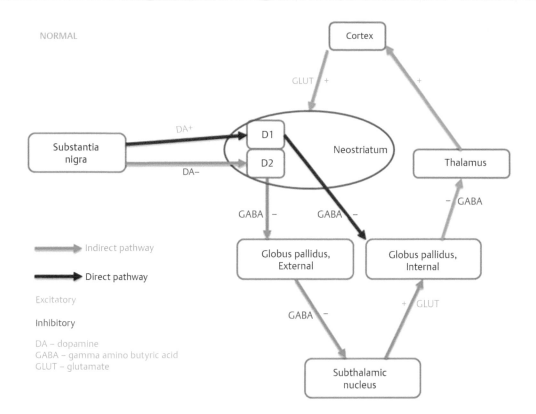

NORMAL

Indirect pathway
Direct pathway

Excitatory
Inhibitory

DA – dopamine
GABA – gamma amino butyric acid
GLUT – glutamate

---

12. Correct: Caudate nucleus; head (A)

Spatial relations of basal ganglia can be identified from the accompanying cross-sectional image:

The head of the caudate nucleus forms the lateral wall of the anterior horn of the lateral ventricle. The tail of the caudate nucleus (**B**) is related to the roof of the inferior horn of the lateral ventricle. The putamen (**C**) is the most lateral nucleus of basal ganglia and

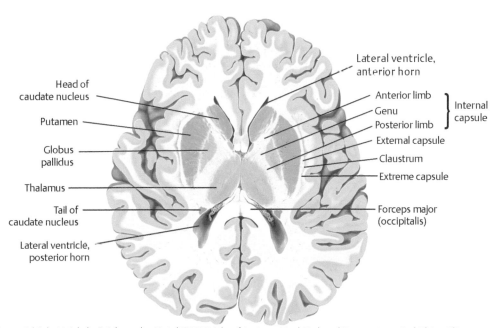

Source: Schünke M, Schulte E, Schumacher U et al. THIEME Atlas of Anatomy: Head, Neck, and Neuroanatomy. 2nd Edition. Thieme; 2016. Illustration by Karl Wesker/Markus Voll.

is separated from the caudate nucleus by the internal capsule. The globus pallidus (**D**) is sandwiched between the internal capsule and the putamen. The dorsomedial nucleus of thalamus (**E**) is related to the lateral wall of the third ventricle.

13. Correct: Hemiballism (A)

The abnormal limb movement described is classical for hemiballism.

Chorea (**B**) is characterized by involuntary, arrhythmic, rapid, and jerky movements that typically involve distal parts of limbs early. Athetosis (**C**) is characterized by slow, sinuous, and purposeless movements that often affect all limbs, neck, face, and tongue. Dystonia (**D**) is characterized by slow, sustained, and involuntary movements or postures that often involve larger trunk or limb girdle muscles. Parkinsonism (**E**) is characterized by the clinical triad of hypokinesia, rigidity, and resting tremor.

14. Correct: STN (E)

Hemiballism is known to occur due to lesion in the contralateral STN.

Unilateral lesions of the caudate nucleus (**A**) cause contralateral choreoathetosis, abulia, and behavioral disinhibition.

Unilateral lesions of the putamen (**B**) cause contralateral hemidystonia, hypophonic dysarthria, and impairment of short-term memory.

Unilateral lesions of globus pallidus (**C** and **D**) cause contralateral hemidystonia, abulia, and short-term memory loss. Bilateral lesions may also cause akinetic mutism.

Unilateral lesions of the substantia nigra (**F**) produce contralateral parkinsonism.

15. Correct: Posterior cerebral artery (D)

The STN and the substantia nigra are supplied by the posterior cerebral and posterior communicating arteries.

Among structures related to basal ganglia, the anterior choroidal artery (**A**, branch of internal carotid) supplies the posterior part of putamen and globus pallidus, and medial striate artery of Heubner (**B**, branch of anterior cerebral/anterior communicating arteries) and the anterior cerebral artery (**E**, branch of internal carotid artery) supply the head of the caudate nucleus. The lateral striate arteries (**C**, branch of middle cerebral artery) supply most of the putamen and globus pallidus.

16. Correct: Loss of excitatory input to globus pallidus, internal (C)

The STN is involved in the indirect pathway of the circuit between basal ganglia and cerebral cortex (see the following flowchart).

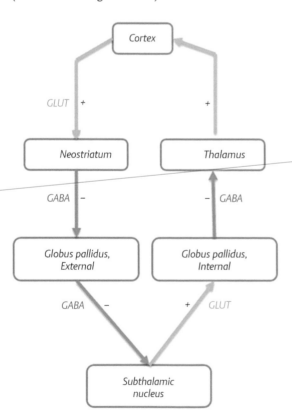

Since activation of STN excites inhibitory neurons from the internal segment of the globus pallidus that project to the thalamus, lesions of STN cause significant reduction of these inhibitory influences on the thalamus. This will cause activation of ipsilateral cortex with consequent increase in movements of contralateral limbs.

As evident from the flow chart, none of the other listed options can explain the pathogenesis of hemiballism.

Refer to the following image key and explanation for answers 17 to 20:

A, head of caudate nucleus; B and D, anterior and posterior limbs of internal capsule; C, putamen and globus pallidus; E, thalamus.

The clinical features are strongly suggestive of Wilson's disease (hepatolenticular degeneration).

17. Correct: Area C (C)

Accumulation of copper in the brain primarily affects the putamen. Atrophy and cavitation of putamen are common findings for the disease.

18. Correct: Impaired copper excretion in bile (A)

Wilson's disease is caused by mutations of the ATP7B gene on chromosome 13, which codes for a membrane-bound copper-transporting ATPase that secretes copper into bile. This impairs incorporation of copper into ceruloplasmin and its eventual secretion into bile. Copper accumulates in the liver (**C**) and is spilled into the circulation in a free, toxic form. This causes pathologic deposition of excess copper in the brain (**D**) and eyes (**E**). Urinary excretion of copper, therefore, is markedly increased (**B**).

19. Correct: Decreased serum ceruloplasmin (B)

Ceruloplasmin is formed in the liver by binding of copper to α-2 globulin. The process is impaired in Wilson's disease, resulting in decreased (and not increased, **A**) secretion of ceruloplasmin in plasma (a diagnostic indicator).

Serum copper levels (**C** and **D**) can be variable depending on the stage of the disease (low in early stage and high in later stages). These are, therefore, not of much value for the diagnosis.

Increased urinary excretion of copper (**E**) is a highly specific screening test for Wilson's disease.

20. Correct: Hemolytic anemia (D)

Excess free copper in the circulation causes hemolysis by its toxicity on the red blood cell membranes. Splenomegaly consequent to hemolytic anemia is a common associated finding in patients with Wilson's disease. None of the other listed features have any known association with Wilson's disease.

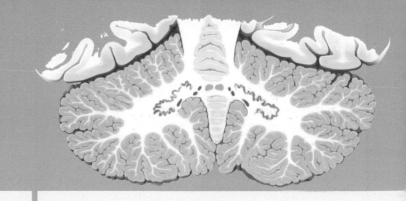

Chapter 16

Cerebellum

LEARNING OBJECTIVES

- ► Identify cerebellar peduncles in gross anatomy specimens. Describe the contents of the cerebellar peduncles.
- ► Describe the internal circuitry of the cerebellum.
- ► Describe the etiopathogenesis and clinical features for Arnold–Chiari malformation.
- ► Describe the blood supply of the cerebellum.
- ► Describe the effects of alcohol on the cerebellum.
- ► Describe the effects of lesions in the various functional areas of cerebellum.
- ► Define the types of appendicular ataxias found in cerebellar disorders.
- ► Describe various forms of input to the cerebellum.
- ► Describe the etiopathogenesis and clinical features for Dandy–Walker syndrome.
- ► Describe the connections for the various functional areas of cerebellum.

16.1 Questions

Easy | Medium | Hard

Consider the following image for questions 1 to 3:

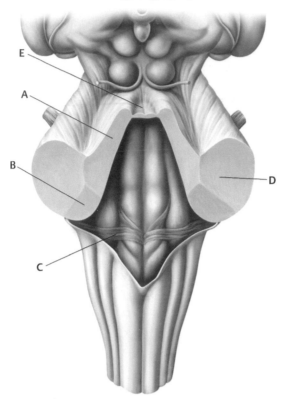

Source: Schünke M, Schulte E, Schumacher U et al. THIEME Atlas of Anatomy: Head, Neck, and Neuroanatomy. 2nd Edition. Thieme; 2016. Illustration by Karl Wesker/Markus Voll.

1. Which of the following areas contains important inputs from the cerebral cortex to the cerebellum?

A. Area A

B. Area B

C. Area C

D. Area D

E. Area E

2. Which of the following areas contains climbing fibers to the cerebellum?

A. Area A

B. Area B

C. Area C

D. Area D

E. Area E

3. Which of the following areas contains important communicating fibers from the cerebellum to the thalamus?

A. Area A

B. Area B

C. Area C

D. Area D

E. Area E

4. A 56-year-old woman presents with intention tremor. Investigation reveals cerebellar hemorrhage that has affected the immediate input pathway for the deep cerebellar nuclei. Which of the following neurons might have been affected?

A. Granule cells within the cerebellum

B. Golgi cells

C. Stellate cells

D. Basket cells

E. Purkinje cells

Consider the following case for questions 5 and 6:

A female newborn presented with flaccid paraplegia of the lower limbs. Neuroimaging revealed Arnold–Chiari (type II Chiari) malformation.

5. Which of the following features might have helped the clinician to diagnose her case?

A. Herniation of cerebellar tonsils through foramen magnum

B. Herniation of lower medulla through foramen magnum

C. Enlarged posterior fossa

D. Atresia of foramen of Luschka

E. Agenesis of cerebellar vermis

6. Which of the following additional features is most likely to be present in this case?

A. Syringomyelia

B. Myelomeningocele

C. Normal skull base

D. Normal supratentorial structures

E. Hydrocephalus due to adhesions occluding the fourth ventricle

Consider the following case for questions 7 and 8:

A 48-year-old woman presents with truncal and limb ataxia, and nystagmus. CT scan reveals evidence of hemorrhage in the left interposed and fastigial nuclei.

7. Which of the following vessels is most likely involved?

A. AICA

B. PICA

C. SCA

D. Pontine branches of basilar

E. Vertebral artery

8. To control bleeding from the involved artery, which of the following vessels should be clamped at surgery?

A. Internal carotid artery

B. Vertebral artery

C. Rostral part of the basilar artery proximal to its bifurcation

D. Caudal part of the basilar artery just distal to its formation

E. Subclavian artery

Consider the following case for questions 9 and 10:

A 62-year-old chronic alcoholic presents with truncal instability, uncoordinated gait, and moderate ataxia of his arms. He has consumed alcohol for 40 years, averaging ~90 mL a day.

9. Which of the following regions might have undergone significant degeneration?

A. Inferior vermis

B. Superior vermis

C. Flocculus

D. Paravermal area

E. Posterior lobe

10. Which of the following cells will most notably be affected?

A. Granule cell

B. Golgi cell

C. Stellate cells

D. Basket cells

E. Purkinje cells

11. A 60-year-old woman presents with an unsteady wide-based stance and nystagmus. Which of the following is the most likely location of a lesion?

A. Superior cerebellar peduncle (SCP)

B. Cortex of the paravermal cerebellar area

C. Cortex of the posterior cerebellar lobe

D. Dentate nucleus

E. Flocculonodular lobe

Consider the following case for questions 12 and 13:

A 69-year-old man is unable to rapidly slap his hand to his knee while alternating pronation and supination of his hand with each movement.

12. Which of the following specifies this particular deficit?

A. Asterixis

B. Dysrhythmia

C. Dysmetria

D. Dysdiadochokinesia

E. Titubation

13. Which of the following structures is most likely lesioned in this patient?

A. Dentate nucleus

B. Fastigial nucleus

C. Flocculonodular lobe of cerebellum

D. Vermal region of cerebellum

E. Ventral spinocerebellar tract

14. Which of the following pairs correctly indicates the exclusive source and nature of climbing fibers to the cerebellar cortex?

A. Ipsilateral inferior olivary nuclei, inhibitory

B. Contralateral inferior olivary nuclei, inhibitory

C. Ipsilateral inferior olivary nuclei, excitatory

D. Contralateral inferior olivary nuclei, excitatory

E. Contralateral pontine nuclei, inhibitory

F. Contralateral reticular nuclei, excitatory

Consider the following case for questions 15 and 16:

A 10-year-old female presents with ataxia, mental retardation, and seizures. Examination reveals an enlarged posterior fossa with cystic dilatation of the fourth ventricle. Atresia of foramens of Luschka and Magendie was considered as the probable etiology for her symptoms.

15. Which of the following is the likely diagnosis?

A. Type I Chiari malformation

B. Type II Chiari malformation

C. Dandy–Walker syndrome

D. Occipital encephalocele

E. Holoprosencephaly

16. Which of the following is a likely associated finding?

A. Syringomyelia

B. Herniation of cerebellar tonsils through foramen magnum

C. Herniation of cerebellar vermis through foramen magnum

D. Agenesis of cerebellar vermis

E. Buckling (Z deformity) of the medulla

Consider the following image for questions 17 to 20:

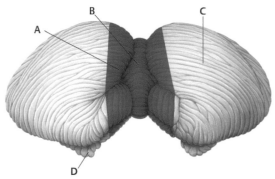

Source: Schünke M, Schulte E, Schumacher U et al. THIEME Atlas of Anatomy: Head, Neck, and Neuroanatomy. 2nd Edition. Thieme; 2016. Illustration by Karl Wesker/Markus Voll.

17. Which of the following areas is the primary destination for fibers conveyed within the MCP?

A. Area A

B. Area B

C. Area C

D. Area D

18. Which of the following areas functions by influencing the MLF?

A. Area A

B. Area B

C. Area C

D. Area D

19. Which of the following areas receives input from the ankle joint?

A. Area A

B. Area B

C. Area C

D. Area D

20. Output from which of the following areas is contained within the uncinate fasciculus?

A. Area A

B. Area B

C. Area C

D. Area D

16.2 Answers and Explanations

Easy	Medium	Hard

Refer to the following image key for answers 1 to 3:

A, SCP; B, inferior cerebellar peduncle; C, stria medullaris of the fourth ventricle; D, MCP; E, superior medullary velum.

1. Correct: Area D (D)

Pontocerebellar fibers contain sensory information from the cerebral cortex (conveyed by corticopontine fibers to pontine nuclei) and travel to the contralateral cerebellum via the MCP (**D**).

2. Correct: Area B (B)

The inferior cerebellar peduncles (**B**) communicate between the cerebellum and the medulla. These carry climbing fibers (from the contralateral inferior olivary nuclear complex) to the cerebellum. All other input to the cerebellum are via mossy fibers.

3. Correct: Area A (A)

The superior (**A**) cerebellar peduncles carry efferent fibers from the cerebellum to the thalamus (dentatothalamic fibers), often via the red nucleus (dentatorubrothalamic tract).

The stria medullaris of the fourth ventricle (**C**) consists of fibers travelling to the cerebellum from the arcuate nuclei (within the medulla) via the inferior cerebellar peduncle.

The roof of the rhomboid fossa is formed by the superior medullary velum (**E**). The trochlear nerve decussates in the rostral aspect of the velum.

4. Correct: Purkinje cells (E)

The internal circuitry of the cerebellum is depicted in the following flowchart:

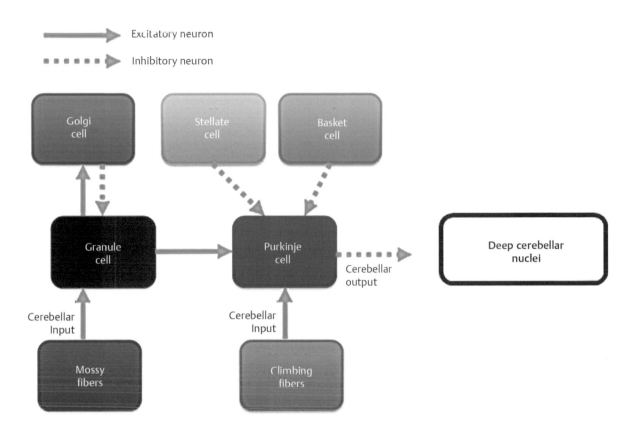

In the cerebellar glomerulus, the mossy fiber afferents synapse with granule cells (**A**). After this first processing stage, the granule cells convey this afferent information through the excitatory parallel fibers to the Purkinje cells and the Golgi cells (**B**). The Golgi cell exerts an inhibitory (feedback) influence on the synapse between the mossy fibers and the granule cells, within the glomerulus. The Purkinje cells also receive direct afferent information (excitatory) through the climbing fibers. Further inhibitory synapses with the Purkinje cells are from stellate cells (**C**) and basket cells (**D**). The Purkinje cells then send its efferent projections (inhibitory) to the deep cerebellar or vestibular nuclei. These nuclei serve as relay and processing stations for information coming from the cerebellar cortex to targets outside the cerebellum.

Consider the following explanation for answers 5 and 6:

Chiari malformations are defined as cerebellar herniation through foramen magnum due to a normal-sized cerebellum developing within an abnormally small posterior fossa.

5. Correct: Herniation of lower medulla through foramen magnum (B)

Chiari type II (Arnold–Chiari) malformation presents in infancy and is characterized by herniation of cerebellar vermis and lower medulla through the foramen magnum.

Isolated herniation of the cerebellar tonsils (**A**) occurs in type I Chiari malformation.

Enlarged posterior fossa (**C**), atresia of the foramens of Luschka and Magendie (**D**), and agenesis of the cerebellar vermis (**E**) occur in Dandy–Walker syndrome.

6. Correct: Myelomeningocele (B)

Myelomeningocele is an inevitable association with Arnold–Chiari malformation. Buckling of the medulla, beaking of the tectum, colpocephaly, lacunar skull, and platybasia are associated signs.

Syringomyelia (**A**) in which a cavity forms within the spinal cord can occur in type II Chiari malformations; however, it is much more frequent in type I.

Platybasia, or flattening of skull base (**C**), is a frequent finding in type II Chiari malformation.

Supratentorial structures (**D**) are often involved in type II Chiari malformation. Hypoplastic and irregular tentorium and falx (Chinese letter sign), enlarged interthalamic adhesion, and agenesis of corpus callosum could occur.

Hydrocephalus, if present in Arnold–Chiari malformation, occurs from cerebral aqueduct stenosis. Hydrocephalus due to adhesions occluding the fourth ventricle (**E**) is commonly seen in type I Chiari malformation.

7. Correct: SCA (C)

The SCAs supply the upper part of the cerebellum, which includes most of the deep cerebellar nuclei (dentate, interposed [globose and emboliform], and fastigial), rostral portion of the MCP, and SCP.

The AICA (**A**) supplies anterior portions of the inferior cerebellum including the flocculus, caudal part of the dentate nucleus, and most of the MCP. The PICA (**B**) supplies majority of the inferior surface including inferior vermis and ICP. Pontine branches of the basilar artery (**D**) supply the pons. A pair of vertebral arteries (**E**) joins to form the basilar artery.

8. Correct: Rostral part of the basilar artery proximal to its bifurcation (C)

The SCAs arise bilaterally near the rostral end of the basilar artery, proximal to its bifurcation. This region will, therefore, need to be clamped to operate on the bleeding SCA.

Clamping the basilar artery just distal to its formation (**D**) will occlude blood supply to vital brainstem and cerebellar structures and should not be considered. The internal carotid (**A**), vertebral (**B**), or subclavian (**E**) arteries are too far and unrelated to the bleeding vessel.

Consider the following explanation for answers 9 and 10:

The most consistently reported structural damage in the cerebellum of alcoholics is tissue volume loss in the anterior superior vermis. Tissue volume loss in this area is due especially to either shrinkage or atrophy of Purkinje cells. Cerebellar shrinkage is most notable in older alcoholics with at least a 10-year duration of alcoholism.

In contrast to alcohol, which exerts its greatest effect on the anterior superior lobules, normal aging primarily affects the posterior lobules.

9. Correct: Superior vermis (B)

10. Correct: Purkinje cells (E)

11. Correct: Flocculonodular lobe (E)

The flocculonodular lobe, via its bidirectional connections with the vestibular nuclei, influences the medial longitudinal fasciculus (MLF) and plays an important role in maintaining balance and vestibulo-ocular reflexes. Lesion to this part of the cerebellum leads to truncal ataxia, vertigo, and nystagmus.

Ventral and rostral spinocerebellar fibers traverse the SCP (**A**) to project to the paravermal (**B**) area within the cerebellum. These structures influence distal limb coordination and their lesion might cause appendicular ataxia, intention tremor, hypotonia, etc.

Output fibers from the posterior cerebellar lobe (**C**) and the dentate nucleus (**D**) form the dentatorubrothalamic tract and traverse the SCP (**A**). These tracts are involved in motor planning for the extremities and their lesion might cause different forms of appendicular ataxia (dysdiadochokinesia, dysmetria, etc.).

12. Correct: Dysdiadochokinesia (D)

The patient is suffering from dysdiadochokinesia, which is a form of appendicular ataxia characterized by abnormalities of rapid alternating movements.

Ataxic movements might have abnormal timing (dysrhythmia, **B**) or abnormal trajectories (dysmetria, **C**).

Asterixis (**A**), or flapping tremor, is a form of brief rapid movement that is often seen in metabolic encephalopathies, particularly in hepatic failure.

Titubation (**E**) is a peculiar tremor of the head or the trunk that occurs with midline cerebellar lesions.

13. Correct: Dentate nucleus (A)

Output from the neocerebellar cortex is primarily to the dentate nucleus, which in turn projects to the red nucleus (parvocellular part) and from there to the VLC of the thalamus, making up the dentatorubrothalamic tract. From the thalamus, information projects back to motor (primary and association) areas of the cortex. This circuit is involved in planning motor programs for the extremities. Lesions to the involved structures cause different forms of appendicular ataxia (dysdiadochokinesia, dysmetria, etc.).

The flocculonodular lobe (**C**), via its bidirectional connections with the vestibular nuclei, influences the MLF and plays an important role in maintaining balance and vestibulo-ocular reflexes. Lesion of this part of the cerebellum leads to truncal ataxia, vertigo, and nystagmus.

Afferents from the vestibular nuclei also project to the vermis (**D**). The midline vermis projects to fastigial nuclei (**B**) and is important in the control of proximal limb and trunk muscles. Lesions of these structures will primarily cause truncal ataxia.

The ventral spinocerebellar tract (**E**) originates from leg interneurons within the spinal cord and projects to the intermediate or paravermal area within the cerebellum. Lesion of this structure is unlikely to cause upper limb ataxia.

14. Correct: Contralateral inferior olivary nuclei, excitatory (D)

Climbing fibers carry excitatory inputs from the contralateral inferior olivary nucleus and synapse directly onto Purkinje cells. The inferior olivary nuclei are fed by several important structures including cerebral cortex, red nucleus, brainstem, and spinal cord.

15. Correct: Dandy–Walker syndrome (C)

The patient has classical features of Dandy–Walker syndrome, which presents with hydrocephalus, ataxia, mental retardation, and/or seizures.

Type I Chiari malformation (**A**) presents in young adults and is characterized by herniation of cerebellar tonsils. Type II Chiari malformation (**B**) presents in infancy and is characterized by herniation of cerebellar vermis and lower medulla. Occipital encephalocele (**D**) is characterized by herniation of brain tissue (enclosed in meninges) through a defect in the occipital bone. Holoprosencephaly (**E**) occurs when the prosencephalon fails to cleave down the midline such that the telencephalon contains a single ventricle.

16. Correct: Agenesis of cerebellar vermis (D)

Components of Dandy–Walker syndrome include enlarged posterior fossa, elevated tentorial attachment, agenesis of cerebellar vermis, and cystic dilation of the fourth ventricle.

Herniation of cerebellar tonsils (**B**) and syringomyelia (**A**) are features of Chiari type I malformation. Herniation of cerebellar vermis (**C**) and buckling of medulla (**E**) are seen in type II Chiari malformation.

Refer to the following image key 17 to 20:

A, intermediate/paravermal area; B, vermis; C, lateral region; D, flocculus.

17. Correct: Area C (C)

Broad areas of cerebral cortex project to the ipsilateral pontine nuclei (corticopontine fibers). From the pontine nuclei, fibers cross the midline (pontocerebellar fibers) and, via the MCP, project to the lateral areas of the cerebellar hemisphere.

18. Correct: Area D (D)

The flocculonodular lobe, via its bidirectional connections with the vestibular nuclei, influences the MLF and plays an important role in maintaining balance and vestibulo-ocular reflexes.

19. Correct: Area A (A)

Unconscious proprioception from lower limb muscles and joints is relayed to Clarke's nucleus in the spinal cord. From there, the fibers travel as dorsal spinocerebellar tract through the ICP to the paravermal or intermediate area of the cerebellum.

20. Correct: Area B (B)

Afferents from the vestibular nuclei project to the vermis. The midline vermis projects to fastigial nuclei. Contralateral fibers from the fastigial nucleus form the uncinate fasciculus and projects back to vestibular nuclei.

Chapter 17

Limbic System

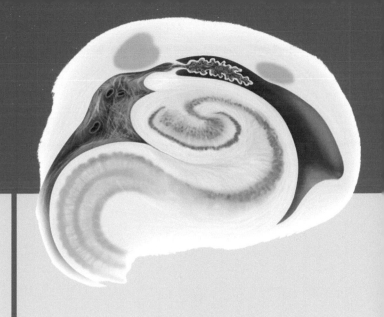

LEARNING OBJECTIVES

► Analyze the role of the parahippocampal gyrus in memory formation.

► Describe the location and functions of the amygdala.

► Analyze the role of the fornix as the primary link between the hippocampus and septal nucleus.

► Locate the commissure of fornix and analyze its role as the primary connection of the two halves of the limbic system.

► Analyze the function of the cingulate cortex, as it pertains to behavioral regulation.

► Analyze the timescale associated with recent memory.

► Analyze the features of remote memory.

► Describe the Papez circuit and related neural pathways.

► Illustrate hippocampal atrophy in an MRI T1 anatomical image.

► Analyze the functional role of the hippocampus in memory formation.

► Analyze the pathological effects of Korsakoff's syndrome on limbic system structures.

► Recognize the effect of prolonged stress on the hippocampus. Describe the anatomy and connections of the hippocampus.

► Describe the components of operant conditioning.

► Describe the role of amygdala lesions in hypersexuality.

► Relate the timescales of memory to anatomical components of the limbic system.

► Analyze the role of the limbic system in modulating aggressive behavior.

► Analyze the link between neurofibrillary tangles and Alzheimer's disease.

17.1 Questions

Easy	Medium	Hard

Consider the following image for questions 1 to 5:

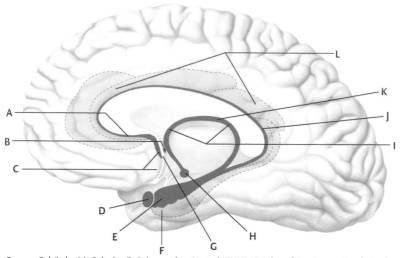

Source: Schünke M, Schulte E, Schumacher U et al. THIEME Atlas of Anatomy: Head, Neck, and Neuroanatomy. 2nd Edition. Thieme; 2016. Illustration by Karl Wesker/Markus Voll.

1. A 22-year-old right-handed male is concerned about his memory over the past few weeks, worrying that he may have developed anterograde amnesia. A structural MRI scan was performed revealing bilateral atrophy to the anatomical structure critical for the formation of remote memories. In which area would you most likely expect to see this damage?

A. Area A

B. Area B

C. Area C

D. Area D

E. Area E

2. A 22-year-old male is experiencing PTSD, and undergoes functional MRI scan to determine areas of increased brain activity relative to normal individuals. He is discovered to have heightened activity within the area of the brain that is involved in emotional responses and fear conditioning, and is connected to the hypothalamus via the stria terminalis. The area in which the abnormal activity was found would be:

A. Area D

B. Area E

C. Area F

D. Area G

E. Area H

3. Which of the following areas of the brain links the hippocampus and the septal nucleus?

A. Area I

B. Area J

C. Area K

D. Area L

E. Area A

4. Which of the following areas of the limbic system allows fibers from one side of the hippocampus to reach the contralateral hippocampus?

A. Area H

B. Area I

C. Area J

D. Area K

E. Area L

5. A 27-year-old woman has been suffering from OCD, comorbid with severe depression. The patient was unresponsive to all available and appropriate psychotropic and behavioral treatments, including three trials of the selective serotonin reuptake inhibitors (clomipramine, fluoxetine, and sertraline) at maximally tolerated doses for 10 weeks, even when augmented with neuroleptics. To alleviate these symptoms, psychosurgery was recommended, in which bilateral lesions of a limbic structure was performed. Which area best correlates with the target of this surgical treatment?

A. Area D

B. Area L

C. Area I

D. Area F

E. Area H

Consider the following case for questions 6 and 7:

An 82-year-old woman is referred to you for neurological testing with a concern that she may be showing the initial features of Alzheimer's disease. When using a word recall test, she is unable to recall any of the presented words without cueing.

6. What capability is being tested at the time of recall, if approximately 5 minutes have elapsed between the time the word list was presented and the time of testing?

A. Habituation

B. Operant conditioning

C. Recent memory

D. Remote memory

E. Immediate recall

7. A second memory test is conducted on the patient in which information about well-known current events and verifiable personal information is asked for. This type of test is assessing the patient's:

A. Recent memory

B. Remote memory

C. Classical conditioning

D. Operant conditioning

E. Immediate recall

8. When examining an MRI scan of a 56-year-old man, you notice damage to the anterior thalamic nucleus. Projections to which of the following structures from the mammillary bodies would be disrupted in this patient?

A. Amygdala

B. Hippocampus

C. Putamen

D. Cingulate gyrus

E. Septal nucleus

Consider the following case for questions 9 and 10:

A 68-year-old male is sent for diagnostic radiology, which revealed atrophy within the area of the limbic system identified in the marked region of the following MRI-T1 image.

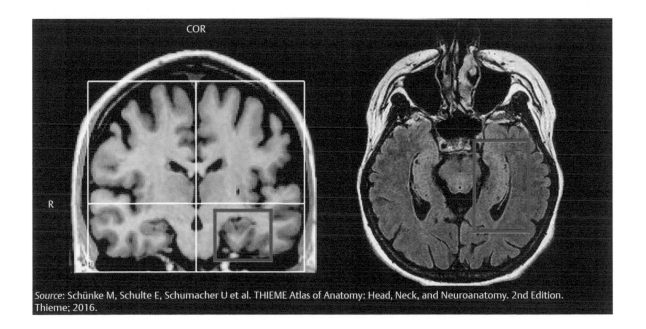

Source: Schünke M, Schulte E, Schumacher U et al. THIEME Atlas of Anatomy: Head, Neck, and Neuroanatomy. 2nd Edition. Thieme; 2016.

9. Which of the following areas is atrophied in him?

A. Cingulate gyrus

B. Hippocampus

C. Putamen

D. Fornix

E. Mammillary bodies

10. Which of the following memory deficit might be found in him?

A. Operant conditioning

B. Classical conditioning

C. Procedural memories

D. Recent memories

E. Remote memories

Consider the following image for questions 11 to 13:

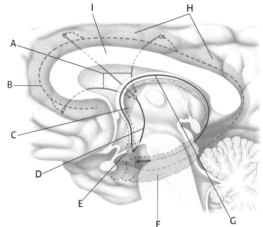

Source: Schünke M, Schulte E, Schumacher U et al. THIEME Atlas of Anatomy: Head, Neck, and Neuroanatomy. 2nd Edition. Thieme; 2016. Illustration by Karl Wesker/Markus Voll.

11. A 68-year-old right-handed male presented to the emergency department after a fall from a first-floor balcony. Upon admission, his blood alcohol level was 0.3 and he scored a 9 on the Glasgow Coma Scale. CT scanning revealed a small right frontal subdural hematoma without mass effect, and no surgical intervention was needed. However, a psychiatric consult was called due to the patient's overall confusion and state of agitation. A diagnosis of Korsakoff's syndrome was made, based on the patients retrograde and anterograde amnesia and the presence of confabulation. An MRI exam was performed. Where might you expect to see atrophy as a result of the thiamine deficiency observed?

A. Area A

B. Area B

C. Area G

D. Area I

E. Area E

12. Several nuclei of the limbic system are interconnected by the Papez circuit. Successive stations of this circuit would be:

A. Areas H→E→F→C

B. Areas H→F→E→C

C. Areas C→E→F→H

D. Areas F→ E→C→H

E. Areas E→C→F→H

13. A patient presents as a neurological consult, displaying significant amnesia. Diagnostic radiology reveals a lesion within the brain region responsible for relaying information from the mammillary bodies to the cingulate gyrus via the thalamocingular radiations. Which area best corresponds with this damage?

A. Area I

B. Area G

C. Area F

D. Area C

E. Area H

14. A 28-year-old woman was referred for a neurology consult following a change in her personality. Specifically, when in situations that would typically elicit fear in most people, she seemed to have little emotional affect. Her emotional response to other stimuli and memory function seems to be normal. Neuroimaging revealed bilateral calcification and atrophy of a specific component within the limbic system. Which of the following structures is likely atrophied in her?

A. Anterior thalamic nuclei

B. Cingulate gyrus

C. Mammillary body

D. Hippocampus

E. Amygdala

15. A 28-year-old woman suffering from post-traumatic stress disorder (PTSD) has been having memory difficulties. Long-term exposure to cortisol as a result of ongoing stress has been linked to producing dendritic retraction within a structure, which has a three-layered archicortex containing pyramidal cells that project via the fornix to the septal area and the hypothalamus. Which of the structures might be involved in this patient?

A. Subiculum

B. Amygdala

C. Dentate gyrus

D. Mammillary body

E. Hippocampus

16. A patient presents to your practice describing very mild symptoms of OCD. To avoid prescribing an SSRI, you suggest the patient may try using principles of operant conditioning to aid in reducing the frequency of unwanted compulsions. You suggest that each time a compulsion arises, the patient snaps a rubber band on their wrist. In this circumstance, the rubber band would be a:

A. Positive punishing stimulus

B. Positive reinforcement

C. Negative reinforcement

D. Conditioned stimulus

E. Negative punishing stimulus

17. A 22-year-old male was referred to a psychiatric unit after presenting signs of nymphomania that began following a bicycle accident in which he was not wearing a helmet. Neuroimaging would most likely reveal a lesion within which of the following structures?

A. Alveus

B. Subiculum

C. Dentate gyrus

D. Amygdala

E. Mammillary bodies

18. Which of the following anatomical structures is uniquely associated with working memory?

A. Brainstem diencephalic activating systems

B. Frontal association cortex

C. Heteromodal association cortex

D. Medial temporal structures

E. Unimodal association cortex

19. A 31-year-old male is admitted to a psychiatric facility following display of very aggressive and violent behavior. Clinical interviews with his family reveal this behavior is very unlike him, and he has no previous history of violent tendencies. As part of his assessment, an MRI scan of the brain is performed, where a tumor was found within his limbic system. Which of the following limbic connections were most likely affected?

A. Limbic system to thalamic nuclei

B. Limbic system to autonomic nuclei

C. Limbic system to septal nuclei

D. Limbic system to hypothalamus

E. Limbic system to orbitofrontal cortex

20. Which of the following is a pathological feature of Alzheimer's disease?

A. Intracellular accumulations of mutant huntingtin protein

B. Presence of Lewy bodies that contain the protein α synuclein

C. Neurodegeneration in the substantia nigra pars compacta

D. Intracellular neurofibrillary tangles consisting of the protein tau

E. Degeneration of the lateral corticospinal tract

17.2 Answers and Explanations

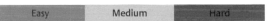

Refer to the following image for answers 1 to 5:

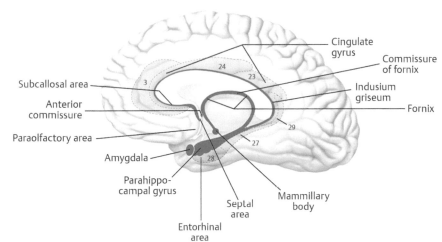

Source: Schünke M, Schulte E, Schumacher U et al. THIEME Atlas of Anatomy: Head, Neck, and Neuroanatomy. 2nd Edition. Thieme; 2016. Illustration by Karl Wesker/Markus Voll. Illustration by Karl Wesker/Markus Voll.

1. Correct: Area E (E)

The parahippocampal gyrus, in conjunction with the entorhinal cortex, is critically involved in the formation of declarative memories. Therefore, damage to this structure, especially when bilateral, is strongly correlated with a loss in the ability to form new memories.

The subcallosal area (**A**) is noteworthy for dense serotonin transporters at the caudal aspect, and as such is considered a pivotal component in a network involved in a wide range of mood and anxiety states, and changes in appetite and sleep (via connections to the hypothalamus, brainstem, amygdala, and insula). Although this region also has connections to the hippocampus, its role in the formation of memories is not as critical as the parahippocampal gyrus.

Atrophy of the anterior commissure (**B**) or the paraolfactory area (**C**) would not be consistent with loss in memory encoding capability. Through its output via the stria terminalis, the amygdala (**D**) is heavily involved in emotional responses and fear conditioning, though damage to this structure is not associated with anterograde amnesia.

2. Correct: Area D (A)

The amygdala, located at the tip of the temporal lobe just anterior to the hippocampus, is heavily involved in emotional responses, and is connected to the hypothalamus via the stria terminalis. Further, this region is known to become hyperactive in patients presenting with PTSD when they are exposed to stimuli related to their trauma.

The parahippocampal gyrus (**B**), in conjunction with the entorhinal cortex (**C**), is critically involved in the formation of declarative memories.

The septal area (**D**, contains extensive reciprocal connections with the hippocampus through fornix) and the mammillary bodies (**E**, important for memory recall) are not known to be affected by PTSD.

3. Correct: Area I (A)

The fornix starts in the hippocampus and terminates in the mammillary bodies, its primary target. It also has reciprocal connections with the septal nucleus and is the source of commissural fibers linking one hippocampus to the other.

The indusium griseum (**B**), also known as the supracallosal gyrus, is a thin layer of gray matter with largely unknown functions.

The commissure of fornix (**C**) connects the left and right fornices.

The cingulate gyrus (**D**) is a part of the limbic lobe that receives input from the thalamus and neocortex, and projects to the entorhinal cortex. This forms an important link between behavior and motivation.

The subcallosal area (**E**) of the limbic system has connections with the hypothalamus, the brainstem, the amygdala, and the insula.

4. Correct: Area K (D)

The hippocampal commissural fibers that allow bilateral communication between hippocampi are contained within the commissure of fornix (also known as the hippocampal commissure).

The mammillary bodies (**A**) are important for options recall via their connections to the anterior thalamus.

The fornix (**B**) starts in the hippocampus and terminates in the mammillary bodies, its primary target.

The indusium griseum (**C**), or supracallosal gyrus, is a thin layer of gray matter with largely unknown functions, and may be an embryological remnant of the developing brain.

The cingulate gyrus (**E**) is a part of the limbic lobe that receives input from the thalamus and neocortex, and projects to the entorhinal cortex.

5. Correct: Area L (B)

In cases of intractable depression and/or OCD, a viable surgical treatment includes the selective lesioning of bilateral anterior cingulate cortex.

Although the amygdala (**A**) is heavily involved in emotional responses, bilateral damage to this structure has been shown to be associated with Klüver–Bucy syndrome, which may result in the individual experiencing a substantially diminished emotional affect. It also may result in problems related to memory, dietary changes, hypersexuality, and visual agnosia.

Damage to the fornix (**C**) results in significant memory impairments. Similarly, the entorhinal cortex (**D**) is critically involved in the formation of declarative memories.

Finally, the mammillary body (**E**) is important for memory recall and is not a target for psychosurgical techniques.

6. Correct: Recent memory (C)

Recent memory is classified as memory used for the storage of information over the span of approximately 5 minutes without rehearsal. It is dependent on functional bilateral medial temporal and diencephalic systems, and its loss is often an early sign of the onset of Alzheimer's disease.

Habituation (**A**) refers to a decrease in response to repetitive stimuli that is not the result of fatigue or sensory adaptation, and is not a timescale of memory.

Operant conditioning (**B**) is the process by which a behavior is paired with a reinforcing stimulus in such a way that the behavior that is being reinforced is more likely to occur.

Remote memory (**D**) is on the timescale of hours, days, months, and years.

Immediate recall (**E**) is memory on the timescale of seconds, without rehearsal, and is a product of reticular formation, frontal cortex, association cortex, and unimodal cortices.

7. Correct: Remote memory (B)

As previously described, remote memory is at the timescale of greater than 5 minutes extending into years, with anatomical substrates consisting of the hippocampus and association cortices.

Recent memory (**A**) is memory on the timescale of minutes.

Classical conditioning (**C**) is the process by which neutral stimuli (neutral) is paired with a stimulus (unconditioned) that elicits an inherent response (unconditioned response). Through multiple pairings, the neutral stimulus can elicit the physiological response in isolation of the unconditioned stimulus, with the formerly neutral stimulus now being described as a conditioned stimulus and the formerly unconditioned response becoming a conditioned response.

Operant conditioning (**D**) is the process by which a behavior is paired with a reinforcing stimulus in such a way that the behavior that is being reinforced is more likely to occur.

Immediate recall (**E**) is memory on the timescale of seconds.

8. Correct: Cingulate gyrus (D)

Information from the mammillary bodies travels via the mammillothalamic tract to the anterior thalamic nucleus. From the thalamus, there are substantial connections to the cingulate gyrus, and these make up a large portion of the Papez circuit, the method by which ontogenically distinct parts of the limbic system are connected together. This results in a connection between information stored in memory and behavior.

The amygdala (**A**), although not part of the conventional Papez circuit, is often included in most contemporary limbic circuits.

The hippocampus (**B**) is also a major component of the limbic circuit, being the ultimate destination of fibers from the cingulate gyrus and the last node within the Papez circuit.

The putamen (**C**) is part of the basal ganglia, an area that is highly connected to the limbic system, but is not considered a part of the limbic system proper.

The septal nucleus (**E**) has reciprocal connections with several limbic structures (including the amygdala, hypothalamus, and cingulate gyrus).

None of the above-mentioned connections for options **A, B, C,** and **E**, however, travel through the anterior thalamic nucleus.

9. Correct: Hippocampus (B)

The area of atrophy is coincident with the hippocampus, which lies at the floor of each lateral ventricle in the region of the inferior or temporal horn.

The cingulate gyrus (**A**) is located immediately superior to the corpus callosum.

The putamen (**C**) is located at the base of the forebrain and, in conjunction with the caudate nucleus, makes up the dorsal striatum. This structure is not visible in the image.

The fornix (**D**), a C-shaped bundle of fibers that is the major output tract of the hippocampus, is also not readily visible within this image.

Lastly, the mammillary bodies (**E**) are located on the undersurface of the brain at the end of the anterior arches of the fornix and are also not visible in this image.

10. Correct: Remote memories (E)

Destruction of the hippocampus has been associated with deficits in both the formation of remote declarative memories. These deficits, however, do not include deficits in conditioning (**A** and **B**), and procedural memories (**C**) usually remain intact. Lastly, recent memories (**D**), on the timescale of minutes, are relative spared with hippocampal damage.

Refer to the following image for answers 11 to 13:

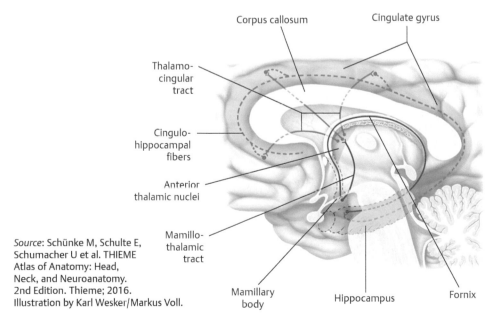

Corpus callosum
Cingulate gyrus
Thalamo-cingular tract
Cingulo-hippocampal fibers
Anterior thalamic nuclei
Mamillo-thalamic tract
Mamillary body
Hippocampus
Fornix

Source: Schünke M, Schulte E, Schumacher U et al. THIEME Atlas of Anatomy: Head, Neck, and Neuroanatomy. 2nd Edition. Thieme; 2016. Illustration by Karl Wesker/Markus Voll.

11. Correct: Area E (E)

Korsakoff's syndrome is the result of thiamine deficiency, common among alcoholics, and has primary presenting symptoms of amnesia and confabulation. Pathological features of Korsakoff's syndrome include atrophy of the cortex, thalamus (dorsomedial and anterior nuclei), and mammillary bodies.

The thalamocingular tract (**A**), cingulohippocampal fibers (**B**), fornix (**C**), and corpus callosum (**D**) are not known to be affected by thiamine deficiency.

12. Correct: Areas F→ E→C→H (D)

The major nuclei of the Papez circuit, in order of succession, are the hippocampus (area F), mammillary body (area E), anterior thalamic nucleus (area C), and cingulate gyrus (area H), before the circuit is completed with a return to the hippocampus. Therefore, the correct order of regions is option **D**.

13. Correct: Area C (D)

The anterior thalamic nucleus, depicted in area C, is responsible for relaying information from the mammillary bodies to the cingulate gyrus via the thalamocingular radiations.

Area I (**A**) corresponds to the corpus callosum, the major white matter pathway connecting the left and right cerebral hemispheres. Area G (**B**) is displaying the fornix, the major output tract of the hippocampus. Area F (**C**) corresponds to the hippocampus, a structure crucial in learning and memory. Area H (**E**) is the cingulate gyrus, an integral part of the limbic system.

14. Correct: Amygdala (E)

Bilateral calcification and atrophy of the amygdala could possibly explain the deficits, since this structure is heavily involved in emotional responses to fear.

Lesions of the anterior thalamic nuclei (**A**), cingulate gyrus (**B**), mammillary body (**C**), and hippocampus (**D**) would all be associated with memory deficits, but would not be expected to have an impact on the experience of fear.

15. Correct: Hippocampus (E)

The hippocampus, a limbic structure with a three-layered archicortex, is crucial in learning and memory, and is particularly sensitive to chronic levels of glucocorticoids arising from stress.

The subiculum (**A**) is known to be involved in working memory, and may show signs of altered structure in PTSD. However, it does not directly connect to the septal areas and hypothalamus via the fornix.

Although the amygdala (**B**) is overactive during PTSD, a reflection of a heightened fear response, it does not fit the anatomical description provided, nor is it known to react to prolonged exposure to cortisol.

The dentate gyrus (**C**) also has a three-layered archicortex, similar to the hippocampus, but it contains granule cells that project to the hippocampus and subiculum.

The mammillary bodies (**D**) project to the anterior nucleus of the thalamus via the mammillothalamic tract, and do not meet the description of the involved structure.

16. Correct: Positive punishing stimulus (A)

Operant conditioning is the process by which a response becomes more or less likely to occur depending on its consequences. In this context, the behavior that is targeted for reduction is the presence of compulsions. In this framework, a punishment is something that makes a response weaker, or less likely to recur. A positive punisher is when an undesired response (in this case, the compulsion) is followed by an unpleasant consequence (snapping of the rubber band), making the response less likely to occur again.

Positive reinforcement (**B**) would be when a pleasant consequence follows a response, making the response more likely to occur again, such as awarding a bonus for scoring highly on a test.

Negative reinforcement (**C**) is when a response is followed by the removal of something unpleasant, making the response more likely to occur again, such as having your friends stop nagging you to do well on a test, after you earn an A.

The term conditioned stimulus (**D**) is used in classical conditioning for a previously neutral stimulus that through repeated exposures has become associated with the unconditioned stimulus and results in the triggering of a conditioned response.

A negative punishing (**E**) stimulus would be a pleasant stimulus that is removed following a response, making that response less likely to occur in the future, such as taking a child's toy away when they misbehave.

17. Correct: Amygdala (D)

Hypersexuality is one of the symptoms of Klüver–Bucy syndrome, which results from damage to the temporal lobes, including the amygdalae.

Damage to the alveus (**A**) of the hippocampus is not known to result in hypersexuality.

The subiculum (**B**) is the most inferior component of the hippocampal formation and is associated with working memory. Clinically, the subiculum has been shown to play a role in some cases of epilepsy and drug addiction.

The dentate gyrus (**C**) is also part of the hippocampus, and is thought to play a large role in the formation of episodic memories.

The mammillary bodies (**E**) are also a critical component of the circuit required for the formation of new memories, but would not be involved with nymphomania.

18. Correct: Frontal association cortex (B)

Frontal association cortex has been shown to be involved in working memory.

Unimodal (E) and heteromodal (C) association cortices are involved in all timescales of memory.

Brainstem-diencephalic activating systems (A) are involved in storage of memories for a second or less.

Medial temporal structures (D) are involved in memory storage at the timescale of minutes to years.

19. Correct: Limbic system to hypothalamus (D)

The limbic system has large outputs to the hypothalamus, a region of the brain that is known to integrate feelings of rage and aggressive behavior. Damage to the limbic system's connection to the hypothalamus, therefore, can have profound impacts on the ability to control emotions and their expression.

The other primary output of the limbic system is to the septal nuclei (C), although this pathway has not been shown to have a role in the expression of violent behavior. It rather plays a role in the linking connections from the hippocampus to the ventral tegmental area as part of the reward pathway of the brain.

The remaining options (A, B, and E) are not significant sources of limbic system output, and further, would not play a role in the behaviors described.

20. Correct: Intracellular neurofibrillary tangles consisting of the protein tau (D)

Neurofibrillary tangles (D), aggregates of hyperphosphorylated tau protein, are primary markers of Alzheimer's disease.

Intracellular accumulations of the mutant protein huntingtin (A) are associated with the development of Huntington's disease.

Presence of Lewy bodies containing the protein α synuclein (B) is associated with the development of Parkinson's disease, as is neurodegeneration in the substantia nigra pars compacta (C).

Degeneration of the lateral corticospinal tract (E) is associated with motor neuron diseases.

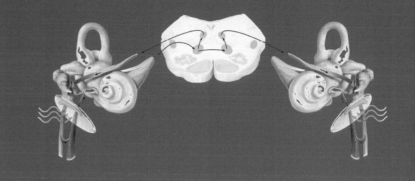

Chapter 18
Auditory System

LEARNING OBJECTIVES

- ▶ Interpret the results of the Weber and Rinne test, and relate those to auditory dysfunction.
- ▶ Correlate the pathogenesis of otitis media with the function of the ossicular chain.
- ▶ Describe the prominent features of the external ear.
- ▶ Define tissue types present in the external ear and relate these to the pathogenesis of auricular hematoma.
- ▶ Describe the function and mechanism of the stapedius reflex.
- ▶ Illustrate the tonotopic representation of primary auditory cortex.
- ▶ Describe the sensory innervation of the auricle.
- ▶ Describe the composition of perilymph and analyze its similarity to extracellular fluid.
- ▶ Analyze the relationship between the malleus, incus, and stapes within the ossicular chain of the middle ear.
- ▶ Analyze the functional roles of inner ear structures.
- ▶ Identify the physiological changes found in the organ of Corti associated with presbycusis.
- ▶ Identify the role of the stria vascularis in maintaining the ionic composition of the endolymph within the scala media.
- ▶ Identify the scala tympani in a cross-section of the cochlea.
- ▶ Describe the functional significance of the medial superior olive.
- ▶ Analyze the common contributing factors in the development of ear infections.
- ▶ Analyze the role of the inner hair cells in hearing loss and locate the inner hair cells on a cross-section of the organ of Corti.
- ▶ Relate lesions of the lateral lemniscus to hearing loss.
- ▶ Interpret the results of an auditory brainstem evoked potential and relate prominent features of the recording to the underlying neural mechanisms.
- ▶ Interpret the results of a Schwabach test.

18.1 Questions

Easy	Medium	Hard

1. A 22-year-old woman presents complaining of hearing loss. During a Weber test, the patient reports the sound is coming from the right ear. During a Rinne test, sound is perceived at a lower threshold when the tuning fork is placed next to the pinna when compared with when the tuning fork is placed on the mastoid of the skull, in both ears. Overall intensity discrimination sensitivity is reduced when testing the right ear. Based on these results, which of the following is most likely?

A. Sensorineural deficits involving the right cochlear nerve

B. Sensorineural deficits involving the left cochlear nerve

C. Conduction loss involving the left middle ear

D. Conduction loss involving the right middle ear

E. Conduction loss involving both ears

2. An 8-month-old infant is brought to a pediatrician by her mother. The mother reports that her daughter seems more fussy than normal and is often tugging on her ears, and she feels her baby is not responding to sounds in her environment as she normally would. Examination reveals bilateral otitis media. Which of the following is most likely involved in the diminished hearing reported?

A. Utricle

B. Saccule

C. Semicircular canals

D. Malleus, incus, and stapes

E. Cochlea

3. A 72-year-old male is undergoing reconstructive helical rim surgery, following tumor extirpation, to his right ear resulting in a 2.2-cm defect. Which area of the presented image best corresponds to the location of this surgery?

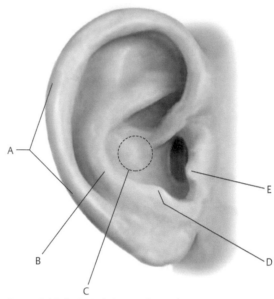

Source: Schünke M, Schulte E, Schumacher U et al. THIEME Atlas of Anatomy: Head, Neck, and Neuroanatomy. 2nd Edition. Thieme; 2016. Illustration by Karl Wesker/Markus Voll.

A. Area A

B. Area B

C. Area C

D. Area D

E. Area E

4. A 16-year-old girl is injured as the result of a high school wrestling match, and suffers direct trauma to the anterior auricle. Which of the following is the most likely effect for such injury?

A. Auricular hematoma forming a localized collection of blood between perichondrium and cartilage

B. Auricular hematoma forming a localized collection of blood between adipose tissue and cartilage

C. Auricular hematoma forming a localized collection of blood between cartilage and osseous tissue

D. Auricular hematoma forming a localized collection of blood between osseous and areolar tissue

E. Auricular hematoma forming a localized collection of blood between perichondrium and adipose tissue

5. A 56-year-old man makes an argument with his audiologist about the necessity for hearing protection while he is hunting. He had read on the internet that there was a reflex within the middle ear that would protect his hearing from high-intensity sounds, such as gunshots. Which of the following should be a reasonable statement for the audiologist to make?

A. The acoustic reflex does not reduce sound at the frequencies associated with gunshots

B. The acoustic reflex is not triggered at the amplitude associated with gunshots

C. The acoustic reflex does not reduce sound at a timescale adequate to protect hearing from the sound of gunshots

D. The acoustic reflex would result in ossicular chain damage at the amplitude associated with gunshots

E. There is no such acoustic reflex

6. A 51-year-old woman undergoes surgery to remove a tumor from the anterior portion of primary auditory cortex within the right superior temporal gyrus. What type of information would this portion of auditory cortex normally respond to best?

A. Auditory information from the left auditory hemifield

B. High-amplitude tones

C. Low-amplitude tones

D. High-frequency tones

E. Low-frequency tones

7. An 82-year-old male is referred to a neurologist after 3 years of increasing left-sided facial weakness, resulting in complete left-sided facial paralysis and hearing loss. MRI studies suggest a schwannoma involving the facial nerve. Which area of sensory innervation identified in the presented image is likely affected by this schwannoma?

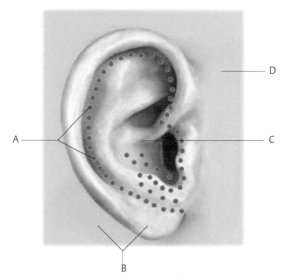

Source: Schünke M, Schulte E, Schumacher U et al. THIEME Atlas of Anatomy: Head, Neck, and Neuroanatomy. 2nd Edition. Thieme; 2016. Illustration by Karl Wesker/Markus Voll.

A. Area A

B. Area B

C. Area C

D. Area D

8. A 28-year-old male is brought to an army medical center following barotrauma experienced on the battlefield resulting in sensorineural hearing loss. Examination reveals the presence of a perilymph fistula, which is causing abnormal communication between the membranous labyrinth and the middle ear resulting in perilymph invading the normally air-filled space of the middle ear. Which of the following statements is true about fluids found within the inner ear?

A. Perilymph is similar to extracellular fluid, high in Na^+ and low in K^+

B. Perilymph is similar to intracellular fluid, high in K^+ and low in Na^+

C. Perilymph is similar to extracellular fluid, high in K^+ and low in Na^+

D. Perilymph is similar to intracellular fluid, high in Na^+ and low in K^+

E. Perilymph is low in Na^+ and K^+

9. A 17-year-old girl is taken to the emergency department after being hit in the side of the head by a softball during a high-school game. Upon examination, it is determined that the incus bone within the right middle ear has been broken as a result of the head trauma, resulting in substantial conductive hearing loss. Which area in the presented image corresponds to the broken bone?

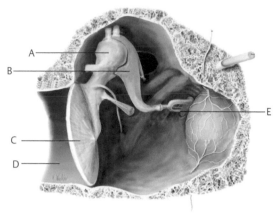

Source: Schünke M, Schulte E, Schumacher U et al. THIEME Atlas of Anatomy: Head, Neck, and Neuroanatomy. 2nd Edition. Thieme; 2016. Illustration by Karl Wesker/Markus Voll.

A. Area A
B. Area B
C. Area C
D. Area D
E. Area E

10. A 52-year-old right-handed male worked in a metal foundry for ~30 years. Recently, he has noticed poorer sensitivity to quiet sounds. Acoustic testing revealed a broader frequency tuning than would be expected in both ears. There is no specific frequency lost. Based on this information alone, which of the following components within the inner ear would you expect to be damaged?

A. Inner hair cells
B. Outer hair cells
C. Inner and outer hair cells
D. Basilar membrane
E. Tectorial membrane

11. A maker of cellular phone applications plans to take advantage of the presbycusis that occurs as a process of natural aging to allow teenagers to send messages without the knowledge of their parents by playing tones at high frequencies. What degenerative process of natural aging are they planning on exploiting?

A. Hearing loss occurring with aging resulting from degeneration of the organ of Corti at the basal coil of the cochlea
B. Hearing loss occurring with aging resulting from degeneration of the organ of Corti at the apical coil of the cochlea
C. Hearing loss occurring with aging resulting from the degeneration of outer hair cells
D. Hearing loss occurring with aging resulting from degeneration of primary auditory cortex
E. Hearing loss occurring with aging resulting from the degeneration of the inferior colliculus

Consider the following image for questions 12 and 13:

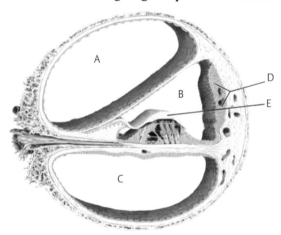

Source: Schünke M, Schulte E, Schumacher U et al. THIEME Atlas of Anatomy: Head, Neck, and Neuroanatomy. 2nd Edition. Thieme; 2016. Illustration by Karl Wesker/Markus Voll.

12. A 27-year-old drummer from a rock band presents to a walk-in clinic complaining of problems with his hearing. Through diagnostic testing, it is revealed that he has edema of the structure responsible for producing endolymph for the scala media, which has resulted in an imbalance in the sodium concentration. Which area in the presented image is responsible for maintaining the ionic composition of the endolymph?

A. Area A
B. Area B
C. Area C
D. Area D
E. Area E

13. A new treatment to combat sensorineural hearing loss as a result of sound damage to the cochlea is being developed. It involves injecting neural stem cells into the scala tympani, with the hope that these migrate through the tunnel of Corti and replace cells within the organ of Corti. Which area of the presented image corresponds to the locations in which stem cells are injected in this promising treatment?

A. Area A

B. Area B

C. Area C

D. Area D

E. Area E

14. A 61-year-old male experiences a stroke which damages the superior olivary complex within the trapezoid body. Diagnostic imaging reveals damage to the medial superior olive (MSO). What kinds of symptoms would you expect this patient to have?

A. Problems in sound localization in the vertical plane

B. Problems in perception of speech

C. Problems hearing high-frequency tones

D. Problems in sound localization in the horizontal plane

E. Problems hearing low-frequency tones

15. A 3-year-old girl experiences several bouts of relatively severe otitis media resulting in conductive hearing loss. During discussions with her pediatrician, her parents learn that children between the ages of 3 months and 3 years of age are especially susceptible to middle ear infections. Which reasons may the pediatrician have provided for these differences between small children and adults in their susceptibility to middle ear infections?

A. Use of pacifier

B. Increased exposure to infection

C. Differences between adult and infant eustachian tubes

D. Increased susceptibility to infection

E. All of the above

16. A famous 46-year-old opera singer makes an appointment with her audiologist after she has noticed difficulties hearing the soprano pieces (the highest voice type), indicating a problem with high-frequency tones. Which of the areas in the presented image is likely related to this hearing loss?

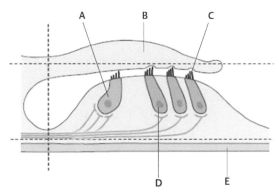

Source: Schünke M, Schulte E, Schumacher U et al. THIEME Atlas of Anatomy: Head, Neck, and Neuroanatomy. 2nd Edition. Thieme; 2016. Illustration by Karl Wesker/Markus Voll.

A. Area A

B. Area B

C. Area C

D. Area D

E. Area E

17. Following trauma, a 22-year-old woman is taken to the emergency department where it is determined that there is damage to the left dorsal acoustic stria within the pons. What type of hearing deficit would be most likely in this patient?

A. Left-sided impairment at low frequencies

B. Left-sided impairment at high frequencies

C. Right-sided impairment at low frequencies

D. Right-sided impairment at high frequencies

E. Bilateral hearing deficits

Consider the following case for questions 18 and 19:

A 2-year-old child is brought to the pediatrician when her parents are concerned that her language has not developed at the rate that it should. As the child is too young to assess hearing capabilities that require verbal response, they are referred to an audiologist to perform a BAER test. The tests for both the right and left ear are displayed.

Left ear

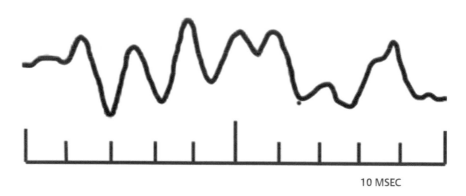

10 MSEC

Right ear

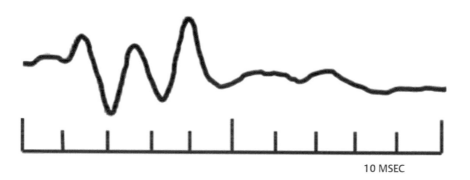

10 MSEC

18. What would be the most likely conclusion of this test?

A. Normal results

B. Left ear abnormal

C. Right ear abnormal

D. Both ears abnormal

E. Unable to determine functioning

19. At what level of the brainstem is the auditory information ceasing to propagate toward primary auditory cortex?

A. Auditory nerve

B. Cochlear nuclei

C. Superior olivary nucleus

D. Lateral lemniscus

E. Inferior colliculus

20. A 17-year-old girl has been aggressively cleaning her ear canals with cotton swabs, and has recently reported that she has trouble hearing out of her right ear. Her primary care physician attempts to determine whether the hearing loss is conductive or sensorineural in nature by performing the Schwabach test on her right ear. The test reveals that there is prolonged duration of tone when compared with that heard by the examiner. This result would point toward:

A. Normal findings

B. Conduction hearing loss

C. Sensorineural hearing loss

D. Sensorineural and conductive hearing loss

E. Patient malingering

18.2 Answers and Explanations

Easy	Medium	Hard

1. Correct: Sensorineural deficits involving the left cochlear nerve (B)

A Weber test that lateralizes to the right is pointing toward either a left sensorineural deficit or a right conduction loss (**D**). The Rinne test in the right ear showed air conduction was greater than bone conduction, indicating the conduction system was functioning properly in the right ear (**D**).

Sensorineural deficit in the right cochlear nerve (**A**) or conduction loss involving the left middle ear (**C**) would both present as a Weber test lateralizing to the left. Lastly, conduction loss in both ears (**E**) would not be consistent with the Weber test lateralizing to the right.

2. Correct: Malleus, incus, and stapes (D)

Otitis media, inflammation of the middle ear, would most likely affect the small bones within the middle ear, resulting in reduction in the flexibility within the ossicular chain and mechanical impairment in conducting sound waves to the cochlea.

The utricle (**A**), saccule (**B**), and semicircular canals (**C**) are all components of the vestibular system, and although they might be affected by infection, these would not affect hearing. Cochlea (**E**) is seldom involved in otitis media.

3. Correct: Area A (A)

The outer ear forms a funnel-shape design to collect acoustic vibrations and funnel them into the auditory canal. The helix of the ear is a common site for reconstructive surgery due to its susceptibility to neoplastic lesions.

Refer to the following image for explanation:

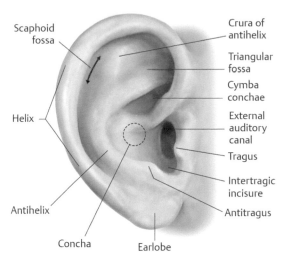

Source: Schünke M, Schulte E, Schumacher U et al. THIEME Atlas of Anatomy: Head, Neck, and Neuroanatomy. 2nd Edition. Thieme; 2016. Illustration by Karl Wesker/Markus Voll.

4. Correct: Auricular hematoma forming a localized collection of blood between perichondrium and cartilage (A)

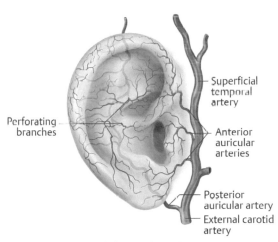

Source: Schünke M, Schulte E, Schumacher U et al. THIEME Atlas of Anatomy: Head, Neck, and Neuroanatomy. 2nd Edition. Thieme; 2016. Illustration by Karl Wesker/Markus Voll.

Auricular hematoma results from trauma and forms a localized collection of blood between the perichondrium and ear cartilage and can result in fibrosis and a deformed auricle—a condition known as wrestler's ear or cauliflower ear. As is evident in the presented image, perforating branches of the anterior and posterior auricular arteries supply the external ear, and these are especially susceptible to the shearing forces experienced when the external ear is compressed and/or twisted.

Adipose (**B** and **E**) or osseous (**C** and **D**) tissue is not found in external ear.

5.   Correct: The acoustic reflex does not reduce sound at a timescale adequate to protect hearing from the sound of gunshots (C)

The acoustic reflex (or stapedius reflex) is an involuntary muscle contraction that occurs within the middle ear both in response to high-intensity sounds and during vocalization. However, the reflex takes ~12 milliseconds to be instituted in response to a high-amplitude sound, which is not fast enough to protect the auditory system from auditory stimuli such as gunshots.

As the stapedius reflex acts to stiffen the ossicular chain by pulling the stapes away from the oval window (via the stapedius muscle) and the malleus toward the middle ear (via the tensor tympani muscle), it would affect a broad range of auditory frequencies (**A**).

A gunshot has a typical decibel rating of ~160 dB, with the stapedius reflex triggered at the 70 to 100 dB level (**B**).

The stapedius reflex would not be of sufficient force, regardless of the amplitude of the auditory stimulus, to cause ossicular chain damage (**D**).

6.   Correct: Low-frequency tones (E)

Primary auditory cortex, located on the superior temporal gyrus of the temporal lobe, is tonotopically organized with the anterior portion responding best to low-frequency tones, and the posterior portion responding most to high-frequency tones (**D**).

Localization (**A**) and amplitude (**B** and **C**) of sound are not coded by anteroposterior location within the primary auditory cortex.

7.   Correct: Area D (D)

As seen in the following image, four cranial nerves contribute to the sensory innervation of the auricle. The facial nerve supplies an ill-defined region of the posterior auricular area.

8.   Correct: Perilymph is similar to extracellular fluid, high in Na$^+$ and low in K$^+$ (A)

Perilymph is similar to extracellular fluid, being high in sodium, Na$^+$, and low in potassium, K$^+$. Endolymph is similar to intracellular fluid, in that it is high in K$^+$ and low in Na$^+$ (**B**). It is this electrochemical gradient between the endolymph and the perilymph that powers the receptor signaling response within the inner hair cells.

No other combinations (**C, D,** and **E**) of potassium and sodium concentrations are correctly matched to either the perilymph or the comparison to intracellular and extracellular fluid.

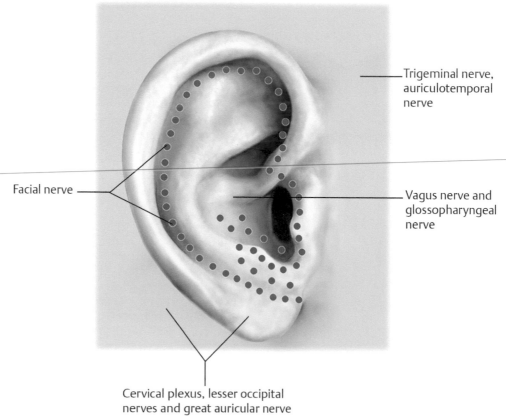

Trigeminal nerve, auriculotemporal nerve

Facial nerve

Vagus nerve and glossopharyngeal nerve

Cervical plexus, lesser occipital nerves and great auricular nerve

Source: Schünke M, Schulte E, Schumacher U et al. THIEME Atlas of Anatomy: Head, Neck, and Neuroanatomy. 2nd Edition. Thieme; 2016. Illustration by Karl Wesker/Markus Voll.

9. Correct: Area B (B)

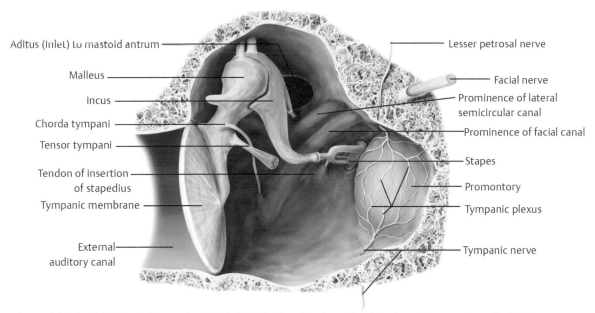

Aditus (Inlet) to mastoid antrum

Malleus

Incus

Chorda tympani

Tensor tympani

Tendon of insertion of stapedius

Tympanic membrane

External auditory canal

Lesser petrosal nerve

Facial nerve

Prominence of lateral semicircular canal

Prominence of facial canal

Stapes

Promontory

Tympanic plexus

Tympanic nerve

Source: Schünke M, Schulte E, Schumacher U et al. THIEME Atlas of Anatomy: Head, Neck, and Neuroanatomy. 2nd Edition. Thieme; 2016. Illustration by Karl Wesker/Markus Voll.

The bones within the middle ear that make up the ossicular chain are the smallest bones in the body, and therefore are quite fragile. Sound waves entering the external auditory canal (**D**) move the tympanic membrane (**C**), which induces movement within the ossicular chain. Movement of the malleus (**A**) is then transferred to the incus bone (**B**), which ultimately causes a tilting movement of the stapes (**E**). This induces waves in the fluid within the inner ear through the oval window.

10. Correct: Outer hair cells (B)

The outer hair cells act as acoustical preamplifiers, non-linearly amplifying low-amplitude sounds more than large-amplitude sounds, and expanding the range of sound pressures perceived by the cochlea through active vibrations of the cell body in response to the receptor potential. This vibration amplifies and tunes the movement of the basilar membrane, as the stereocilia are embedded in the tectorial membrane. Therefore, outer hair damage results in poorer sensitivity and broader frequency tuning, as is described in this patient case.

The deflection of the inner hair cells (**A and C**) causes graded and biphasic potentials in response to sound waves due to both the electrical and chemical gradients between the endolymph and perilymph. The release of neurotransmitters binds to receptors and triggers action potentials within the nerve, which ultimately is perceived as sound. Damage to the inner hair cells would result in a loss in frequency perception, rather than the scenario described.

Damage to either the basilar (**D**) or the tectorial membrane (**E**) is not a likely result of exposure to factory sounds, as reported in this case. Further, damage to either of these structures would most likely result in sensorineural deafness within the affected ear(s).

11. Correct: Hearing loss occurring with aging resulting from degeneration of the organ of Corti at the basal coil of the cochlea (A)

Presbycusis, hearing loss occurring with aging, results from degenerative disease of the organ of Corti within the first few millimeters of the basal coil of the cochlea, corresponding to loss of high-frequency tones.

As the cochlea is tonotopically organized with higher frequency tones at the basal end, degeneration at the apical coil of the cochlea (**B**) would result in a deficit in perceiving low-frequency tones. Additionally, this type of degeneration is not observed with natural aging.

There is no known process by which aging affects the outer hair cells of the inner ear (**C**), and further, such degeneration would not result in a specific deficit in the perception of high-frequency tones.

Degeneration of primary auditory cortex (**D**), within the superior temporal gyrus, would not result in specific frequency deficits, but rather in difficulty in processing complex sounds such as speech.

Lastly, damage limited to the inferior colliculus (**E**) has been shown to result in errors in sound localization with the illusion that sound sources from within the contralesional hemifield being perceived as coming from the ipsilesional auditory hemifield.

Refer to the following image for answers 12 and 13:

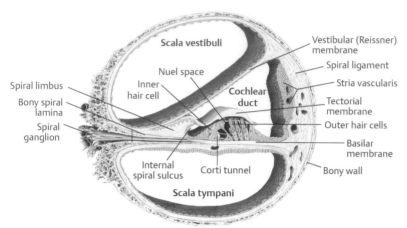

Source: Schünke M, Schulte E, Schumacher U et al. THIEME Atlas of Anatomy: Head, Neck, and Neuroanatomy. 2nd Edition. Thieme; 2016. Illustration by Karl Wesker/Markus Voll.

12. Correct: Area D (D)

The presented image is a cross-section through the cochlea in the petrous bone. The outer wall of the cochlear duct (upper portion of the spiral ligament) contains the stria vascularis, which, as the name suggests, is heavily vascularized. The primary function of the stria vascularis is to produce endolymph for the scala media (**B**), the fluid-filled cavity which contains the tectorial membrane (**E**). If the ionic composition of the scala media is not maintained, hair cells within the organ of Corti can be damaged, resulting in deficits in hearing.

Areas A and C in the presented image represent the other two fluid-filled membranes of the cochlea, the scala vestibuli (**A**) and scala tympani (**C**). These two compartments are filled with perilymph, as opposed to endolymph.

13. Correct: Area C (C)

In the described treatment, neural stem cells are injected into the scala tympani, which is area C, as can be identified from the image.

14. Correct: Problems in sound localization in the horizontal plane (D)

The medial superior olive is thought to help locate sound within the horizontal plane (whether the sound source is located to the left or right, relative to the listener).

Sound localization in the vertical plane (**A**) is thought to be a function of fusiform cells of the dorsal cochlear nucleus, and bypasses the superior olivary complex directly projecting to the inferior colliculus. Problems with perceiving complicated auditory signals like speech (**B**) are common with damage to many levels of the auditory system, but not the MSO. Problems with high- (**C**) and low-frequency (**D**) tones would most likely result from damage to the base or apex of the cochlea, respectively.

15. Correct: All of the above (E)

Although differences in the size (larger), length (longer), and angle (greater) of the adult eustachian tube compared with an infant are the often cited reasons for increased occurrences of otitis media in young children (**C**), all of the factors listed are involved. Use of a pacifier has been linked to increased risk of ear infections (**A**), though there is some debate as to the causal nature of this relationship. Infants have both increased exposure (**B**) and susceptibility (**D**) to infection.

16. Correct: Area A (A)

Hearing loss at specific frequencies is most commonly associated with inner hair cell damage, represented in area A of the presented image.

Area C represents stereocilia, the mechanosensing organelles of hair cells. The stereocilia respond to fluid motion of the endolymph.

Area D represents the outer hair cells, which are involved in acoustic preamplification. Areas B and E represent the tectorial and basilar membranes, respectively.

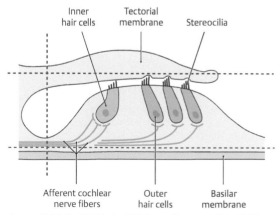

Source: Schünke M, Schulte E, Schumacher U et al. THIEME Atlas of Anatomy: Head, Neck, and Neuroanatomy. 2nd Edition. Thieme; 2016. Illustration by Karl Wesker/Markus Voll.

17. Correct: Bilateral hearing deficits (E)

Similar to lesions at the level of cortex, unilateral damage to the lateral lemniscus (consisting of the intermediate acoustic stria, trapezoid body, and dorsal acoustic stria) will result in bilateral hearing deficit.

Impairment at specific frequencies (**A, B, C,** and **D**) would require damage to the cochlea. Further, unilateral hearing deficits (**A, B, C,** and **D**) would most likely require damage to the cochlea or in close proximity to the cochlear nuclei.

Refer to the following image for answers 18 and 19:

Left ear

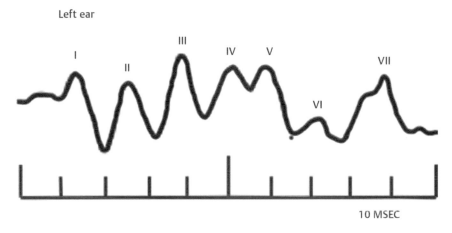

10 MSEC

Right ear

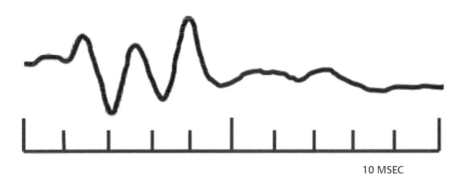

10 MSEC

18. Correct: Right ear abnormal (C)

When performing a brainstem auditory evoked potential test, unilateral ear stimulation (typically a clicking stimulus) is used to elicit electrical potentials in the CNS.

Activities are measured within the brainstem and the cerebral cortex. Seven waves (labeled in ascending order I–VII) correspond to activities within the auditory nerve, cochlear nuclei, superior olivary nucleus, lateral lemniscus, inferior colliculus, medial geniculate body, and auditory radiations. In the left ear, there are seven identifiable peaks in the sweep, indicating normal electrical potentials (**A, B, D,** and **E**). However, in the right ear there are only three identifiable peaks, indicating a dysfunction.

19. Correct: Lateral lemniscus (D)

Since there are three peaks for the right ear, it appears that sensorineural functioning is normal at the levels of the auditory nerve (**A**), cochlear nuclei (**B**), and superior olivary nucleus (**C**). Therefore, the

169

information is ceasing to propagate from the level of the lateral lemniscus and cannot make it to the inferior colliculus (**E**).

20.   Correct: Conduction hearing loss (B)

The Schwabach test compares the patient's bone conduction to that of a known normal sample (typically the examiner). If the patient hears the tuning fork longer than the examiner, this would suggest conductive hearing loss. Use of cotton swabs to clean the external auditory canal can result in conductive hearing loss due to an impaction of cerumen (ear wax).

Normal findings (**A**) would consist of both the examiner and the patient hearing the tuning fork for the same duration.

Sensorineural hearing loss (**C**) would be evidenced by the patient ceasing to hear the tone before the examiner.

If the hearing deficit is a result of both sensorineural and conductive processes (**D**), a Schwabach test will be inconclusive and further testing must be performed.

Lastly, if the patient is malingering (**E**), the Schwabach test will again provide inconclusive results and additional testing, not requiring patient compliance, would have to be performed.

Chapter 19
Vestibular System

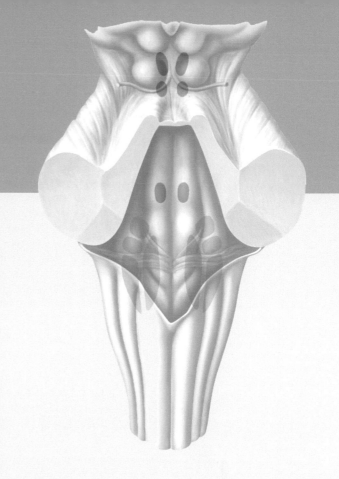

LEARNING OBJECTIVES

► Analyze features of Dix–Hallpike positional testing that is consistent with a peripheral lesion causing vertigo.

► Analyze features of Dix–Hallpike positional testing that is consistent with a central lesion causing vertigo.

► Analyze symptoms associated with the diagnosis of benign paroxysmal positional vertigo.

► Identify the nuclei receiving afferent input from the saccular macula.

► Illustrate the location and functions of the lateral vestibulospinal tract.

► Describe the location and functions of the ampullary crests.

► Identify the location of the otolith organs within the inner ear, and analyze their functional significance.

► Identify the location of the anterior semicircular canal.

► Identify the CN responsible for innervation of the vestibular system.

► Analyze the features of oculocephalic testing.

► Interpret normal test results for a postrotational nystagmus test.

► Interpret normal caloric irrigation test results utilizing cold water.

► Interpret caloric nystagmus test results in a comatose patient.

► Analyze symptoms associated with decerebrate rigidity and relate this condition to probable lesion location.

► Identify the symptoms associated with benign positional vertigo.

► Describe the pathophysiology and clinical features of Meniere's disease.

► Analyze the role of calcium carbonate within the utricle and saccule.

► Identify the symptoms commonly associated with acoustic schwannoma.

19.1 Questions

Easy	Medium	Hard

1. A 51-year-old male presents to the emergency department, complaining of excessive vertigo. After verifying there is no damage to cervical sections of the spinal cord, you begin Dix–Hallpike positional testing to determine whether the vertigo is a result of central or peripheral dysfunction. Following the completion of your testing, you determine the type of lesion to be peripheral in nature. Which of the following results of the positional testing would point toward this finding?

A. Onset of nystagmus was delayed by ~3 seconds

B. Adaptation/habituation was observed when the same maneuver was repeated

C. Horizontal nystagmus was observed

D. Nystagmus occurred in the absence of vertigo

E. Rotary nystagmus was observed

2. A 22-year-old female presents to the emergency department with the primary complaint of vertigo and nausea. After ruling out contraindications, you perform Dix–Hallpike positional testing on both the left and right sides. On completion of the testing, you determine the vertigo to be a result of a central lesion. Which of the following pieces of information would be consistent with this diagnosis?

A. Horizontal nystagmus was present

B. Onset of nystagmus was delayed

C. Rotary nystagmus was observed

D. Vertical nystagmus was present

E. Nystagmus was present at the same time as a sensation of vertigo

3. 38-year-old male presents to his primary care physician after he experienced intense vertigo for 3 hours after bending over to tie his shoe. Since his initial symptoms, which appeared 2 days ago following a mild bump to his head, he has had brief episodes of vertigo which last for a few seconds if he moves his head too quickly, at which point he has to brace himself for fearing he will fall over. He says his symptoms are worst when he is trying to lie down at the end of the day. Which of the following diagnosis is most consistent with this patient's symptoms?

A. Vestibular neuronitis

B. Acoustic neuroma

C. Vertebrobasilar ischemia

D. Benign paroxysmal positional vertigo

E. Meniere's disease

Consider the following image for questions 4 and 5:

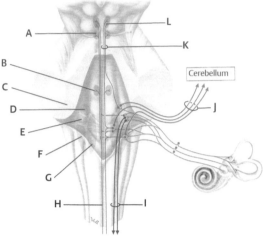

Source: Schünke M, Schulte E, Schumacher U et al. THIEME Atlas of Anatomy: Head, Neck, and Neuroanatomy. 2nd Edition. Thieme; 2016. Illustration by Karl Wesker/Markus Voll.

4. A 77-year-old male is taken to the emergency department after collapsing at a restaurant. Upon examination, it is determined that there is damage to the vestibular nuclei. Specifically, the lesion is affecting the nuclei onto which afferent fibers of the saccular macula terminate. The lesioned area would affect:

A. Area D

B. Area G

C. Areas D and G

D. Area E

E. Area F

F. Areas E and F

5. A 92-year-old female is having difficulty maintaining her posture. In particular, it is determined that the vestibular system is no longer capable of providing input to increase the tone of extensor muscles that are used to combat gravity, despite a normal vestibular ocular response. Which pathway in the presented figure is most related to the efferent fibers that would normally provide this capability?

A. Area H

B. Area I

C. Area J

D. Area K

E. Area L

Consider the following image for questions 6 to 8:

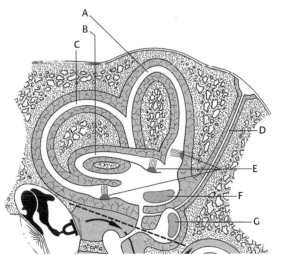

Source: Borsody M. Comprehensive Board Review in Neurology. 2nd Edition. Thieme; 2009.

6. A 19-year-old male presents to the hospital after drinking an excessive amount of alcohol. At his blood alcohol concentration, there is a specific change in the buoyancy of the ampullary cupula, creating a density gradient between the cupula and the surrounding endolymph, resulting in vertigo. The ampullary cupula are related to which labeled area in the presented image?

A. Area A

B. Area B

C. Area C

D. Area D

E. Area E

7. A 17-year-old girl presents to the emergency department after attending a rock concert with complaints of dizziness. Through ocular vestibular-evoked myogenic potential (oVEMP) testing, it is determined that exposure to excessive sound levels has damaged one of the otolith organs responsible for detecting horizontal linear accelerations. Which area of the image best corresponds with this damage?

A. Area D

B. Area E

C. Area F

D. Area G

E. Area A

8. A 26-year-old woman presents to her primary care physician following the development of autophony and dizziness. In particular, she states that her dizziness is worsened by certain sounds (Tullio phenomenon), and her voice sounds like it is being relayed through a loudspeaker in her head. Further testing revealed that she is not suffering from a patulous eustachian tube, which is the most common cause of autophony. Diagnostic radiology revealed that there was substantial thinning of the temporal bone overlaying area A in the presented image, resulting in her symptoms. What part of the vestibular system is likely being affected by this temporal bone thinning resulting in this patient's symptoms?

A. Anterior semicircular canal

B. Lateral semicircular canal

C. Posterior semicircular canal

D. Utricle

E. Saccule

9. A 17-year-old girl is suspected of having damage to the CN which is responsible for the innervation of the ampullae within the semicircular canals, the utricle, and the saccule. The CN responsible for the innervation of vestibular system end organs is:

A. CN III

B. CN IV

C. CN V

D. CN VI

E. CN VIII

10. A 28-year-old woman is brought to emergency department following a hit-and-run accident. After verifying there was no cervical spinal trauma through radiological examination, the oculocephalic reflex was tested to examine the functional status of the brainstem eye movement pathways. The patient was unconscious at the time of testing, and doll's eyes were present. To make this conclusion, the examiner observed:

A. The eye lids opened upon movement of the head.

B. The eyes moved in the direction opposite to head movements.

C. The eyes moved in the same direction as the head movements.

D. The eye lids closed upon movement of the head.

E. Oculocephalic testing cannot be performed on an unconscious patient.

11. A 44-year-old male presents to his primary care physician with complaints of dizziness. A simple test of visual function is performed in the office in which the patient sits in a rotating chair and is asked to close his eyes. Next, the physician spins the chair at a rate of 0.5 Hz, for a total of 10 rotations. Immediately following the 10th rotation, the spinning is stopped and the patient is asked to open their eyes. When observing the eyes, if the patient's vestibular system is functioning you would expect:

A. The fast phase of nystagmus to be against the direction of rotation

B. The slow phase of nystagmus to be against the direction of rotation

C. No nystagmus should be present

D. The fast phase of nystagmus to be in the upward direction

E. The fast phase of nystagmus to be in the downward direction

12. An 8-year-old girl is suspected of having damage to the hair cells within the left semicircular canal. To test functioning of the left labyrinth, the external auditory meatus is irrigated with cold water, while the patient tilts her head back 60 degrees. A normal test result was observed. Which of the following eye movements would be expected?

A. In the same direction as the irrigated ear

B. The left eye moving in the direction of the irrigated ear

C. Upward

D. Opposite to the direction of the irrigated ear

E. The right eye moving in the direction opposite of the irrigated ear

13. A 66-year-old comatose male is suspected of having brainstem lesion. To localize the lesion, a cold-water caloric irrigation test is performed by irrigating the left external acoustic meatus with cold water. The results of the irrigation test revealed no movement of the eyes. What is the most likely conclusion based on the results of this test?

A. Unilateral left-sided damage to the MLF

B. Unilateral right-sided damage to the MLF

C. Bilateral damage to the MLF

D. Lower brainstem damage

E. Brainstem intact

14. A 66-year-old male presented to the emergency department following 3 days of nervousness and a subjective feeling of numbness in all four limbs which progressed to the point of weakness and decreased visual acuity. Upon admission, miotic pupils were observed, as were bilateral patellar and ankle clonus, and bilateral Babinski's responses. Soon after admission, he began to display opisthotonos (muscle spasms causing a backward arching of the spine, neck, and head). If this patient underwent diagnostic radiology, where would a lesion most likely be found?

A. At the vestibular nuclei

B. Between the red nucleus and the vestibular nuclei

C. At the internal capsule

D. Within the cerebral hemisphere

E. Within the vestibulospinal tract

15. A 45-year-old woman presents to her primary care physician with complaints of dizziness. In particular, she says that when she gets out of bed or stands up from a chair, she gets "the spins." During the patient interview, it is revealed that she gets dizzy on occasions if she turns her head too quickly or sometimes when she is in a crowd. She had similar symptoms, a year ago, which resolved on their own. Her current symptoms seem worse, and she does not feel like they are getting better. During her periods of dizziness, she does not report any changes in hearing. What is the most likely cause of her condition?

A. Meniere's disease

B. Labyrinthitis

C. Benign positional vertigo

D. Acoustic schwannoma

E. Multiple sclerosis

Consider the following case for questions 16 and 17:

A 48-year-old male was admitted to the emergency department with severe vertigo and right sensorineural hearing loss. He had suffered from fluctuating right sensorineural hearing loss with vertigo for the preceding 8 years, often accompanied by nausea and vomiting. Audiogram revealed prominent loss of hearing, predominantly within the low-frequency range. Neurological examination revealed a horizontal nystagmus, with the fast phase toward the left ear.

16. What is the most likely explanation for the patient's symptoms?

A. Increased endolymphatic pressure

B. Dislocation of the utricular macular otoliths

C. Bacterial infection of the inner ear

D. Compression of CN VIII

E. Loss of hair cells within the semicircular canals

17. What would be a suitable treatment course to combat the hearing loss observed in this patient?

A. Diazepam

B. Gentamicin

C. Vestibular nerve section

D. Labyrinthectomy

E. None of the above

18. A 7-year-old girl is brought to the emergency department after drinking a toxin that is known to dissolve calcium carbonate crystals within the inner ear. What effect would you expect this chemical to have on vestibular function?

A. There would be no effect on the vestibular system

B. The semicircular canals will cease to function properly

C. The utricle will cease to function, but the sacculus would be unaffected

D. The saccule will cease to function, but the utricle would be unaffected

E. Both the utricle and the saccule would cease to function properly

19. A 22-year-old woman presented to a walk-in clinic with complaints of progressive hearing loss, facial weakness, and headaches, all felt more on the right side. When examining the patient's gait, it was noted to be somewhat unsteady and the patient felt dizzy. She had no bouts of vomiting or nausea. What is the most likely diagnosis for this patient?

A. Meniere's disease

B. Labyrinthitis

C. Benign positional vertigo

D. Acoustic schwannoma

E. Multiple sclerosis

19.2 Answers and Explanations

Easy	Medium	Hard

1. Correct: Adaptation/habituation was observed when the same maneuver was repeated (B)

When performing Dix–Hallpike positional testing, for peripheral lesions, adaptation should occur in successive maneuvers.

Both peripheral and central lesions may be associated with a 2- to 5-second delay from maneuver to nystagmus (**A**). However, immediate onset of nystagmus would point toward a central lesion location. Nystagmus should not occur in the absence of vertigo (**D**) with a peripheral lesion. Lastly, the presence of horizontal (**C**) or rotary nystagmus (**E**) does not differentiate between peripheral and central causes of vertigo.

2. Correct: Vertical nystagmus was present (D)

The presence of vertical nystagmus (**D**) would be diagnostic of brainstem or cerebellar cause (central lesion).

Horizontal (**A**), rotary (**C**), or delayed-onset (**B**) nystagmus can be observed with either central or peripheral lesions. Similarly, nystagmus present with a sensation of vertigo (**E**) can occur with both central and peripheral lesions.

3. Correct: Benign paroxysmal positional vertigo (D)

The symptoms reported are most consistent with a diagnosis of benign paroxysmal positional vertigo. The sudden onset of symptoms following a minor blow to the head and the initial symptom lasting several hours followed by much shorter bouts following positional changes are all suggestive of this diagnosis.

Vestibular neuronitis (**A**) is a result of a viral infection or idiopathic inflammation of the vestibular ganglia and/or nerve. In these cases, several days of severe vertigo is most common, followed by a feeling of general unsteadiness that can last for months.

An acoustic neuroma (**B**) would be expected to present with hearing loss and tinnitus, and the vertigo would present with a general unsteadiness rather than discrete episodes.

A vertebrobasilar ischemia (**C**) with involvement of the vestibular nuclei or cerebellum can also cause vertigo; however, additional symptoms consistent with vertebrobasilar disease would be expected (such as disconjugate gaze, headache, or paresis).

With a diagnosis of Meniere's disease (**E**), one would expect the additional symptoms of fluctuating hearing loss, tinnitus, and often a feeling like the "ear is full."

Refer to the following image for answers 4 and 5:

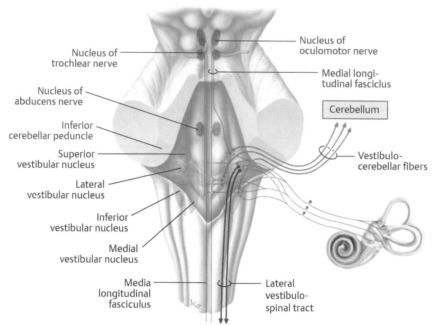

Source: Schünke M, Schulte E, Schumacher U et al. THIEME Atlas of Anatomy: Head, Neck, and Neuroanatomy. 2nd Edition. Thieme; 2016. Illustration by Karl Wesker/Markus Voll.

4. Correct: Areas E and F (F)

The afferent fibers of the saccular macula terminate in the lateral (area **E**) and the inferior (area **F**) vestibular nuclei.

The superior vestibular nuclei (area D [**A** and **C**]) receive input from the ampullary crests of the semicircular canals. The medial vestibular nuclei (area G [**B** and **C**]) receive input from the utricular macula and the semicircular canals.

5. Correct: Area I (B)

Efferent fibers from the lateral vestibular nuclei (area E in the figure) pass to the lateral vestibulospinal tract (area I in the figure). The primary function of this pathway is to keep the body upright by increasing muscle tone in response to vestibular stimulation.

Area H (**A**), area K (**D**), and area L (**E**) correspond to the MLF, its rostral continuation, and its termination at the nucleus of CN III, respectively. The MLF is a collection of ascending and descending pathways that form the main connections between the nuclei of CN III, CN IV, and CN VI, and is related to ocular motility and gaze.

Area J (**C**) is indicating vestibulocerebellar fibers, which act through the cerebellum to modulate muscular tone.

6. Correct: Area E (E)

The ampullary cupula are located within the ampullary crests, denoted as area E in the presented image.

The areas A, B, and C represent the anterior, lateral, and posterior semicircular canals, respectively. Although movement within the semicircular canals can result in vertigo, it is not the mechanism by which it is introduced in the current case. Area D represents the endolymphatic duct, a nonsensory component of the membranous labyrinth that leads from the utricular and saccular ducts within the vestibule to the endolymphatic sac on the posterior surface of the petrous portion of the temporal bone.

7. Correct: Area F (C)

The otolith organs (areas F and G) are responsible for detecting displacements and linear accelerations of the head, such as what is observed by tilting or translational movements. Further, the utricle (area F; [**C**]) is positioned in such a way to respond to movements of the head in the horizontal plane, and the saccule (area G; [**D**]) is positioned to respond to movements of the head in the vertical plane.

Area D (**A**) represents the endolymphatic duct, a nonsensory component of the membranous labyrinth that leads from the utricular and saccular ducts within the vestibule to the endolymphatic sac on the posterior surface of the petrous portion of the temporal bone. Area E (**B**) is displaying the ampullary crests. Area A (**E**) represents the anterior semicircular canal, which is sensitive to angular acceleration.

8. Correct: Anterior semicircular canal (A)

This patient is displaying signs of superior canal dehiscence syndrome (SCDS). Common symptoms include autophony and sound-induced vertigo, as reported here. This rare medical condition is caused by thinning or absence of the part of the temporal bone that overlays the anterior semicircular canal. Due to the proximity of the anterior semicircular canal to the temporal bone, it is especially sensitive.

As options **B, C, D,** and **E** are contained further from the surface of the skull, they are not likely to be affected by the thinning.

9. Correct: CN VIII (E)

The end organs of the vestibular system are innervated by the vestibular part of CN VIII. Bipolar afferent neurons whose peripheral processes form synaptic contact with the hair cells are known as Scarpa's ganglion.

CN III (**A**), the oculomotor nerve, is responsible for eye movements. The trochlear (CN IV; **B**) nerve is also responsible for eye movements, but is specific to control of the superior oblique muscle. The trigeminal nerve (CN V; **C**) provides sensation to the skin of the face, while providing motor innervation of the muscles involved in mastication. The abducens nerve (CN VI; **D**) is involved in eye movements, but is limited to control of the lateral rectus muscle, which is responsible for abduction movements of the eye.

10. Correct: The eyes moved in the direction opposite to head movements (B)

During oculocephalic testing, a positive doll's eye consists of the eyes moving in the direction opposite to head movements. This test can be useful if the patient cannot follow commands to move their eyes, and instead relies on the vestibulo-ocular reflex.

Importantly, when dealing with a conscious patient, doll's eyes are usually not present as visual fixation and voluntary eye movements mask the reflex, making it only appropriate to test brainstem dysfunction in the unconscious patient (**E**).

Although ptosis can be indicative of damage to CN III, which supplies innervation for the levator palpebrae superioris, the eye lids opening (**A**) or closing (**D**) upon movement of the head is not part of the doll's eye response.

If the eyes move in the same direction as the head movement (**C**), this would suggest negative "doll's eyes," and be indicative of damage to the brainstem.

11. Correct: The fast phase of nystagmus to be against the direction of rotation (A)

The postrotational nystagmus test, also known as rotary chair testing, involves rotating the patient at a speed within the range of 0.5 and 2.0 Hz for ~10 rotations. Immediately following the rotation, a normal vestibular response would consist of the fast phase of nystagmus in the opposite direction to that of rotation. The slow phase of nystagmus, therefore, would be consistent with the direction of rotation, ruling out (**B**).

An abnormal or absent nystagmus (**C**) would indicate improper function of the vestibular system. It is possible to have a vertical nystagmus (**D** and **E**); however, as the rotation plane was along the horizontal axis, the nystagmus should also be along the horizontal axis.

12. Correct: Opposite to the direction of the irrigated ear (D)

When performing the caloric nystagmus test, both hot and cold water can be used to irrigate the external auditory meatus. The advantage of using a caloric test, as opposed to a postrotational nystagmus test, is each labyrinth can be tested individually, and tests can be performed on the comatose patient. The direction of nystagmus (defined by the direction of the fast phase) elicited by irrigation can be remembered through the use of the mnemonic COWS—cold, opposite; warm, same. With this mnemonic in mind, since cold water was used, nystagmus would be expected in the direction opposite to the irrigated ear. However, if warm water had been used for the testing, one would expect the movement to be in the same direction as the irrigated ear (**A**). It is important to remember that this mnemonic only applies for the awake patient, as the fast phase of nystagmus is absent in a comatose patient.

An upbeating nystagmus (**C**) is most likely indicative of brainstem damage, and would not be expected with a normal caloric irrigation test. A normal test result would also not consist of monocular eye movements (**B** and **E**).

13. Correct: Lower brainstem damage (D)

When performing cold water caloric nystagmus testing in a comatose patient, no movement of the eyes would indicate lower brainstem damage, due to disruption of the vestibular nuclei.

Unilateral damage to the MLF on either side (**A** and **B**) would not result in an absence of movement as described. Similarly, bilateral damage to the MLF (**C**) would also not prevent movement of the eyes, but instead would result in the abducting eye deviating to the side of cold irrigation.

A normal result in a comatose patient, indicating the brainstem was intact (**E**), would consist of both eyes performing a conjugate deviation toward the side of the cold irrigation.

It is important to note that in the comatose patient the COWS (cold, opposite; warm, same) mnemonic is not appropriate as nystagmus is not present.

14. Correct: Between the red nucleus and the vestibular nuclei (B)

This patient is displaying the classic signs of decerebrate rigidity. This type of posturing, characterized by opisthotonos (extension, adduction, hyperpronation of the arms, and extension of the feet with plantar flexion), is caused by a lesion that transects the brainstem between the red nucleus and the vestibular nuclei. With such a lesion, the tonic activity of the reticular formation and the lateral vestibular nuclei results in abnormal innervation of the extensor muscles responsible for antigravity tone.

Lesions of the vestibular nuclei (**A**) and the vestibulospinal tract (**E**) would not result in decerebrate rigidity; in fact, their ablation would likely abolish decerebrate rigidity in a patient. A lesion within the internal capsule (**C**) or the cerebral hemisphere (**D**) is more likely to result in decorticate rigidity, rather than decerebrate rigidity.

15. Correct: Benign positional vertigo (C)

This patient is displaying common symptoms associated with benign positional vertigo. Benign positional vertigo, the most common cause of vertigo, is usually elicited by certain head positions. The paroxysm of vertigo is usually accompanied by nystagmus, but is not associated with hearing loss or tinnitus. It is believed to result from cuprolithiasis of the posterior semicircular duct, in which the utricular macular otoliths are dislocated.

Although Meniere's disease (**A**) often presents with episodic attacks of vertigo, symptoms usually include tinnitus, hearing loss, vomiting, nausea, and a sensation of fullness and pressure in the ear.

Similarly, labyrinthitis (**B**) presents with many of the same symptoms as in Meniere's disease, but is the result of an inflammation of the labyrinth, usually resulting from toxic (alcohol, salicylates, quinine, etc.), viral, or bacterial causes.

Acoustic schwannoma (**D**) most often results in vertigo in combination with tinnitus and unilateral hearing loss.

Multiple sclerosis (**E**) is most commonly associated with internuclear ophthalmoplegia, consisting of medial rectus paresis on attempted lateral gaze in conjunction with monocular nystagmus in the abducting eye with intact vergence.

16. Correct: Increased endolymphatic pressure (A)

This patient is displaying symptoms consistent with Meniere's disease, an inner ear disease associated with an increase in endolymphatic fluid pressure. Of particular diagnostic importance is the combined presence of hearing loss, nausea, nystagmus, and vertigo.

Dislocation of the utricular macular otoliths (**B**) is associated with benign positional vertigo, a condition that would not include hearing loss.

Bacterial infection of the inner ear, or labyrinthitis (**C**), would have many of the same symptoms as seen in Meniere's disease, but the persistent nature of the condition would be counter-indicative of an infection of the middle ear, as most resolve without intervention on the timescale of weeks.

Compression of CN VIII (**D**), as what may be observed with an acoustic schwannoma, may present with hearing loss, tinnitus, and vertigo, but would very rarely be associated with nystagmus.

Loss of hair cells within the semicircular canal (**E**) would result in the balance disorder reported, but would not account for the hearing deficits.

17. Correct: None of the above (E)

There is currently no viable treatment for the hearing loss associated with Meniere's disease, leaving supportive devices such as a hearing aid the best option. All of the presented options are possible treatments for the vestibular symptoms associated with this condition.

Diazepam (**A**) can help control the nausea and vomiting often experienced.

Gentamicin (**B**) is an antibiotic that can be injected into the middle ear (and ultimately absorbed into the inner ear). It is toxic to the inner ear, and therefore reduces (or abolishes) the affected ear's vestibular system. The nonaffected ear can provide vestibular information to maintain a sense of balance.

A vestibular nerve section (**C**) involves ablation of the vestibular section of the vestibulocochlear nerve (CN VIII) on the affected side, while avoiding the cochlear portion. This treatment, though more invasive than the use of nonsurgical treatments, offers the possibility of preserving whatever hearing function is left within the affected ear.

Labyrinthectomy (**D**) is a very effective treatment for vertigo and is most appropriate for patients in whom there is no preserved hearing.

18. Correct: Both the utricle and the saccule would cease to function properly (E)

Within the macula of both the utricle and the saccule, the kinocilium and stereocilia are surrounded by a gelatinous matrix. On top of the matrix is the otolithic membrane, which contains crystals of calcium carbonate, known as otoconia. Therefore, if calcium carbonate crystals were dissolved in the inner ear, this would have an effect on both the utricle and saccule (ruling out **A, C,** and **D**).

The semicircular canals do not utilize calcium carbonate crystals for their sensory function (**B**).

19. Correct: Acoustic schwannoma (D)

This patient is displaying symptoms associated with an acoustic schwannoma, which most often results in vertigo in combination with tinnitus and unilateral hearing loss. Facial weakness can be observed due to involvement of the facial nerve as the schwannoma expands.

Meniere's disease (**A**) and labyrinthitis (**B**) often present with episodic attacks of vertigo; symptoms usually include tinnitus, hearing loss, vomiting, and nausea. Benign positional vertigo (**C**) is not associated with hearing loss or tinnitus. Multiple sclerosis (**E**) is most commonly associated with internuclear ophthalmoplegia, consisting of medial rectus paresis on attempted lateral gaze in conjunction with monocular nystagmus in the abducting eye with intact vergence.

Chapter 20

Visual System and Eye Movements

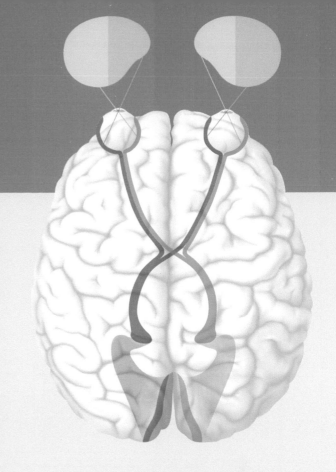

LEARNING OBJECTIVES

► Identify the effects of damage to the optic chiasm, and define the location of the optic chiasm relative to the pituitary gland.

► Identify the likely location of a lesion based on eye movement deficits.

► Define the location of the frontal eye fields (FEFs) and analyze the clinical findings associated with damage to the FEFs.

► Describe the brainstem components for eye movement and relate their damages to gaze patterns.

► Locate the rostral interstitial nucleus of the medial longitudinal fasciculus (riMLF) and relate its damage to deficits in eye movements.

► Distinguish between paramedian pontine reticular formation (PPRF) and abducens nuclear lesions.

► Relate lesions of the primary visual pathway to visual field defects.

► Analyze the function of the occipital eye fields.

► Analyze the role of iodopsin in phototransduction.

► Describe the pathophysiology and funduscopic changes of papilledema.

20.1 Questions

Easy	Medium	Hard

1. A 63-year-old woman presents to her primary care physician reporting visual difficulties. Based on the results of a visual field confrontation test, the physician refers her for neuroimaging, where a pituitary tumor greater than 1 cm is noted to be pressing on the base of the brain. What were the most likely results of the visual field confrontation test?

A. Total blindness of both eyes

B. Right lower homonymous quadrantanopia

C. Right homonymous hemianopsia

D. Bitemporal hemianopsia

E. Binasal hemianopsia

2. A 42-year-old man presents to the emergency department with difficulty moving his eyes. While he has no difficulty looking straight ahead or to the right, when asked to look to the left, the right eye cannot adduct, and the left eye displays a nystagmus when abducted. Convergence movements of both eyes is intact. Based on this exam, where is a likely location of the lesion?

A. Right CN III

B. Right CN II

C. Left CN VI

D. Pontine reticular formation

E. MLF

3. A 42-year-old right-handed male is involved in an automobile accident that has resulted in a traumatic brain injury. Neuroimaging reveals he has suffered damage to the caudal part of the middle frontal gyrus (area 8). What type of eye movement symptoms would you expect this patient to display?

A. Monocular horizontal nystagmus in the contralateral eye

B. Transient ipsilateral conjugate deviation of the eyes

C. Anisocoria

D. Medial rectus palsy

E. Difficulty following a slow-moving object

Consider the following case for questions 4 to 8:

Gaze patterns obtained from five different patients from an ophthalmology clinic on a given day are presented below:

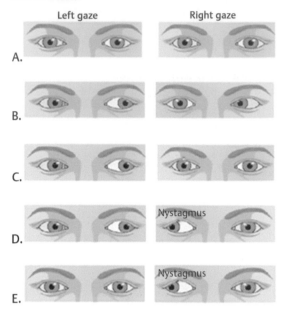

4. Which of the patients was suffering from right abducens nerve palsy?

5. Which of the patients was suffering from left MLF palsy?

6. Which of the patients was suffering from right abducens nucleus palsy?

7. Which of the patients was suffering palsy of left MLF and left abducens nucleus?

8. Which of the patients was suffering from bilateral abducens nucleus palsy?

9. A 60-year-old right-handed woman had been under treatment for hypertension for approximately 10 years before being admitted to the emergency department after experiencing transient dysarthria, dizziness, vomiting, and diplopia. Brain CT scans showed progressive stenosis of the basilar artery, and damage was specifically noted at the rostral interstitial nucleus of medial longitudinal fasciculus (riMLF). What deficit in eye movements would you most likely expect following damage to this structure?

A. Bilateral horizontal gaze palsy

B. Left horizontal gaze palsy

C. Right horizontal gaze palsy

D. Bilateral vertical gaze palsy

E. Left vertical gaze palsy

10. A 73-year-old woman presents to the emergency department following a suspected cerebrovascular accident. Following neurological exam, she is found to have right lateral gaze palsy. The physicians believe that she may have damage to either the paramedian pontine reticular formation (PPRF) or to the abducens nucleus. Which of the following tests could be performed to distinguish between these two lesions?

A. A test of lens accommodation

B. A test of pupil constriction

C. A test of horizontal saccades

D. A test of vertical saccades

E. A test of vestibular movements

Consider the following case and options for questions 11 to 17:

Visual field charts obtained from seven different patients from an ophthalmology clinic on a given day are presented here (black indicating impaired vision).

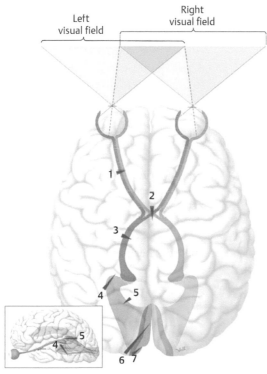

Source: Schünke M, Schulte E, Schumacher U et al. THIEME Atlas of Anatomy: Head, Neck, and Neuroanatomy. 2nd Edition. Thieme; 2016. Illustration by Karl Wesker/Markus Voll.

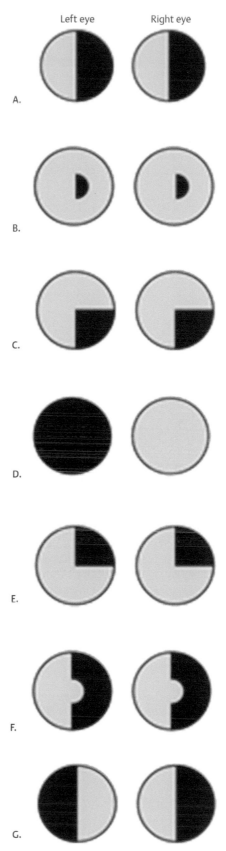

Source: Schünke M, Schulte E, Schumacher U et al. THIEME Atlas of Anatomy: Head, Neck, and Neuroanatomy. 2nd Edition. Thieme; 2016. Illustration by Karl Wesker/Markus Voll.

11. Which is most likely the chart for patient with lesion in area 1?

12. Which is most likely the chart for patient with lesion in area 2?

13. Which is most likely the chart for patient with lesion in area 3?

14. Which is most likely the chart for patient with lesion in area 4?

15. Which is most likely the chart for patient with lesion in area 5?

16. Which is most likely the chart for patient with lesion in area 6?

17. Which is most likely the chart for patient with lesion in area 7?

18. A 15-year-old male suffers a mild-traumatic brain injury in a soccer game when his head collided with an opposing team mate's, as they both attempted to hit the ball with their heads. After displaying signs of eye movement difficulty, he is sent for further evaluation. During neurological exam, it is determined that he has trouble performing tracking movements with both eyes. Based on this information, where would you expect brain damage to have occurred?

A. PPRF

B. FEFs

C. Occipital eye fields

D. riMLF

E. Bilateral abducens nerve

19. A 19-year-old army recruit is undergoing her entrance physical when it is determined that she has a genetic mutation affecting the iodopsins within her eyes. What is the most likely effect of this genetic mutation?

A. Poor spatial sensitivity

B. Poor daylight vision

C. Poor color discrimination

D. Poor night vision

E. No known effects of this mutation

20. Following a subdural hematoma, a 66-year-old male complains of headache, nausea, vomiting, and diplopia. Funduscopic examination reveals prominent papilledema in the left eye. Which area of the presented image is most likely to show earliest changes?

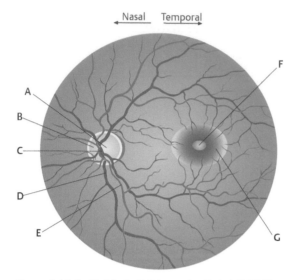

Source: Schünke M, Schulte E, Schumacher U et al. THIEME Atlas of Anatomy: Head, Neck, and Neuroanatomy. 2nd Edition. Thieme; 2016. Illustration by Karl Wesker/Markus Voll.

A. Area B

B. Area D

C. Area E

D. Area F

E. Area G

20.2 Answers and Explanations

Easy	Medium	Hard

1. Correct: Bitemporal hemianopsia (D)

A pituitary tumor may put pressure on the optic chiasm, which will predominantly affect the crossover of fibers responsible for visual information from the nasal retina of each eye. Since these fibers are responsible for temporal visual fields of both eyes, the patient will suffer from bitemporal hemianopsia.

Total blindness of both eyes (**A**) would require complete bilateral damage of either the optic pathways or the primary visual cortices, both unlikely in the case of a pituitary tumor.

A right lower homonymous quadrantanopia (**B**) would most likely result from damage to the left superior projections of the retinal ganglion cells as they travel through the parietal lobe.

A right homonymous hemianopsia (**C**) is most likely following damage to the left optic tract past the optic chiasm or left unilateral visual cortex.

A binasal hemianopsia (**E**) results from damage to the lateral retinal nerve fibers that do not cross in the optic chiasm, such as is seen in cases of calcification of the internal carotid arteries.

2. Correct: MLF (E)

Damage to the right MLF best explains the impairments observed. The right medial rectus muscle is no longer active during left horizontal gaze, resulting in the adduction deficit for the right eye.

A lesion to right CN III (**A**) would not allow for convergence movement of the right eye (due to medial rectus palsy), and would be associated with ptosis and the eye being in a down and out position.

A lesion to right CN II (**B**) would result in visual loss for the right eye.

A lesion to the left CN VI (**C**) would affect the left lateral rectus, resulting in the left eye being pulled medially when the patient looks straight ahead.

Lastly, damage to the pontine reticular formation (**D**) would result in impairment in conjugate movement in both eyes.

3. Correct: Transient ipsilateral conjugate deviation of the eyes (B)

The frontal eye fields (FEFs) are located within area 8 of the middle frontal gyrus, and are responsible for voluntary saccadic eye movements. Therefore, lesions to this region result in transient ipsilateral conjugate deviation of the eyes.

Monocular horizontal nystagmus (**A**) is commonly observed following damage to the MLF, especially in an internuclear ophthalmoplegia (INO).

Anisocoria (**C**) is a condition where the two pupils are not equal in diameter, commonly seen in CN III palsies and Horner's syndrome.

Medial rectus palsy (**D**) is most commonly observed following damage to the subcortical center for lateral conjugate gaze, the PPRF.

Lastly, difficulty following a slow-moving object (**E**) is correlated with damage to the occipital eye fields (areas 18 and 19), the cortical center for involuntary pursuit and tracking movements.

Consider the following explanation for answers 4 to 8:

Patient with gaze pattern **A** has bilateral deficits in rightward and leftward gaze. This can occur with bilateral abducens nuclear palsy.

Patient with gaze pattern **B** has impaired abduction of the right eye, but intact movement of the left eye and leftward gaze. This could happen with right abducens nerve palsy.

Patient with gaze pattern **C** has right lateral gaze palsy consisting of impaired abduction of the right eye and impaired adduction of the left eye. Leftward gaze is intact. This could happen with right abducens nucleus palsy.

The pattern of gaze observed in **D** would result from damage to the left MLF, consisting of impaired adduction of the left eye and nystagmus in the right eye on right gaze. Leftward gaze is intact.

Lastly, as seen in gaze pattern **E,** if both the left abducens nucleus and left MLF are damaged, left internuclear ophthalmoplegia (INO) and left gaze palsy will occur. The left eye would not abduct, and the right eye would not adduct during left gaze (left abducens nuclear lesion). The left eye would not adduct and the right eye will have nystagmus during right gaze (left MLF lesion).

4. Correct: (B)

5. Correct: (D)

6. Correct: (C)

7. Correct: (E)

8. Correct: (A)

9. Correct: Bilateral vertical gaze palsy (D)

The riMLF is located in the midbrain and helps with vertical saccades. It normally has bilateral effects on the elevator muscles (i.e., the superior rectus and inferior oblique muscles) and unilateral effects on depressor muscles (i.e., the inferior rectus and superior oblique muscles). Lesion to this area will, therefore, result in vertical gaze palsy.

A bilateral horizontal gaze palsy (**A**) would be expected following damage to the horizontal gaze center, the PPRF. Left (**B**) and right (**C**) horizontal gaze palsies would be expected following damage to the left and right abducens nuclei, respectively.

Left vertical gaze palsy (**E**) could be the result of damage to the superior rectus muscle of the left eye.

10. Correct: A test of vestibular movements (E)

Although lesions of the PPRF and abducens nuclei will present with very similar gaze deficits, tests of vestibular movements (such as through tests of vestibulo-ocular reflex) will distinguish these two etiologies. Specifically, with lesions of the PPRF, pursuit and vestibular movements may remain intact, since these do not rely on the horizontal gaze centers.

Lens accommodation (**A**) or pupillary constriction (**B**) relies on the autonomic nervous system, and are likely intact in both PPRF and abducens nuclear lesions.

Horizontal saccades (**C**) would reveal identical deficits, while vertical saccades (**E**) are likely to be intact in both abducens nuclear and PPRF lesions.

Refer to the following image for answers 11 to 17:

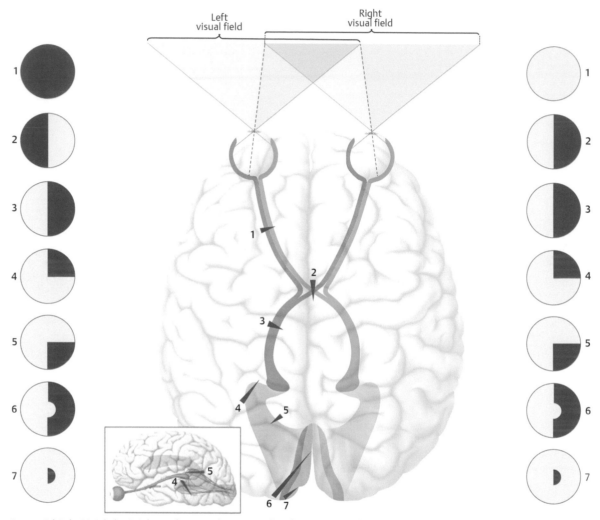

Source: Schünke M, Schulte E, Schumacher U et al. THIEME Atlas of Anatomy: Head, Neck, and Neuroanatomy. 2nd Edition. Thieme; 2016. Illustration by Karl Wesker/Markus Voll.

Lesion 1: unilateral optic nerve—complete blindness in the ipsilateral eye (**D**).

Lesion 2: optic chiasm—bitemporal hemianopia since it interrupts fibers from the nasal portions of the retina, which represent the temporal visual fields (**G**).

Lesion 3: unilateral lesion of the optic tract—contralateral homonymous hemianopia because it interrupts fibers from the temporal portions of the retina on the ipsilateral side and the nasal portions on the opposite side (**A**).

Lesion 4: unilateral lesion of the optic radiation in the anterior temporal lobe (Meyer's loop)—contralateral upper quadrantanopia (**E**).

Lesion 5: unilateral lesion in the medial part of the optic radiation in the parietal lobe—contralateral lower quadrantanopia (**C**).

Lesion 6: unilateral lesion of the occipital lobe—contralateral homonymous hemianopia, with macular sparing; observed due both to the extensive amount of primary visual cortex that is dedicated to foveal vision, and the collateral circulation by the middle cerebral artery to foveal regions in addition to supply by the posterior cerebral artery (**F**).

Lesion 7: unilateral lesion confined to the cortical areas of the occipital pole, which represent the macula—contralateral homonymous hemianopic central scotoma (**B**).

11. Correct: (D)

12. Correct: (G)

13. Correct: (A)

14. Correct: (E)

15. Correct: (C)

16. Correct: (F)

17. Correct: (B)

18. Correct: Occipital eye fields (C)

Involuntary pursuit and tracking movements are performed by the occipital eye fields in areas 18 and 19 of cortex near the junction of the occipital lobe, posterior parietal cortex, and temporal lobe.

Damage within the PPRF (**A**) would result in deficits in horizontal voluntary saccades. FEF damage (**B**) would also result in deficits in programming saccades, as well as contralateral conjugate deviation of the eyes. Damage to the riMLF (**D**) would result in impairment in voluntary vertical saccades. Bilateral abducens nerve (**E**) damage would be expected to eliminate abduction movements of both eyes during horizontal gaze.

19. Correct: Poor color discrimination (C)

Iodopsin is the photopigment found within the cones of the eye. Cones only operate at high illumination levels, are concentrated within the fovea, and are responsible for vision within the day, color vision, and high visual acuity. Mutations resulting in changes in the iodopsins result in abnormalities in color vision. In most cases of color vision deficiencies (protanopia and deuteranopia), poor color discrimination is present.

Poor spatial sensitivity (**A**) and poor daylight vision (**B**) may result from defective cone function, but these are not due to mutations of iodopsin.

Vision in low ambient light settings is largely a product of rod photoreceptors, which utilize opsin as a photopigment. Iodopsin alterations, therefore, is not likely to result in poor night vision (**D**).

20. Correct: Area B (A)

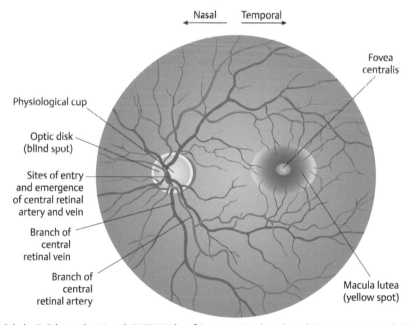

Source: Schünke M, Schulte E, Schumacher U et al. THIEME Atlas of Anatomy: Head, Neck, and Neuroanatomy. 2nd Edition. Thieme; 2016. Illustration by Karl Wesker/Markus Voll.

Papilledema is a noninflammatory congestion of the optic disc that is caused by increased ICP, such as what is often observed following subdural hematomas. Increased ICP causes the cerebrospinal fluid to compress the optic nerve within its sheath resulting in axoplasmic flow stasis and ischemia. Early papilledema causes a nerve fiber edema that surrounds the optic disc.

Areas D (**B**) and E (**C**) represent the branches of the central retinal vein and artery, respectively. These are involved (obscured) in advanced stages of papilledema.

Area F (**D**) represents the fovea centralis and area G (**E**) represents the macula lutea. None of these regions would be altered in papilledema.

Chapter 21
Olfactory and Gustatory Systems

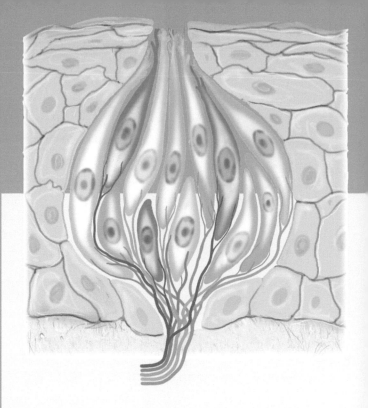

LEARNING OBJECTIVES

▶ Identify the olfactory bulb and analyze the role of progenitor cells within this region.

▶ Identify the medial and lateral olfactory striae and describe their projections.

▶ Illustrate the relative organization of the olfactory system anatomy.

▶ Identify cortical regions associated with olfactory hallucination.

▶ Identify the link between depression and reduced olfactory capability.

▶ Relate a common cause of anosmia to the most likely anatomical substrate.

▶ Discuss the etiopathogenesis and clinical features of Foster–Kennedy syndrome.

▶ Analyze the role of basal cells in olfactory cell regeneration.

▶ Define the role of ammonia as a trigeminal nerve stimulator and identify the presence of trigeminal nerve receptors within the olfactory epithelium.

▶ Illustrate the connections within the olfactory system.

▶ Analyze the pathological alteration of taste buds following chronic viral infection.

▶ Identify the chorda tympani nerve, and analyze its relation with the tympanic membrane.

▶ Identify primary gustatory cortex.

▶ Identify cortical regions associated with olfactory discrimination ability.

▶ Identify the role of the vomeronasal organ in humans and other animal species.

▶ Illustrate the structure of the olfactory mucosa and correlate it with its functions; critique its structure/ultrastructure in histological sections; discriminate it from normal respiratory mucosa.

21.1 Questions

Easy	Medium	Hard

Consider the following image for questions 1 and 2:

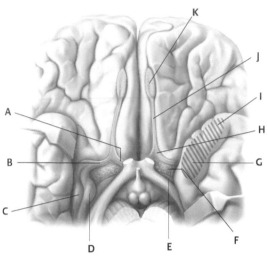

Source: Schünke M, Schulte E, Schumacher U et al. THIEME Atlas of Anatomy: Head, Neck, and Neuroanatomy. 2nd Edition. Thieme; 2016. Illustration by Karl Wesker/Markus Voll.

1. A 34-year-old male visits his general practitioner after 4 months of congestion, difficulty breathing through his nose, and tenderness around his eyes. He also reports a reduced sense of smell and taste. Diagnostic testing reveals he has been suffering from chronic sinusitis. Which area in the presented figure, which contains progenitor cells that differentiate on olfactory stimulation, would be reduced in size in this patient?

A. Area G

B. Area H

C. Area I

D. Area J

E. Area K

2. A 42-year-old patient suffers traumatic brain injury following a motorcycle accident. Diagnostic radiology reveals damage to the portion of the olfactory tract that relays to the nuclei within the septal area (part of the limbic system). Where was the damage observed?

A. Area A

B. Area B

C. Area C

D. Area D

E. Area J

3. A 22-year-old male is brought to the emergency department after colliding with another player during a game of soccer. In the collision, it is believed the patient's head was struck by the other player's knee. Diagnostic radiology reveals signs of impact to the uncus of the parahippocampal gyrus. Which olfactory structure would most likely be spared from the impact of the injury?

A. Ambient gyrus

B. Semilunar gyrus

C. Prepiriform area

D. Medial olfactory stria

E. Lateral olfactory stria

4. A 51-year-old left-handed woman is brought to an urgent care clinic after she experienced what her family thought was a seizure. The night before, while watching television, she became quite alarmed that something was burning. None of the other family members could smell anything, and after an hour of internet searching became convinced it was a seizure-related aura. Which part of the olfactory system is most associated with olfactory hallucinations?

A. Olfactory bulb

B. Olfactory tract

C. Medial olfactory stria

D. Parahippocampal gyrus

E. Orbitofrontal cortex

5. A relatively healthy 39-year-old woman visits her primary care physician as she is concerned about what she perceives as food tasting blander than she believes it should. Which of the following conditions might have an impact on her ability to perceive odors?

A. Generalized anxiety disorder

B. Major depressive disorder

C. Seasonal affective disorder

D. Sleep–wake disorder

E. Somatic symptom disorder

6. A 22-year-old woman is brought to the emergency department following an automobile collision of sufficient force to deploy the airbags. Following the trauma, it is determined that she has completely lost her ability to smell (anosmia). Where on the following image was the damage most likely to have been sustained?

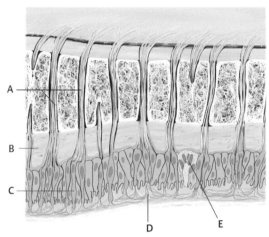

Source: Schünke M, Schulte E, Schumacher U et al. THIEME Atlas of Anatomy: Head, Neck, and Neuroanatomy. 2nd Edition. Thieme; 2016. Illustration by Karl Wesker/Markus Voll.

A. Area A
B. Area B
C. Area C
D. Area D
E. Area E

Consider the following case for questions 7 and 8:

A 27-year-old right-handed woman from a rural town in Nebraska, in the 35th week of her pregnancy, presented to the emergency department after experiencing labor contractions. Although the contractions stopped, she mentioned she had been suffering from headaches for the previous 2 years that have gotten worse since she was pregnant, and she had begun to have difficulty seeing out of her left eye. On neurological exam, it was determined she had bilateral anosmia, reduced vision in the left eye, and normal vision in her right eye. Funduscopy revealed pallor and swelling of the left optic disk. Blood work was within the normal range for a pregnant woman. A T1 MRI of the brain revealed a suprasellar mass, 2.8 cm × 3.1 cm × 1.4 cm, which was isointense.

7. What is the most likely diagnosis in this patient?

A. Olfactory reference syndrome
B. Olfactory delusional syndrome
C. Foster–Kennedy syndrome
D. CHARGE syndrome
E. Kallmann's syndrome

8. Where is the most likely location of the observed tumor?

A. Olfactory bulb
B. Olfactory groove
C. Outer sphenoid wing
D. Medial (inner) sphenoid ridge
E. Tuberculum sellae

9. A 34-year-old male factory worker is exposed to a noxious chemical that results in bilateral anosmia. Unlike other sensory systems, the primary olfactory cells have a normal lifespan of approximately 60 days. Which of the following cells related to the system, being precursors of olfactory cells, could restore olfaction in him?

A. Granule cells
B. Light cells
C. Dark cells
D. Mitral cells
E. Basal cells

10. Following a traumatic brain injury, a 41-year-old male has function of the olfactory nerve tested by smelling common odors through each nostril in isolation. When smelling coffee, cloves, and tobacco, the patient is unable to report the odors. However, when smelling ammonia, the patient is able to report a response. Which mechanism best explains this result?

A. The strong smell of ammonia compensates for the sensory deficit.
B. The nitrogen within the ammonia has a high affinity to olfactory receptors.
C. Trigeminal nerve fibers within the olfactory epithelium are sensitive to ammonia.
D. The patient is malingering.
E. Sensory habituation does not occur for ammonia.

Consider the following image for questions 11 and 12:

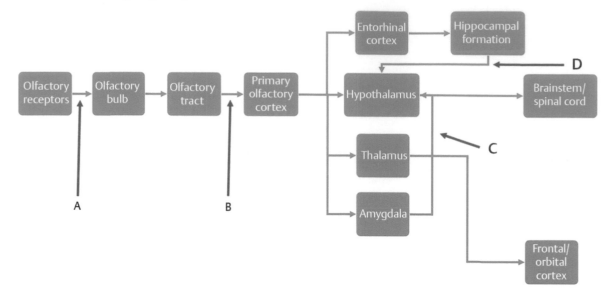

11. A patient is suffering from bilateral hyposmia due to degeneration of the lateral olfactory stria. In the presented chart, which identified pathway is affected?

A. Pathway A

B. Pathway B

C. Pathway C

D. Pathway D

12. A 3-year-old male infant has been shown to have a malformation of the fornix. In the presented image, what pathway of the olfactory system may be affected?

A. Pathway A

B. Pathway B

C. Pathway C

D. Pathway D

13. A 29-year-old male makes an appointment with his general practitioner as a follow-up appointment concerning a viral encephalitis that he had been suffering from for a prolonged period of time. He says that he feels like he has generally recovered, but some of his favorite foods have lost their taste. What is the most likely cause of this alteration in taste sensation?

A. Damage to the solitary nucleus

B. Inflammation of the geniculate ganglion

C. Infection of the chorda tympani

D. Damage to the lingual nerve

E. Changes in the function of taste buds

14. A 52-year-old woman partially loses sensation of taste following minor surgery to the tympanic membrane. Which of the identified pathways best corresponds to the location of damage resulting in her loss of sensation?

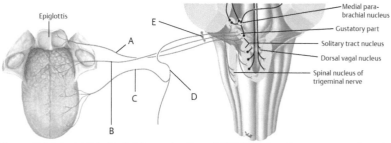

Source: Schünke M, Schulte E, Schumacher U et al. THIEME Atlas of Anatomy: Head, Neck, and Neuroanatomy. 2nd Edition. Thieme; 2016. Illustration by Karl Wesker/Markus Voll.

A. Pathway A

B. Pathway B

C. Pathway C

D. Pathway D

E. Pathway E

15. Following a traumatic brain injury, a 41-year-old male has an impaired sense of taste. Which areas of the brain are involved in the central processing of taste?

A. Frontal operculum and anterior insular cortex

B. Frontal operculum and posterior insular cortex

C. Parietal operculum and anterior insular cortex

D. Parietal operculum and posterior insular cortex

E. Frontal and parietal opercula

16. Following a bicycle accident, a 22-year-old male mail courier is brought to the emergency department where it is discovered that he has lost the ability to discriminate odors. Which of the following brain regions were likely injured resulting in this impaired perceptually ability?

A. Posterior parietal cortex

B. Precentral gyrus

C. Postcentral gyrus

D. Superior temporal gyrus

E. Prefrontal cortex

17. A perfume company is hoping to design a product that will positively influence its wearer's sexual appeal through mechanisms known to be present in many subhuman species. Specifically, the desired response could be achieved by eliciting olfactory impulses that are in response to various sex steroids contained within the engineered scent. What component of the human olfactory system will this new perfume attempt to activate?

A. Olfactory bulb

B. Olfactory mucosa

C. Dorsal vagal nucleus

D. Vomeronasal organ

E. Salivatory nuclei

Consider the following case for questions 18 to 20:

A 16-year-old girl presents with voice changes and anosmia. She has a history of viral infection that affected her upper respiratory tract over the past 2 weeks. She was treated with antibiotics to prevent secondary infection. A tissue biopsy obtained from her is examined under the electron microscope (see accompanying image.)

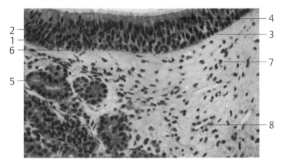

Source: Kühnel W. Color Atlas of Cytology, Histology, and Microscopic Anatomy. 4th Edition. Thieme; 2003.

18. Which of the following might be a probable source for the tissue?

A. Maxillary sinus

B. Vocal cord

C. Roof of nasal cavity

D. Trachea

E. Alveoli

19. Which of the following might be damaged and is responsible for some of her symptoms?

A. Area 1

B. Area 2

C. Area 3

D. Area 5

E. Area 7

20. Which of the following is true for area 5?

A. These are the primary sensory cells within the structure

B. These are the primary supporting cells within the epithelium

C. These are the primary regenerating cells within the epithelium

D. These are secretory serous cells within the epithelium

E. These are secretory mucus cells within the epithelium

21.2 Answers and Explanations

Easy	Medium	Hard

Refer to the following image for answers 1 and 2:

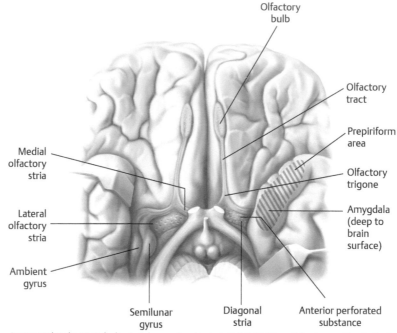

Olfactory
bulb

Olfactory
tract

Prepiriform
area

Olfactory
trigone

Amygdala
(deep to
brain
surface)

Medial
olfactory
stria

Lateral
olfactory
stria

Ambient
gyrus

Semilunar
gyrus

Diagonal
stria

Anterior perforated
substance

Source: Schünke M, Schulte E, Schumacher U et al. THIEME Atlas of Anatomy: Head, Neck, and Neuroanatomy. 2nd Edition. Thieme; 2016. Illustration by Karl Wesker/Markus Voll.

1.   Correct: Area K (E)

The sensory olfactory epithelium and the olfactory bulb (area K) contain progenitor cells that differentiate into neurons well into adulthood, unlike the majority of cells within the central nervous system that develop in the embryonic and early postnatal periods. However, this differentiation is dependent on olfactory stimulation. Therefore, during conditions of olfactory stimulus deprivation, the size of the olfactory bulb may be reduced.

The amygdala (**A**) is responsible for the linking between memory and olfaction.

The olfactory trigone (**B**) is an important location as damage rostral to this region results in unilateral and damage caudal to this region results in bilateral loss of olfaction.

Prepiriform area (**C**) is considered to be the primary olfactory cortex and contains the third-order neurons of the olfactory pathway.

The olfactory tract (**D**), a bundle of axons connecting the mitral and tufted cells of the olfactory bulb, makes up the second-order neurons of the olfactory pathway.

2.   Correct: Area A (A)

Axons of the olfactory tract (**E**, area J) that run in the medial olfactory stria (area A) project to nuclei in the septal region of the brain, and are concerned with emotional responses elicited by olfactory stimuli.

The lateral olfactory stria (**B**), in contrast, runs to the amygdala, ambient gyrus (**C**), and the semilunar gyrus (**D**).

3.   Correct: Medial olfactory stria (D)

The medial olfactory stria arises from the olfactory tract and projects on the septal area (medial olfactory area), which is located on the medial surface of the frontal lobe. This pathway is not anatomically related to the uncus.

The lateral olfactory stria (**E**) projects to the primary olfactory cortex of the temporal lobe, which is located within the uncus of the temporal lobe and is composed of prepiriform cortex (**C**), periamygdaloid area, and part of the entorhinal area. Ambient (**A**) and semilunar (**B**) gyri are protrusions on the anterior part of the uncus, covering the amygdala.

4.   Correct: Parahippocampal gyrus (D)

Lesions and seizing of the parahippocampal uncus have been associated with the experience of olfactory hallucinations (phantosmia).

Activity within the olfactory bulb (**A**) or tract (**B**) does not seem to directly impart the sensation of odor, as even direct electrical stimulation of these does not result in olfactory hallucinations.

Axons of the olfactory tract that run in the medial olfactory stria (**C**) project to nuclei in the septal region of the brain, and are concerned with emotional responses elicited by olfactory stimuli. With relation to olfaction, orbitofrontal cortex (**E**) contains the secondary and tertiary olfactory cortical areas, in which information about the identity and also about the reward value of odors is represented. Neither **C** nor **E** has been implicated in the experience of olfactory hallucinations, despite their prominent roles in the olfactory system.

5.   Correct: Major depressive disorder (B)

Research has demonstrated that patients suffering from major depressive disorder have reduced olfactory sensitivity. Though the exact mechanisms are still not known, it is believed both reduced ability to encode olfactory information and reduced volume of the olfactory bulb may be partially responsible.

General anxiety disorders (**A**), seasonal affective disorder (**C**), sleep–wake disorder (**D**), or somatic symptom disorder (**E**) has not been associated with decrease in olfactory sensitivity or ability to perceive odors.

6.   Correct: Area A (A)

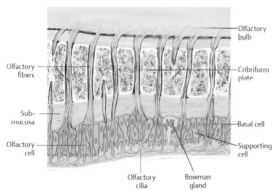

Source: Schünke M, Schulte E, Schumacher U et al. THIEME Atlas of Anatomy: Head, Neck, and Neuroanatomy. 2nd Edition. Thieme; 2016. Illustration by Karl Wesker/Markus Voll.

One of the leading causes of anosmia is head trauma. The olfactory system is especially susceptible to this type of injury, as a crushing or cutting motion can be applied to the olfactory nerve fibers from the cribriform plate, making this the most likely area of damage

The other labeled regions (area B, submucosa; area C, olfactory cell; area D, olfactory cilia; area E, Bowman's gland) form part of the olfactory epithelium and are not as susceptible to traumatic injury.

7.   Correct: Foster–Kennedy syndrome (C)

Foster–Kennedy syndrome consists of a clinical triad of optic atrophy in one eye, papilledema in the contralateral eye, and anosmia, caused by space-occupying anterior fossa masses.

Olfactory reference syndrome (**A**) is a condition in which people have an excessive and irrational fear that they are emitting a foul or unpleasant odor; anosmia is not reported.

Olfactory delusional syndrome (**B**) is a condition where the person develops an insidious onset of firm, unshakeable, false belief of odors; however, it typically does not include anosmia.

CHARGE syndrome (**D**) is a genetic disorder that presents with multiple birth defects including coloboma, congenital heart disease, choanal atresia, growth retardation, genital abnormalities, and ear abnormalities, with deafness.

Kallmann's syndrome (**E**) results from defective hypothalamic GnRH synthesis and is associated with anosmia or hyposmia due to olfactory bulb agenesis or hypoplasia. Classically, the syndrome may also be associated with color blindness, optic atrophy, and nerve deafness. However, this is a congenital disorder where females present with primary amenorrhea and failure of secondary sexual development.

8.   Correct: Olfactory groove (B)

Foster–Kennedy syndrome results from a meningioma of the olfactory groove, which compresses both the olfactory tract and the optic nerve.

Meningioma affecting the olfactory bulb (**A**) would not affect vision.

The outer sphenoid wing meningiomas (**C**) are usually accompanied by epilepsy, focal weakness, and trouble with language function when present on the left side.

The tumors of the medial (inner) sphenoid ridge (**D**) usually compress the optic nerve and present with early unilateral visual loss. They also may involve the cavernous sinus to cause double vision and numbness of the face.

Meningiomas affecting the tuberculum sellae (**E**) usually arise in the midline from the region of the tuberculum sellae and planum sphenoidale. As the tumor enlarges, it compresses the optic nerves and chiasm. The most common initial symptom is asymmetric loss of vision followed by progression to bilateral involvement.

9.   Correct: Basal cells (E)

Resting on or near the basal lamina of the olfactory epithelium, basal cells are stem cells that are capable of division and differentiation into olfactory supporting cells and olfactory cells themselves.

Granule cells (**A**) are contained within the olfactory bulb, and receive collateral axons from mitral cells and are involved in inhibitory processes believed to heighten olfactory contrast.

Light (**B**) and dark (**C**) cells are located within the vomeronasal organ, a little understood component of the olfactory system that has unknown neural connections. This region in many animal species is involved in mate selection, and is known to respond to steroids and may evoke unconscious reactions in human subjects.

195

Mitral cells (**D**) within the olfactory bulb form the apical dendrites that receive synaptic innervations from the primary sensory cells.

10. Correct: Trigeminal nerve fibers within the olfactory epithelium are sensitive to ammonia (C)

Ammonia (any irritant for that matter) is a trigeminal nerve stimulator, which is responsible for conveying general sensation from the nasal cavity.

Although ammonia has a strong distinct odor (**A**), it is not the strength of the odor that is likely causing detection in this case, as coffee and tobacco also have very strong, identifiable odors.

Nitrogen within ammonia (**B**) is not known to have a higher affinity for olfactory receptors.

If the patient was malingering (**D**), he would not report perception of any of the presented odors.

Lastly, sensory habituation (**E**) will occur for all persistent odors.

Consider the following explanation for answers 11 and 12:

Pathway A represents the portion of the olfactory nerve (CN I) that passes through the cribriform plate of the ethmoid bone.

Axons of the olfactory tract run within the lateral olfactory stria (pathway B) and project to the primary olfactory cortex of the temporal lobe.

Pathway C represents stria terminalis, the connection between the amygdala and the hypothalamus.

Pathway D represents the fornix, a connection between the hippocampal formation and the hypothalamus.

11. Correct: Pathway B (B)

12. Correct: Pathway D (D)

13. Correct: Changes in the function of taste buds (E)

All of the above structures are involved in the sensation of taste; however, only pathological changes in the function of the taste buds have been reported following chronic viral infections.

The rostral part of the solitary nucleus (**A**) receives taste information from the tongue (anterior two-thirds, CN VII; posterior one-third, CN IX) and a small area of the epiglottis (CN X).

The geniculate ganglion (**B**) is a collection of fibers and sensory neurons of facial nerve (CN VII) and includes special sensory cell bodies for taste.

The chorda tympani (**C**) is a branch of the facial nerve that originates from the anterior taste buds in the tongue.

The lingual nerve (**D**) is a branch of the trigeminal nerve (CN V) that chorda tympani nerve utilizes to hitchhike to travel to and from the tongue.

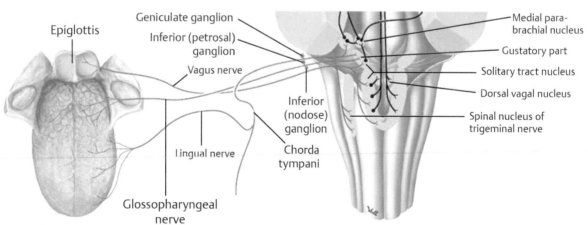

Source: Schünke M, Schulte E, Schumacher U et al. THIEME Atlas of Anatomy: Head, Neck, and Neuroanatomy. 2nd Edition. Thieme; 2016. Illustration by Karl Wesker/Markus Voll.

14. Correct: Structure D (D)

The anterior two-thirds of the tongue are supplied by the facial nerve (CN VII). The afferent fibers first pass through the lingual nerve (**C**) and then the chorda tympani (**D**), which runs from anterior to posterior across the tympanic membrane. Therefore, the nerve could be damaged consequent to surgery on the tympanic membrane.

Vagus nerve (**A**), glossopharyngeal nerve (**B**), or the inferior (petrosal) ganglion of the glossopharyngeal nerve (**E**) is not related to the tympanic membrane.

15. Correct: Frontal operculum and anterior insular cortex (A)

The primary gustatory cortex, the region of brain that is primarily responsible for the sensation of taste, includes the anterior insular and the frontal operculum. None of the other combinations include both substructures which make up the primary gustatory cortex. The posterior insular cortex (**B** and **D**) has been implicated in a number of processes, including pain, temperature, and itch. The parietal operculum (**C, D,** and **E**) is involved in multisensory processing, due to the presence of secondary somatosensory cortex within it.

16. Correct: Prefrontal cortex (E)

The prefrontal cortex is largely involved in the conscious perception of smell, as it contains major inputs from the olfactory bulb, and lesions to this area is known to impair odor discrimination ability.

Posterior parietal cortex (**A**) is involved in planning movements, spatial reasoning, and attention. The precentral gyrus (**B**) is the site of primary motor cortex and the postcentral gyrus (**C**) is home to primary somatosensory cortex. The superior temporal gyrus (**D**) is largely involved in auditory processing and social cognition.

17. Correct: Vomeronasal organ (D)

The vomeronasal organ is located within the anterior nasal septum, and is known to respond to steroids and elicit unconscious reactions in subjects. Further, this area is known to influence mate selection in many subhuman species.

The olfactory bulb (**A**) and mucosa (**B**) will certainly respond to fragrant aspects of the perfume, but such a response would not be consistent with the goals of the perfume manufacturer.

Both the dorsal vagal (**C**) and the salivatory (**E**) nuclei receive input from the olfactory system indirectly from the medial forebrain bundle. Therefore, both these regions would respond to olfactory stimulation, again, without achieving the goal of the manufacturer.

Consider the following explanation for answers 18 to 20:

Upper respiratory infections, usually viral in nature, are the most common cause of permanent hyposmia or anosmia. Such infections inflict damage to olfactory cells within the olfactory epithelium.

18. Correct: Roof of nasal cavity (C)

The olfactory epithelium, specialized for smell, lines the roof of the nasal cavity. This region may be recognized by the tall epithelium (ciliated pseudostratified columnar) that lacks goblet cells. The maxillary sinus (**A**) and trachea (**D**) are lined by respiratory epithelium (ciliated pseudostratified columnar with goblet cells); the vocal cord (**B**) is lined by nonkeratinized stratified squamous epithelium; alveoli (**E**) are lined by type I (squamous) and type II (cuboidal) cells.

19. Correct: Structure 1 (A)

Anosmia is primarily caused by damage to olfactory cells, identified by the location of their nuclei in the middle tier. Nuclei in the top tier (area 2, **B**) belong to supporting cells and those in the bottom tier (area 3, **C**) belong to the stem cells within the epithelium. Area 5 is olfactory (Bowman's) gland (**D**), while area 7 represents plasma cell (**E**, activated lymphocyte, component of MALT).

20. Correct: These are secretory serous cells within the epithelium (D)

Areas 5 are specialized olfactory (Bowman's) glands, secretions from which are serous rather than mucus. The secretions dissolve odorants to facilitate their detection.

Chapter 22

Autonomic Nervous System

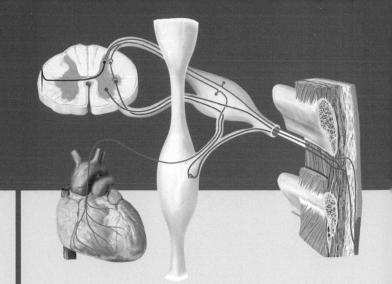

LEARNING OBJECTIVES

- ▶ Describe the origination and primary function of the sympathetic nervous system.
- ▶ Describe the etiopathogenesis and diagnosis of pheochromocytoma.
- ▶ Analyze the symptoms associated with Horner's syndrome, and relate them to functional components of the sympathetic autonomic nervous system.
- ▶ Identify the transmitter released from preganglionic endings of the sympathetic nervous system.
- ▶ Identify the role of the dorsal funiculus in the parasympathetic nervous system.
- ▶ Analyze the symptoms and characteristics of familial dysautonomia.
- ▶ Identify the components of the carotid sinus reflex.
- ▶ Identify presynaptic and postsynaptic neurotransmitters within the autonomic nervous system.
- ▶ Analyze the etiopathogenesis and the clinical features of Raynaud's disease.
- ▶ Identify the location of descending autonomic pathways from the medulla.
- ▶ Identify the four parasympathetic nuclei within the brainstem.
- ▶ Analyze referred pain from organs involving specific spinal segments.
- ▶ Trace referred pain from diaphragm involvement.
- ▶ Identify the role of the autonomic nervous system in innervation of the trachea and bronchi.
- ▶ Relate intestinal motility to function of the enteric nervous system.
- ▶ Analyze the hierarchy of control of the autonomic nervous system.
- ▶ Identify the upper motor neuron, sympathetic, and parasympathetic control of bladder function.
- ▶ Identify the neurotransmitters involved in innervation of sweat glands and arrector pilorum muscles.

22.1 Questions

Easy | Medium | Hard

1. A neurology resident was reviewing the basic organization and functions of the autonomic nervous system with her intern. She understands that the sympathetic nervous system arises from the _____ and is mainly involved in _____ functions.

A. T1–L2 spinal levels; "rest and digest"

B. T1–L2 spinal levels; "fight or flight"

C. CN nuclei and S2–S4 spinal levels; "rest and digest"

D. CN nuclei and S2–S4 spinal levels; "fight or flight"

2. A 31-year-old male presented with symptoms related to recurrent episodes of headache, profuse sweating, and palpitation. During the initial phase of the physical exam, his blood pressure, heart rate, and electrocardiogram were all within normal limits. Near the end of the exam, the patient reported that he had another episode. You noticed that he began to sweat, and had an elevated heart rate and blood pressure. Further diagnostic testing reveals a tumor of the right adrenal gland. Which of the following substances would you expect to be elevated in his peripheral circulation?

A. Thyroxine

B. Melatonin

C. Glutamate

D. Choline

E. Vanillylmandelic acid

3. A 42-year-old female was referred to your clinic by her primary care physician for an ongoing headache and feeling of pain and pressure behind her left eye. She had a CT scan performed earlier that was read as normal with no structural abnormalities. Neurological exam revealed miotic left pupil, slight drooping of her left upper eyelid, and anhidrosis on the left side of her face. Which of the following structures might be the site of lesion for her?

A. Ciliary ganglion

B. Submandibular ganglion

C. Otic ganglion

D. Superior cervical ganglion

E. Pterygopalatine ganglion

4. A pharmaceutical company is attempting to design a new drug to combat hypertension. They wish to selectively block synaptic transmission in autonomic ganglia to reduce blood pressure levels. Which type of drug would the company be most interested in developing?

A. Dopaminergic antagonist

B. Serotonergic antagonist

C. GABAergic antagonist

D. Cholinergic antagonist

E. Noradrenergic antagonist

5. A 58-year-old male presents to his primary care physician with the concern that his mouth feels dry all the time, even when eating. When examining his previous history, you realize he is on a number of medications that may cause dry mouth. To produce the coordinated stimulation of various glands that result in increased salivation during eating, information from the mammillary bodies is required. Which of the following tracts is involved in carrying such information from the diencephalon?

A. Dorsal longitudinal fasciculus

B. Medial longitudinal fasciculus

C. Superior longitudinal fasciculus

D. Inferior longitudinal fasciculus

E. Dorsolateral fasciculus

6. A 7-month-old male infant is brought to a pediatrician as the family is concerned about his development. Case history reveals persistent bilateral eye irritations and what appears to be the absence of tears with emotional crying. Deep tendon reflex testing is not possible, due to the child's age, but the rooting reflex is reduced. Upon questioning, it is determined that the child's grandfather had bouts of abnormal sweating, orthostatic hypotension, and progressive sensory loss, and died at approximately 30 years of age. Based on this information alone, what is your most likely diagnosis?

A. Hirschsprung's disease

B. Raynaud's disease

C. Familial dysautonomia

D. Botulism

E. Autoimmune autonomic ganglionopathy

7. A 68-year-old male presents to the emergency department with recurrent bouts of dizziness and syncope. Gentle neck massage elicited asystole and bradycardia. Based on this information, it is concluded that the patient has a hypersensitive carotid sinus. Which of the following is initially involved in the carotid sinus reflex?

A. Vagal afferent fibers

B. Glossopharyngeal afferent fibers

C. Solitary nucleus

D. Dorsal vagal nucleus

E. Interneurons within the nucleus ambiguus

Consider the following diagram for questions 8 and 9:

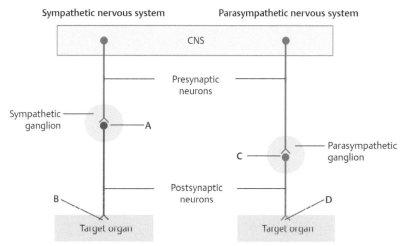

Source: Schünke M, Schulte E, Schumacher U et al. THIEME Atlas of Anatomy: Head, Neck, and Neuroanatomy. 2nd Edition. Thieme; 2016. Illustration by Karl Wesker/Markus Voll.

8. A 22-year-old male is suspected of being exposed to the botulinum toxin, which is known to block the release of acetylcholine. In the presented circuit diagram of both the sympathetic and parasympathetic divisions of the autonomic nervous system, which of the following synapses use acetylcholine as a transmitter?

A. Areas A, B, and C

B. Areas A, C, and D

C. Areas C, D, and B

D. Areas A and B

E. Areas B and D

9. A 33-year-old woman presents to the emergency department after collapsing at the company picnic. Testing reveals she is suffering from a drug reaction that has an antiadrenergic action. Which of the following might be the site of action for the drug?

A. Area A

B. Area B

C. Area C

D. Area D

E. Areas C and D

Consider the following case for questions 10 and 11:

A 17-year-old girl presents to your practice. She had recently started working at a grocery store, and was stocking meat in one of the large freezers in the back of the store. Her hands lost color, changing to white, and she said it was very painful. The color change was only distal to the wrist. Her grip strength remained intact, with her fingers turning red when she came back into the warmth. Upon further questioning, it is determined that her mother suffers from the same condition. She is not under any regular medication. There was no significant difference in arterial pressure recorded between the upper and lower limbs. Abduction and external rotation of her upper limb did not cause alteration of her radial pulse. There was no other abnormality detected on physical examination and routine blood workup came back as normal.

10. What condition is most likely the cause of the patient's symptoms?

A. Peripheral vascular disease

B. Thoracic outlet syndrome

C. Diabetes mellitus

D. Raynaud's disease

E. Familial dysautonomia

11. If warranted in severity and frequency, what treatment may be useful for her?

A. Propranolol

B. Oral contraceptives

C. Pseudoephedrine

D. Digital sympathectomy

E. Insulin

12. A 36-year-old woman experiences orthostatic hypotension after standing up quickly to answer the telephone. Diagnostic radiology reveals that a tumor, located within the CNS, was responsible for her fainting. Where would you most likely expect the tumor to be?

A. Insular cortex

B. Medial dorsal nucleus of thalamus

C. Posterior cranial fossa

D. Inferior colliculus

E. Precentral gyrus

13. A 28-year-old male presents to the emergency department following an accident in which he slipped on ice and fell down, striking the base of his skull on the arm rail of a flight of stairs. The injury is suspected to have affected one of the parasympathetic nuclei within the brainstem. Which of the following cranial nerves could be spared during his neurological examination?

A. CN III

B. CN VII

C. CN VIII

D. CN IX

E. CN X

Consider the following image for questions 14 and 15:

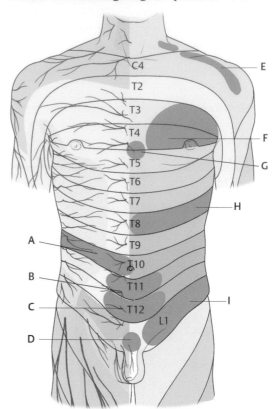

Source: Schünke M, Schulte E, Schumacher U et al. THIEME Atlas of Anatomy: Head, Neck, and Neuroanatomy. 2nd Edition. Thieme; 2016. Illustration by Karl Wesker/Markus Voll.

14. A 20-year-old male with abdominal pain is brought in to the emergency department. His vital signs are all normal, with the exception of shallow breathing at a rate of 20. The patient describes his pain originating from the umbilicus, and is an 8 on a 1 to 10 pain scale. The pain started in the morning, and has been a constant ache since. Further localization reveals the pain to originate from the dermatome indicated by the area H on the presented figure. What is the most likely internal organ affected?

A. Liver

B. Gallbladder

C. Large intestine

D. Heart

E. Stomach

15. A 28 year old woman presents to the emergency department with ruptured spleen. Which of the following dermatomes in her would be affected due to irritation of the diaphragm by contaminated peritoneal fluid?

A. Area E

B. Area F

C. Area G

D. Area H

E. Area I

16. As a routine preoperative medication for bronchoscopy in a 54-year-old male patient, atropine is administered. What will be the effects of administration of this drug?

A. Promote secretion of the bronchial glands and narrowing of the bronchial passages via parasympathetic stimulation

B. Promote secretion of the bronchial glands and narrowing of the bronchial passages via sympathetic stimulation

C. Reduce secretion of the bronchial glands and widen the bronchial passages via parasympathetic blockage

D. Reduce secretion of the bronchial glands and widen the bronchial passages via sympathetic blockage

E. Reduce secretion of the bronchial glands and widening of the bronchial passages via sympathetic stimulation

17. A 55-year-old male is suffering from disorders of intestinal motility after a surgery involving manipulation of the digestive tube. Which of the following is primarily responsible to increase the motility of the intestine?

A. Parasympathetic innervation of the internal submucosal plexus

B. Parasympathetic innervation of the myenteric plexus

C. Parasympathetic innervation of the external submucosal plexus

D. Sympathetic innervation of the myenteric plexus

E. Sympathetic innervation of the external submucosal plexus

18. Control of the peripheral actions of the autonomic nervous system is subject to a hierarchy of control from various levels. The correct order, from the top down would be:

A. Hypothalamus; limbic system; medulla oblongata; spinal cord; target organs

B. Medulla oblongata; limbic system; hypothalamus; spinal cord; target organs

C. Hypothalamus; medulla oblongata; limbic system; spinal cord; target organs

D. Limbic system; medulla oblongata; hypothalamus; spinal cord; target organs

E. Limbic system; hypothalamus; medulla oblongata; spinal cord; target organs

19. A 14-year-old boy suffers spinal damage to the S2–S3 spinal segments when he jumped into shallow water. Which of the following best describes the type of loss of bladder control for him?

A. Removal of sympathetic input preventing reflexive control of bladder

B. Removal of sympathetic input preventing voluntary control of bladder

C. Removal of sympathetic control preventing voluntary and reflexive control of bladder

D. Removal of parasympathetic control preventing voluntary and reflexive control of bladder

E. Removal of upper motor neuron control preventing voluntary and reflexive control of bladder

20. A 22-year-old male patient returned from military operations suffering from posttraumatic stress disorder. When describing his symptoms, he states that the sight of military camouflage makes him start to sweat and gives him goosebumps. This response is most likely a result of:

A. Preganglionic sympathetic cholinergic fibers

B. Preganglionic parasympathetic cholinergic fibers

C. Postganglionic sympathetic adrenergic fibers

D. Postganglionic parasympathetic adrenergic fibers

E. Preganglionic sympathetic adrenergic fibers

22.2 Answers and Explanations

Easy	Medium	Hard

1. Correct: T1–L2 spinal levels; "fight or flight" (B)

The sympathetic division of the autonomic nervous system arises from the T1–L2 spinal levels and is involved in preparing the body for immediate action by increasing heart rate and blood pressure, increasing pupil size, and bronchodilation (known as the fight or flight response).

In contrast, the parasympathetic division of the autonomic nervous system arises from CN nuclei and S2–S4 spinal levels (**C** and **D**), and is involved in the maintenance of vegetative functions such as digestion and urination, slowing the heart rate, and decreasing pupil size (known as the rest and digest response, **A** and **C**).

2. Correct: Vanillylmandelic acid (E)

Symptoms for the patient are most consistent with pheochromocytoma. Pheochromocytomas synthesize and store catecholamines, which include norepinephrine, epinephrine, and dopamine. Elevated serum and urinary levels of catecholamines or their metabolic byproducts (like vanillylmandelic acid) is the cornerstone for diagnosis of pheochromocytomas.

Elevated levels of thyroxine (**A**), melatonin (**B**), glutamate (**C**), or choline (**D**) have not been observed in pheochromocytomas.

3. Correct: Superior cervical ganglion (D)

The patient is displaying the classic triad of symptoms consistent with Horner's syndrome, which results from interruption of sympathetic input to the eye at any level. Superior cervical ganglion contains the cell bodies of the postganglionic sympathetic neurons that innervate the eye and face. Paresis of dilator pupillae (miosis) and Muller's muscle (ptosis), and dysfunction of sweat glands (anhidrosis), therefore, result from a lesion of the superior cervical ganglion.

The ciliary (**A**), submandibular (**B**), otic (**C**), and pterygopalatine (**E**) ganglia are all part of the parasympathetic division of the autonomic nervous system.

4. Correct: Cholinergic antagonist (D)

Preganglionic endings of both the sympathetic and parasympathetic fibers release acetylcholine; therefore, to selectively block synaptic transmission at this level, a cholinergic antagonist would need to be developed.

None of the other listed antagonists would have any effect on synaptic transmission within the autonomic ganglia.

5. Correct: Dorsal longitudinal fasciculus (A)

Increased salivation during eating results from stimulation of the salivary glands, a function of the parasympathetic nervous system. To produce this response, parasympathetic nuclei require excitatory input from higher centers, such as the mammillary bodies. These fibers are carried through the dorsal longitudinal fasciculus.

The medial longitudinal fasciculus (**B**) is composed of ascending and descending fibers arising from the vestibular nuclei that serve as central connections for the oculomotor, trochlear, and abducens nerve and, accordingly, plays a large role in eye movement.

The superior longitudinal fasciculus (**C**) is a fiber tract found in both cerebral hemispheres passing from the frontal lobe to the occipital and anterior portions of the temporal lobe.

The inferior longitudinal fasciculus (**D**) connects the temporal lobe and occipital lobe.

The dorsolateral fasciculus (**E**) is a small tract found throughout the spinal cord and contains axons projecting from the dorsal root ganglion cells to the spinothalamic tract.

6. Correct: Familial dysautonomia (C)

Familial dysautonomia (Riley–Day syndrome) is an autosomal recessive trait involving reduction of autonomic and sensory ganglionic neurons, with primary symptoms consisting of abnormal sweating, orthostatic hypotension, inadequate tone in the gastrointestinal tract, and progressive sensory loss. Lack of tears during emotional crying, reduced rooting reflex, and a positive family history provide evidence for the diagnosis.

Hirschsprung's disease (**A**), also known as congenital megacolon, is a developmental abnormality that results from failure of migration of neural crest cells, which results in the absence of ganglion cells in Auerbach's plexus of a segment of distal colon.

Raynaud's disease (**B**) is an autonomic dysfunction characterized by pallor and cyanosis of the digits consequent to cold-induced vasoconstriction.

Botulism (**D**) occurs when a neurotoxin (produced by the bacterium Clostridium botulinum) blocks the release of acetylcholine from presynaptic vesicles. This effect can be seen in both motor end plates and synapses of autonomic ganglia. Although dry eyes would be a symptom consistent with botulism, paralysis of striated muscles (the primary clinical finding in botulism) was not observed in this patient.

Lastly, autoimmune autonomic ganglionopathy (**E**) is an autoimmune disorder in which autoantibodies against ganglionic acetylcholine receptors impair transmission in autonomic ganglia. Dry eyes would be consistent; however, a positive family history is highly unlikely due to the immune nature of the damage caused.

7. Correct: Glossopharyngeal afferent fibers (B)

The first step in the carotid sinus reflex involves baroreceptors on the terminals of the peripheral branches of the glossopharyngeal nerve, which provide the afferent signals corresponding to changes in pressure within the carotid sinus. This information is then passed to the neurons in the solitary nucleus (**C**) and nucleus ambiguus (**E**), which then synapse on neurons in the dorsal motor nucleus (**D**) of the vagus nerve which innervate the heart. Stimulation of the reflex (or in this case overstimulation) results in a decrease in cardiac output and drop in blood pressure.

Vagal afferent fibers (**A**) contain the signals from baroreceptors within the aortic arch, rather than the carotid sinus.

8. Correct: Areas A, C, and D (B)

The parasympathetic nervous system uses acetylcholine as a transmitter in both the presynaptic (area C) and postsynaptic neurons (area D). In the sympathetic nervous system, acetylcholine is used by the presynaptic neuron (area A). However, the postsynaptic neuron of the sympathetic nervous system (area B) utilizes norepinephrine.

9. Correct: Area B (B)

Postganglionic sympathetic neurons exhibit adrenergic activity, the primary neurotransmitters involved being epinephrine and norepinephrine. This would, therefore, be the most likely site of action for an anti-adrenergic drug.

Areas A, C, and D all utilize acetylcholine as the transmitter.

10. Correct: Raynaud's disease (D)

Raynaud disease is a painful disorder that is characterized by sequential pallor, cyanosis, and rubor of digits after exposure to cold. Vasoconstriction without underlying vascular pathology produces these changes.

Typically, peripheral vascular disease (A) affects the legs more than the arms, and there is a difference in arterial pressure recorded between the upper and lower limbs.

Thoracic outlet syndrome (B) may also present with similar symptoms; however, negative Adson's sign (abduction and external rotation of upper limb not causing diminution of radial pulse) makes it a less likely diagnosis.

Diabetes mellitus (C) may also present symptoms similar to those described by this patient; however, the age of the patient and normal bloodwork in absence of medication make it a less likely diagnosis.

Lastly, familial dysautonomia (E) is associated with abnormal sweating, blood pressure instability, loss of tone in the gastrointestinal tract, and progressive sensory loss.

11. Correct: Digital sympathectomy (D)

Digital sympathectomy involves stripping the adventitial layer from the affected common and proper digital arteries. This may be the only alternative to amputation when medical therapy (with calcium channel blockers, a2 adrenergic antagonists, warfarin, plasminogen activator, etc.) has failed.

Propranolol (A), oral contraceptives (B), and pseudoephedrine (C) are all associated with increased vasospasm, thereby increasing the symptoms of Raynaud's disease.

Insulin (E) has no known effects in Raynaud's disease.

12. Correct: Posterior cranial fossa (C)

Descending autonomic pathways from the medulla could be affected by the presence of a tumor within the posterior fossa and result in the inability to modulate blood pressure with positional changes.

Insular cortex (A) plays an important role in the sympathetic control of cardiovascular tone. However, tumors within this region are more likely to be associated with induction of seizures than with orthostatic hypotension.

The medial dorsal nucleus (B) of the thalamus relays input from the amygdala and olfactory cortex to prefrontal and limbic structures, and therefore would not likely affect blood pressure in the manner described.

As the inferior colliculus (D) is the principal midbrain nucleus of the auditory pathway, a tumor within this region would have little impact on changes in blood pressure.

Lastly, the precentral gyrus (E) is the location of primary motor cortex. Although tumors here may result in movement deficits that could result in a fall, it would not likely impact control mechanisms involved with blood pressure.

13. Correct: CN VIII (C)

CN VIII is involved in the transmission of sound and balance information from the inner ear, and is not associated with the parasympathetic nervous system.

CN III (A, accommodation and miosis of the eye), CN VII (B, lacrimation, mucus secretion from palate and nose, and salivation from submandibular and sublingual glands), CN IX (D, salivation from the parotid gland), and CN X (E, innervation to the thoracic and abdominal viscera) are involved with parasympathetic functions.

14. Correct: Stomach (E)

Referred pain from the stomach is most consistent with the left T8 dermatome.

Although pain originating from both the liver (A) and gallbladder (B) can appear at the T8 dermatome, these will usually be localized to the right side. Pain from the large intestine (C) is most often localized in central T12–L1 dermatomes. Pain from the heart (D) most commonly localizes to the left T3–T4 dermatome.

15. Correct: Area E (A)

Rupture of the spleen will irritate the left diaphragm by peritoneal fluid contaminated with blood. Since the diaphragm is supplied by the phrenic nerve (C3, C4, and C5), pain would be referred to the tip of the left shoulder.

Pain from irritation of the diaphragm will not refer to the other listed areas.

16. Correct: Reduce secretion of the bronchial glands and widen the bronchial passages via parasympathetic blockage (C)

Parasympathetic stimulation of the local ganglia promotes secretion of mucus from the bronchial glands and promotes bronchoconstriction. Atropine, a competitive antagonist of muscarinic acetylcholine receptors (thereby acting as parasympatholytic), reduces secretion of the bronchial glands and causes bronchodilation.

Atropine does not act by stimulating or inhibiting the sympathetic system (**B, D,** and **E**). It is not a parasympathomimetic drug (**A**), and certainly does not promote bronchial secretion.

17. Correct: Parasympathetic innervation of the myenteric plexus (B)

Intestinal motility is primarily increased by parasympathetic innervation of the myenteric plexus (**B**). It is not enhanced by sympathetic innervation (**D** and **E**). Both the internal (**A**) and external (**C**) submucosal plexi are primarily concerned with control of the secretory functions of the gut.

18. Correct: Limbic system; hypothalamus; medulla oblongata; spinal cord; target organs (E)

The limbic system acts upon the hypothalamus, which in turn acts upon the medulla oblongata. From the medulla, activity is sent to the spinal cord and then ultimately to the target organs. This hierarchy is what allows for higher level cognition (such as fear or excitement) to have a direct impact on the autonomic nervous system function.

19. Correct: Removal of parasympathetic control preventing voluntary and reflexive control of bladder (D)

Control of the bladder is largely a function of parasympathetic innervation, which is controlled by the S2–S4 segments of the spinal cord. Removal of parasympathetic control of the bladder at this level would prevent both voluntary and reflexive control resulting in an atonic bladder.

Sympathetic input to the bladder is from T12–L3 spinal segments, and damage to these fibers has no appreciable effect on bladder function (**A, B,** and **C**).

Upper motor neuron input (**E**) controls volitional micturition via the corticosacral tract. Bilateral transection of this pathway would result in loss of voluntary control, but reflexive control of bladder function would remain intact.

20. Correct: Preganglionic sympathetic cholinergic fibers (A)

Innervation of the sweat glands and arrector pilorum muscles (muscles responsible for making the hair stand on end [goose bumps]) utilizes acetylcholine at both the pre- and postganglionic synapses.

This is in contrast to most other sympathetic systems that utilize acetylcholine for the preganglionic (**E**) and epinephrine and norepinephrine for the postganglionic (**C**) neurons.

Parasympathetic innervation (**B** and **D**) is not responsible for sweating or goosebumps.

Chapter 23

Neuroimaging

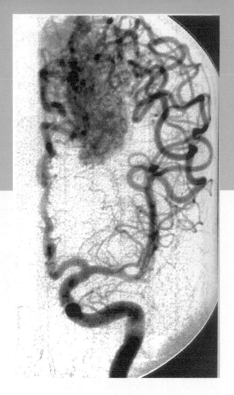

LEARNING OBJECTIVES

▶ Analyze the properties of a T2-weighted MRI scan.

▶ Identify abnormal findings on four commonly used MRI sequences.

▶ Interpret common presentation of global hypoxia in a small child in the MRI modality.

▶ Relate clinical symptoms to lesion location on a T1-weighted MRI.

▶ Identify a CT bone windowed scan.

▶ Interpret herniation types from neuroimaging.

▶ Differentiate traumatic subarachnoid hemorrhage from other related causes based on the presence of a contrecoup injury.

▶ Identify the optimal MRI scanning sequence for imaging subarachnoid hemorrhage.

▶ Identify common scenarios in which contrast is preferred in CT scanning.

▶ Analyze the normal enlargement of ventricles and sulci observed in natural aging in a T2-weighted MRI scan.

▶ Describe the process to which 18F-FDG tracers are sensitive.

▶ Analyze the timing of imaging findings related to noncontrast CT scans when evaluating MCA embolus and infarction.

▶ Interpret diffusion weighted image (DWI) MRI and T2-weighted FLAIR MRI scans, and analyze significant clinical findings arising from an MCA embolus and infarction.

▶ Identify cerebral blood flow (CBF) findings consistent with an MCA embolus and infarction.

▶ Describe the contraindications to MRI scanning.

▶ Describe the contraindications to CT scanning with and without contrast.

▶ Identify subdural hematoma based on noncontrast CT scanning.

▶ Distinguish between types of skull fractures in a CT scan without contrast.

▶ Identify epidural hematoma based on noncontrast CT scanning.

23.1 Questions

Easy | Medium | Hard

Consider the following case for questions 1 to 3:

A previously healthy 4-year-old infant is brought to the emergency department after being found unresponsive in the crib. Diagnostic imaging is performed, with the following results:

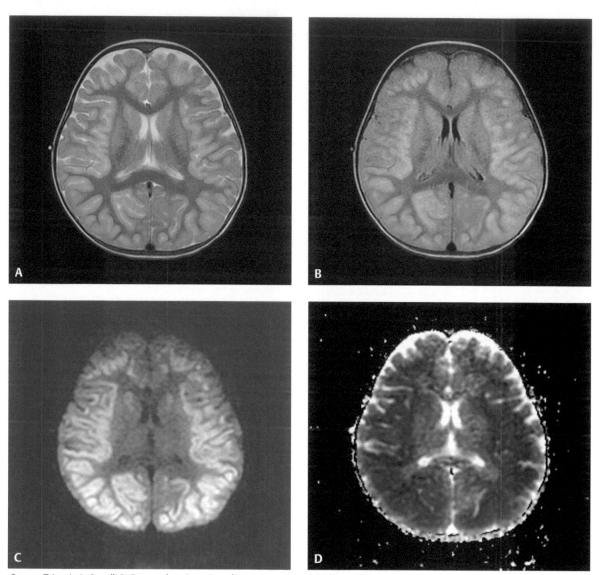

Source: Tsiouris A, Sanelli P, Comunale J. Case-Based Brain Imaging. 2nd Edition. Thieme; 2013.

1. What imaging modality is the image in A?

A. CT with contrast
B. CT without contrast
C. T2-weighted MRI
D. T2-weighted FLAIR MRI
E. Diffusion weighted image (DWI)

2. Which scans best demonstrate abnormal hyperintensity within the cortex of the cerebral hemispheres?

A. Images A and B
B. Images A and C
C. Images A and D
D. Images B and C
E. Images C and D

3. What condition most likely resulted in this pattern of imaging results?

A. Watershed injury

B. Cavernous malformation

C. Arteriovenous malformation

D. Primary angiitis of the CNS

E. Global anoxic brain injury

Consider the following case for questions 4 and 5:

A 77-year-old man awakens on a Saturday morning and has difficulty speaking. His wife rushes him to the emergency department. His medical history reveals that he takes medication for high blood pressure, but it is controlled. The results of the examination suggest a small stroke, with weakness of facial muscles on the lower right side of the face (see accompanying image).

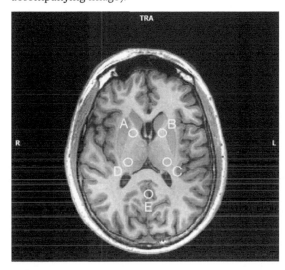

4. Where would you expect to see a lesion?

A. Area A

B. Area B

C. Area C

D. Area D

E. Area E

5. What type of imaging modality was used to acquire the presented image?

A. T1-weighted MRI

B. T2-weighted MRI

C. T2-FLAIR MRI

D. CT contrast

E. CT angiogram

Consider the following case for questions 6 and 7:

A 25-year-old male is brought to the emergency department following a motorcycle/school bus collision. From the time that he was initially brought in, his mental status has been progressively declining, and a fixed dilated pupil was present in his right eye.

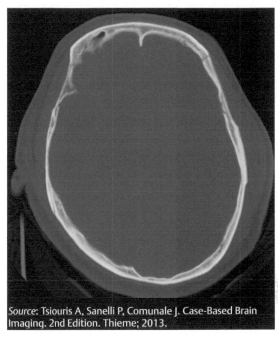

Source: Tsiouris A, Sanelli P, Comunale J. Case-Based Brain Imaging. 2nd Edition. Thieme; 2013.

6. What type of scan was performed on this patient to produce the presented image?

A. CT angiogram

B. CT brain window

C. CT bone window

D. Proton density MRI

E. Plain film X ray

7. The scan presented in the case demonstrates a left anterior frontal bone fracture. Combined with the ipsilateral dilated pupil, herniation is suspected. The following images show the CT scan with brain window applied at two axial locations. In the presented images, what type(s) of herniation is/are present?

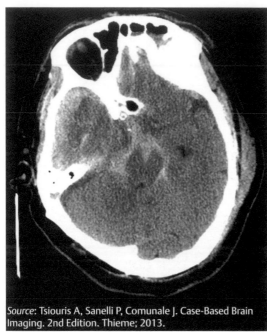

Source: Tsiouris A, Sanelli P, Comunale J. Case-Based Brain Imaging. 2nd Edition. Thieme; 2013.

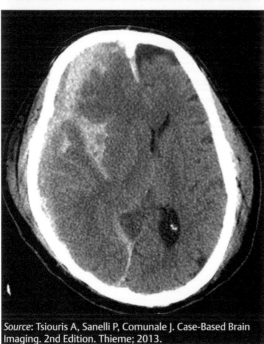

Source: Tsiouris A, Sanelli P, Comunale J. Case-Based Brain Imaging. 2nd Edition. Thieme; 2013.

A. Subfalcine
B. Uncal
C. Central
D. Transcalvarial
E. Subfalcine and uncal

Consider the following case for questions 8 and 9:

You are working in the radiology department when the following image is sent from the ER. The electronic records system is currently offline, so you do not receive any additional information.

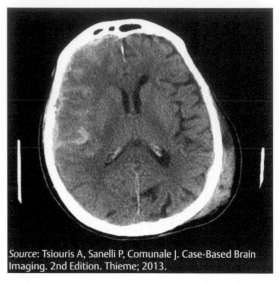

Source: Tsiouris A, Sanelli P, Comunale J. Case-Based Brain Imaging. 2nd Edition. Thieme; 2013.

8. Based on the CT scan sent, which of the following conditions would be most consistent with the observed image?

A. Aneurysm rupture
B. Spontaneous hemorrhage related to anticoagulant use
C. Benign subarachnoid hemorrhage
D. Traumatic subarachnoid hemorrhage
E. Arteriovenous malformation

9. You wish to perform further diagnostic imaging with this patient. Which MR sequence would be the most useful for a definitive diagnosis?

A. T2-weighted
B. T2-weighted FLAIR
C. T1-weighted
D. Proton density MR
E. MRI is not sensitive to subarachnoid hemorrhage

10. A family has scheduled an appointment with their family physician, as they are concerned about a procedure that was recommended in the course of treatment for their 7-year-old child. They were advised that a CT scan with contrast would be the imaging method of choice, but they were concerned about the radiation associated with this procedure. To set their mind at ease, you explain that a CT scan with contrast is preferred in which of the following scenarios?

A. Tumor
B. Infection
C. Demyelinating processes
D. Angiographic studies
E. All of the above

Consider the following case for questions 11 and 12:

A 76-year-old man presents to their primary care provider concerned about recent problems with memory. The Alzheimer's and dementia rating scale reveal memory impairment, and he is referred for further testing.

11. Radiological exam using T2-weighting was performed (see accompanying images). What are the radiologic findings of this exam?

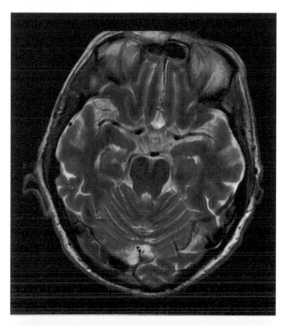

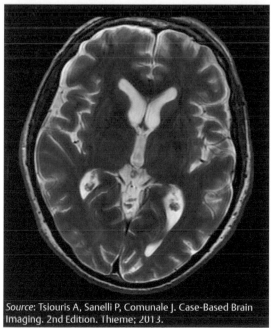

Source: Tsiouris A, Sanelli P, Comunale J. Case-Based Brain Imaging. 2nd Edition. Thieme; 2013.

A. There are no abnormalities

B. Increased prominence of ventricles and sulci consistent with aging

C. Increased prominence of ventricles and sulci indicative of Alzheimer's dementia complex

D. Compression of the medial temporal lobes

E. Tumor within the right medial temporal lobe

12. A second radiologic study is performed using PET scanning and the tracer 18F-FDG (fluorodeoxyglucose, a glucose analog), where moderate symmetric decreases in the signal density in the region of the temporal lobes were found. What is this decrease signal in the PET scan (see accompanying image) indicating?

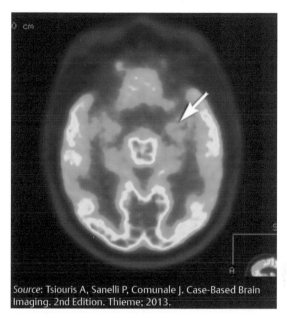

Source: Tsiouris A, Sanelli P, Comunale J. Case-Based Brain Imaging. 2nd Edition. Thieme; 2013.

A. Buildup of amyloid beta plaques

B. Decrease in functional activity

C. Decrease in cortical metabolism

D. Decrease in dopamine (D1 and D2) receptors

E. Decrease in serotonin transporters

Consider the following case for questions 13 to 15:

A 76-year-old woman is brought to the emergency department immediately following acute onset of left-sided hemiparesis. Although she shows signs of a right MCA embolus and acute infarction, diagnostic radiology is performed.

13. What would you expect to see on a noncontrast CT scan?

A. Prominent loss of gray–white matter distinction
B. Faint loss of gray–white matter distinction
C. Hypodensity within vascular territory of the MCA
D. Gyral swelling
E. Hemorrhagic transformation (parenchymal/petechial)

14. To aid in the diagnosis of this patient, DW and T2-weighted FLAIR MRI scans were ordered (see accompanying images). Which of the following findings is consistent with the images?

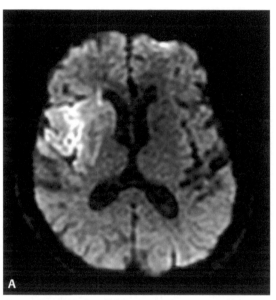
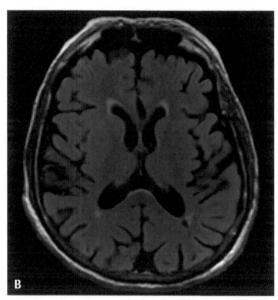

Source: Tsiouris A, Sanelli P, Comunale J. Case-Based Brain Imaging. 2nd Edition. Thieme; 2013.

A. No significant signal abnormality
B. No significant signal abnormality on the DWI MRI scan and hypointense signal on the T2-weighted FLAIR scan
C. No significant signal abnormality on the DWI MRI scan and hyperintense signal on the T2-weighted FLAIR scan
D. Hypointense DWI signal and no significant signal abnormality on the T2-weighted FLAIR scan
E. Hyperintense DWI signal and no significant signal abnormality on the T2-weighted FLAIR scan

15. Advanced MRI techniques were employed in this patient, using a gadolinium contrast agent in an MRI scan to examine cerebral blood flow (CBF). Which of the following images would be consistent with MRI scan examining CBF in this patient?

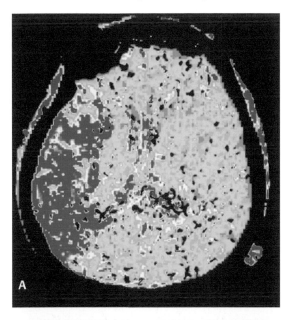

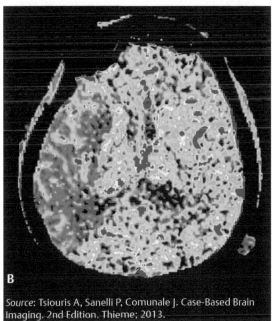

Source: Tsiouris A, Sanelli P, Comunale J. Case-Based Brain Imaging. 2nd Edition. Thieme; 2013.

A. Both images could be consistent

B. Image A is consistent

C. Image B is consistent

D. Neither image would be consistent

16. A 26-year-old girl is referred for an MRI scan, and she is being evaluated for contraindications. Which of the following is a safe option for her to undergo an MRI?

A. Insulin pump

B. Hearing aid

C. Intracranial metal clip

D. Pregnancy

E. Metallic body within the eye

17. A 10-year-old male is referred to diagnostic radiology for a CT scan, with contrast. Which of the following conditions would absolutely preclude this study from being performed?

A. Weight

B. Young age

C. Claustrophobia

D. Contrast allergy

E. None of the above

18. A 54-year-old woman is brought to the emergency department after she slipped and fell while descending an icy stairway. She is unconscious at the time of admission. A CT scan without contrast is performed (see accompanying image). What is the most likely diagnosis in this case?

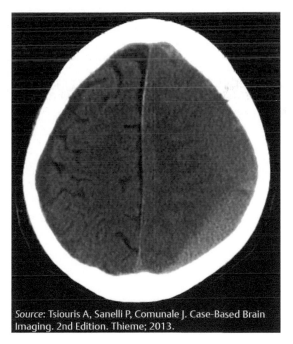

Source: Tsiouris A, Sanelli P, Comunale J. Case-Based Brain Imaging. 2nd Edition. Thieme; 2013.

A. Subdural hematoma

B. Epidural hematoma

C. Dural based neoplasm

D. Thrombosis

E. No evidence of pathology

Refer to the following case for questions 19 and 20:

A 24-year-old male is taken to the emergency department following an altercation in a local nightclub. He was reportedly struck on the side of the head with a heavy, blunt object. Immediately following the impact he was unconscious, but at the time of admission he had regained consciousness. A noncontrast CT scan is performed with the following results:

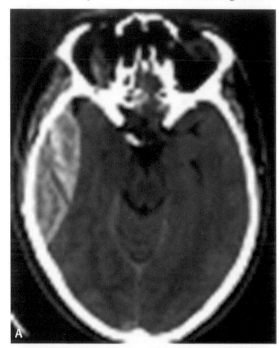

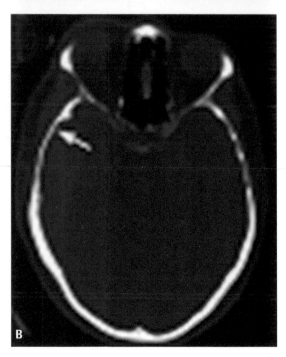

19. The CT scan with bone window applied (image B) is denoting what type of pathology at the arrow head?

A. Displaced skull fracture

B. Nondisplaced skull fracture

C. Depressed skull fracture

D. Diastatic skull fracture

E. Basilar skull fracture

20. What is the most likely diagnosis in this case?

A. Subdural hematoma

B. Epidural hematoma

C. Thrombosis

D. No evidence of pathology

23.2 Answers and Explanations

Easy	Medium	Hard

1. Correct: T2-weighted MRI (C)

The presented images are T2-weighted MRI images.

Since the image in question has CSF within the ventricles as bright, this rules out both types of CT scans (**A** and **B**).

A T2-weighted FLAIR scan (**D**) has many properties similar to a T2-weighted image (white matter is dark and gray matter is light); however, unlike a traditional T2-weighted scanning, the signal from fluid is attenuated, resulting in the ventricles imaging as dark. In fact, the acronym FLAIR stands for fluid-attenuated inversion recovery, denoting the impact this sequence has on the appearance of fluids.

A DWI (**E**) would also have CSF within the ventricles come up as dark (as seen in image C).

2. Correct: Images A and B (A)

Both of the T2-weighted images, scans A and B (**A**), reveal diffuse hyperintensity involving bilateral cortex. This hyperintensity is most apparent at the deep margins of the cortex at the corticomedullary junction, with traces of increased intensity within the bilateral caudate nuclei.

Scan C, a DWI, and scan D, an apparent diffusion coefficient (ADC) scan image, both show hypodensity in the corresponding areas—ruling out all other response options (**B, C, D,** and **E**).

3. Correct: Global anoxic brain injury (E)

This patient is showing signs of a global anoxic brain injury, consistent with their age. In infants and young children, hypoxia results in damage primarily to the lateral geniculate nuclei, corpora striata, hippocampi, and cerebral cortex (in particular anterior frontal and parieto-occipital areas). For unknown reasons, in comparison to adults, the sparing of thalami during this type of injury is a consistent finding.

A watershed injury (**A**) occurs at the distal boundary of the major arterial territories. Although neuroimaging may reveal similarities between a watershed injury and global anoxic brain injury, due to the age of this patient (young child), absence of significant risk factors (hypertension, smoking, high cholesterol, and diabetes mellitus), and the location of damage, a watershed injury is much less likely to be the cause.

A cavernous malformation (**B**) would typically present with a well-defined hyperintense lesion when examined with a T2-weighted image that is hypointense on T1-weighted scans, which was not observed in this case.

An arteriovenous malformation (**C**) would present as a wedge-shaped, compact mass of enlarged tangled vessels visible through a CT angiogram that would be observed as a hyperdense or isodense lesion on CT images and as abnormal flow voids associated with dilated cortical veins and a tightly packed mass visible on a T1-weighted anatomical image.

Lastly, primary angiitis (**D**) typically presents on T2-weighted FLAIR MRIs as scattered areas of abnormal hyperintensities involving the supratentorial white matter.

4. Correct: Area B (B)

Weakness of the facial muscles on one side and difficulty speaking are, in this case, a result of disruption of the corticonuclear fibers as they traverse the genu (**A** and **B**) of the internal capsule. Corticonuclear fibers at this level are mainly contralateral to the portion of the facial nucleus that innervates the lower face, so a left-sided lesion (**B**) will result in a weakness of the lower face on the right.

As there are no appreciable weaknesses of the extremities, damage to the posterior limb of the internal capsule (**C** and **D**) is unlikely. Damage to area E (**E**, bilateral striate cortex) would most likely result in visual deficits.

5. Correct: T1-weighted MRI (A)

The presented image is a T1-weighted MRI. The superior anatomical resolution of soft tissue and distinction between gray and white matter is indicative of MRI as the modality utilized, ruling out CT scanning (**D** and **E**).

As the fluid in the ventricle is dark, we can eliminate a T2-weighted MRI (**B**). The white matter is bright, and the gray matter is dark, eliminating a T2-FLAIR MRI (**C**).

6. Correct: CT bone window (C)

CT scans can adjust the way in which radiodensity information is displayed to be optimized for detection of various forms of pathology. At a very basic level, these settings may be adjusted and optimized for viewing soft tissue within the brain (CT brain window) or for viewing bone within the skull (CT bone window). The presented image is readily identifiable as a CT bone window, as all of the soft tissue within and outside of the skull appears a low-contrast gray. In comparison, a CT brain window (**B**) would show soft tissue at a much greater level of detail than what is presented.

A CT angiogram (**A**) is used to produce detailed images of blood vessel and tissues through the use of an iodine-rich contrast agent that is injected into the patient. As neither soft tissue nor vasculature is observable, it can be ruled out.

Proton density MRI scans (**D**) are an intermediate sequence sharing some features of both T1-weighted and T2-weighted contrasts. Due to its ability to offer excellent signal distinction between fluid and different forms of cartilage, this sequence is now more commonly employed in the assessment of joints and has largely been replaced by T2-weighted FLAIR sequences for neuroimaging uses.

A plain film X-ray (**E**) is unable to show the different densities of tissue material present in the image, and is inherently two-dimensional.

7. Correct: Subfalcine and uncal (E)

In a subfalcine (cingulate) herniation (**A**), the cingulate gyrus is forced under part of the falx cerebri, as is observed here. In an uncal herniation (**B**), the innermost part of the temporal lobe (the uncus) is pushed toward the tentorium and puts pressure on the midbrain, as can also be seen. This increased pressure on the brainstem can cause dysfunction of the oculomotor nerve (CN III), causing the fixed and dilated pupil observed.

In central herniation (**C**), the diencephalon, including parts of the temporal lobes (bilaterally), is forced through the tentorium cerebelli by forces causing the brain to move up or down across the tentorium (an ascending or descending transtentorial herniation).

A transcalvarial herniation (**D**) occurs when the brain is pushed through a fracture or surgical opening in the skull, a condition that may be observed following craniectomy.

8. Correct: Traumatic subarachnoid haemorrhage (D)

All of the answer options provided would be included in the differential diagnosis, due to similarities in how each presents. In particular, all would result in extravasation of blood into the subarachnoid space, sulcal hyperdensity, and midline shift, as seen in the CT scan. However, only traumatic subarachnoid hemorrhage would explain the prominent left parietal scalp hematoma. The sulcal hyperdensity observed, therefore, is most likely a contrecoup injury corresponding to an impact on the left of the skull.

9. Correct: T2-weighted FLAIR (B)

As diagnosing subarachnoid hemorrhage requires identifying fluid in regions of the brain where it should not be present, a T2 scan is going to be preferred over a T1-weighted (**C**) or proton density (**D**) scan, due to its increased signal intensity to fluid. Further, with a regular T2-weighted MRI sequence (**A**), a subarachnoid hemorrhage would be roughly the same signal intensity as CSF, making a T2-weighted FLAIR sequence preferred, as it would provide the most contrast between CSF and extravasated blood.

10. Correct: All of the above(E)

All of the above scenarios would likely benefit from the inclusion of a contrast agent. If a tumor (**A**) is suspected, CT scanning may be performed both with and without contrast to assess for metastatic disease. Many tumors will show enhancement following contrast administration.

Similarly, if there is suspicion of infection (**B**), a CT with contrast may reveal meningeal enhancement suggesting inflammation and/or infection.

Demyelinating processes (**C**) usually result in isodense or hypodense lesions in noncontrast CT scans, with acute lesions possibly showing enhancement post contrast administration, increasing diagnostic value of the test.

Lastly, all angiographic studies (**D**) in CT require the use of contrast.

11. Correct: Increased prominence of ventricles and sulci consistent with aging (B)

Although this patient is displaying symptoms consistent with probable Alzheimer's disease, the presented T2-weighted MRI does not show disproportionate atrophy within the temporal lobes (or any other brain region). There is an increase in the prominence of the ventricles and sulci that is consistent with aging, as longitudinal characterization of MRI images has shown increases in the size of ventricles and sulci as part of the natural aging process. As these increases are not region specific, the prominence of ventricles and sulci are not indicative of Alzheimer's dementia complex (**C**).

12. Correct: Decrease in cortical metabolism (C)

Standard 18F-FDG PET is a glucose analog, taken up by glucose using cells. The brain utilizes glucose as part of the metabolic process, and therefore a decrease in the uptake of 18F-FDG is indicative of a decrease in cortical metabolism within that region.

Recent PET tracer development has allowed for the imaging of the neuro-aggregate amyloid (**A**), such as 18F-FDDNP. However, these imaging probes are only beginning to be brought into clinical use, and 18F-FDG is not sensitive to this pathological process.

Although glucose is related to functional activity, a more direct tracer such as O-15 would be better suited to measure functional activity (**B**). It is important to note that, similar to functional MRI, O-15 PET scanning is only an indirect measure of activity, as it simply maps oxygenated blood flow (unlike in vivo electrical recordings).

PET tracers have been created to image both dopamine receptors (**D**) and serotonin transporters (**E**)—11C-raclopride and 11C-DASB, respectively. However, 18F-FDG is insensitive to both these processes.

13. Correct: Faint loss of gray–white matter distinction (B)

Within the first 6 hours of onset of symptoms, noncontrast CT scanning may reveal a faint, but not prominent (**A**), loss of the gray–white matter distinction.

Hypodensity within the vascular territory of the MCA (**C**) and gyral swelling (**D**) would not be expected until 12 to 24 hours, and hemorrhagic transformation (**E**) would not be expected until 24 to 48 hours, following onset of symptoms.

14. Correct: Hyperintense DWI signal and no significant signal abnormality on the T2-weighted FLAIR scan (E)

Image A can be identified as a DWI MRI scan, as we have a lower resolution of anatomical features through the inclusion of diffusion values on the typical T2 signal. Image B is identifiable as a T2-weighted FLAIR scan, as it shows prominent features of a traditional T2-weighted scan, but CSF within the ventricles is giving a low signal intensity. There is a prominent area of hyperintensity in the left (DWI

MRI scan) image, but no apparent signal abnormalities in the right image, ruling out a normal scan result (**A**). As noted, the signal for the DWI MRI scan is neither normal (**B** and **C**) nor hypointense (**D**).

15. Correct: Image B is consistent (C)

As the scan was examining CBF, one would expect a decrease in CBF within the territory of the right MCA, as demonstrated in Image B. Image A is showing an increase within the territory of the right MCA, and is therefore not consistent with the symptoms.

16. Correct: Pregnancy (D)

Most of human studies have demonstrated MRI as safe for the developing fetus, and therefore pregnancy is not a contraindication. However, MRI should only be used in pregnant women if other forms of nonionizing radiation studies are inadequate and if the procedure is medically necessary for the proper care of the mother or fetus.

Due to use of a strong magnetic field (typically 1T to 3T in a clinical setting), patients with certain conditions are contraindicated for MRI procedures. Electronic devices that may be destroyed or otherwise malfunction (**A** and **B**) should not be brought into the MRI room. An intracranial metal clip (such as an aneurysm clip; **C**) may undergo subtle movement due to strong torsional forces and is a common contraindication for MRI procedures. Similarly the presence of a metallic foreign body within the eye (**E**) would eliminate someone from this procedure as there is the possibility of the foreign body reacting to the magnetic field, causing movement that could damage the eye.

17. Correct: None of the above (E)

Absolute contraindications to CT scanning are relatively few. Even in the case of a known allergy to the contrast (**D**), medication to prevent reaction can be utilized or a non-IV contrast can be selected. None of the other parameters listed absolutely prevent the use of this scanning technique.

18. Correct: Subdural hematoma (A)

This scan shows typical signs associated with an acute subdural hematoma. In particular, there is a large heterogeneously hyperdense area within the left hemisphere, with a crescentic shaped configuration that spans across the sutural margins. Additionally, there is a mass effect with sulcal effacement and changes in the gray–white matter junction in both the frontal and parietal lobes.

An epidural hematoma (**B**) would not cross suture margins. A dural-based neoplasm (**C**) or thrombosis (**D**) may present with similar signs on a noncontrast CT scan; however, considering the patient history of a recent fall, a hematoma is a much more likely diagnosis.

19. Correct: Nondisplaced skull fracture (B)

The presented scan is displaying a nondisplaced skull fracture, as the skull fragments are still within normal alignment.

A displaced skull fracture (**A**) would consist of the bone no longer being in alignment. Depressed (**C**) and diastatic (**D**) skull fractures are two specific types of displaced skull fractures. In depressed skull fracture, broken bones are displaced inward. In diastatic skull fracture, the break line traverses the sutures, causing a widening of the suture. Diastatic breaks are more commonly observed in young children, as sutures have not yet fused in this population. A basilar skull fracture (**E**) refers to linear fractures (nondisplaced) that occur in the floor of the cranial vault.

20. Correct: Epidural hematoma (B)

The noncontrast CT scan with brain window applied (image A) demonstrates a hyperdense collection with biconvex shape within the right temporal lobe, in line with the fracture observed in the bone window (image B). Additionally, there is apparent soft tissue swelling in the temporalis muscle, indicating the probable site of impact. Such findings are consistent with an epidural hematoma, where the pressure from the bleeding vessel within the epidural space has stripped the dura away from the skull.

A subdural hematoma (**A**) is typically crescentic and crosses suture lines. Although thrombosis (**C**) should be part of the differential diagnosis for epidural hematoma, the presence of skull fracture and case history rule thrombosis out in this case.

Chapter 24

Comprehensive Review

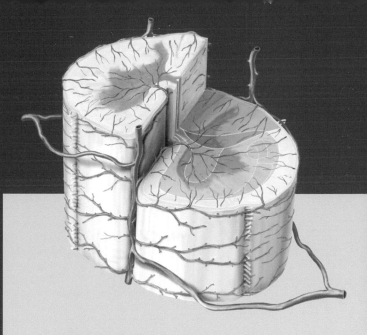

LEARNING OBJECTIVES

- ► Describe the effect of lesion to corticobulbar fibers within the crus cerebri.
- ► Describe the role of autonomic nervous system in male sexual function.
- ► Describe the normal physiological variants in pupil diameter.
- ► Analyze the role of the tectospinal tract in reflexive postural movements of the head in response to external auditory and visual stimuli.
- ► Define different types of appendicular ataxias found in cerebellar disorders. Describe the effects of lesions of functional areas of the cerebellum.
- ► Describe the effects of lesion of the trochlear nucleus.
- ► Describe the connections and functions of thalamic nuclei. Describe the blood supply of thalamus.
- ► Analyze the symptoms of vestibular neuronitis and distinguish it from similar disorders of the vestibular system.
- ► Describe the clinical features associated with lesions of the pontine tegmentum.
- ► Describe the etiopathology and clinical and radiological features for Chiari type II malformation.
- ► Analyze the role of the olfactory glomeruli in olfactory discrimination.
- ► Interpret Weber and Rinne test.
- ► Describe the etiopathology and clinical features of Wernicke's encephalopathy and Korsakoff's psychosis.
- ► Analyze the sidedness for brain lesions.
- ► Localize brainstem lesions based on symptomology; correlate clinical symptoms with damage to major structures within the pons.
- ► Describe the location and function of glomus choroideum. Describe the arteries that feed the choroid plexus within the ventricles.
- ► Analyze the effects of damage to the medial longitudinal fasciculus on eye movements.
- ► Identify the location of the olfactory glomera within the olfactory bulb.
- ► Relate lesions of the primary visual pathway to visual field defects.

- ► Analyze the etiology and clinical features of Parinaud's syndrome.
- ► Analyze the effects of unilateral lesions to primary auditory cortex.
- ► Analyze features of oculomotor nerve paralysis as occurs in transtentorial herniation.
- ► Describe the role of hypothalamus in maintaining homeostasis.
- ► Illustrate the fiber pathway connecting the hippocampus to the mammillary bodies.
- ► Describe the internal circuitry of the cerebellum.
- ► Interpret caloric stimulation results in the comatose patient.
- ► Analyze the symptoms of detached retina and relate these to its functions.
- ► Analyze the etiology of uncinate seizures resulting in olfactory hallucinations.
- ► Identify the constituents of the cerebellar peduncles.
- ► Identify muscles innervated by the oculomotor nerve in a gross specimen.

24.1 Questions

Easy	Medium	Hard

1. A 60-year-old woman's tongue deviates to the left on protrusion and the angle of her mouth deviates to the right on an attempt to smile. Damage to which of the following areas would most likely explain this woman's deficits?

A. Right ventromedial medulla

B. Left ventromedial medulla

C. Right caudal pontine tegmentum

D. Left caudal pontine tegmentum

E. Middle third of the right crus cerebri in the midbrain

F. Middle third of the left crus cerebri in the midbrain

2. A 58-year-old male presents to his primary care provider with problems related to sexual function. In particular, this patient is having difficulty both maintaining an erection and with ejaculation. Which of the following features of autonomic nervous system functions is true for these acts?

A. Erection mediated by parasympathetic fibers of the L2–L4 spinal cord; ejaculation mediated by sympathetic fibers of the S2–S4 spinal cord

B. Erection mediated by parasympathetic fibers of the S2–S4 spinal cord; ejaculation mediated by sympathetic fibers of the L2–L4 spinal cord

C. Erection mediated by sympathetic fibers of the L2–L4 spinal cord; ejaculation mediated by the parasympathetic fibers of the S2–S4 spinal cord

D. Erection mediated by the sympathetic fibers of the S2–S4 spinal cord; ejaculation mediated by parasympathetic fibers of the L2–L4 spinal cord segment

E. Erection mediated by the parasympathetic fibers of the L2–L4 spinal cord; ejaculation mediated by parasympathetic fibers of the S2–S4 spinal cord

3. A 22-year-old woman makes an appointment with her primary care physician when she realizes her left and right pupils are of different diameters. After googling the symptoms, she became increasingly concerned that she might have brainstem dysfunction. Ophthalmic examination revealed right and left pupillary diameters to be 5 and 5.8 mm, respectively. Both eyes reacted to light. Which of the following is the most likely diagnosis for this patient?

A. Horner's syndrome

B. Normal physiological variant

C. Mechanical anisocoria

D. Adie (tonic) pupil

E. Pharmacological usage–related anisocoria

4. A 36-year-old man presents with lesion of fibers that arise from the superior colliculus and then course in the contralateral ventral white column to provide synaptic inputs to ventral gray interneurons. Which of the following might be a presenting symptom?

A. Ataxia and postural instability

B. Diplopia

C. Intention tremor

D. Maintenance of gaze reflex

E. Deficits in orienting responses to stimuli

Consider the following case for questions 5 and 6:

A 28-year-old woman has difficulty in touching the physician's fingers with her index finger, as he slowly moves it from left to right in her visual field.

5. Which of the following conditions might she be suffering from?

A. Asterixis

B. Dysrhythmia

C. Dysmetria

D. Dysdiadochokinesia

E. Titubation

6. Which of the following structures is most likely lesioned in this woman?

A. Dentate nucleus

B. Fastigial nucleus

C. Flocculonodular lobe of cerebellum

D. Vermal region of cerebellum

E. Ventral spinocerebellar tract

7. Which of the following will be a likely finding in a 45-year-old man with a lesion affecting the paramedian area of his caudal left midbrain tegmentum?

A. Mydriasis affecting left eye

B. Mydriasis affecting right eye

C. Vertical diplopia affecting left eye

D. Vertical diplopia affecting right eye

E. Loss of pain sensation from left arm

F. Loss of pain sensation from right arm

Consider the following case for questions 8 and 9:

A 66-year-old woman presents with pain and paresthesia of her right upper limb. She has age-appropriate strength in the limb and no other notable neurodeficit.

8. Which of the following structures might be lesioned in her?

A. VPL nucleus, right thalamus

B. VPL nucleus, left thalamus

C. VPM nucleus, right thalamus

D. VPM nucleus, left thalamus

E. Right paracentral lobule

F. Left paracentral lobule

9. Given the structure damaged, which of the following vessels is most likely to be involved in her case?

A. Left anterior cerebral artery

B. Right anterior cerebral artery

C. Thalamogeniculate branch of left posterior cerebral artery (P2)

D. Thalamogeniculate branch of right posterior cerebral artery (P2)

E. Thalamoperforating branch of left posterior cerebral artery (P1)

F. Thalamoperforating branch of right posterior cerebral artery (P1)

10. A generally healthy 32-year-old female presented to the emergency department with severe rotatory vertigo, nausea, vomiting, and headache. Symptoms had started approximately a week earlier, and they have been continuous for the previous 2 days, which is what prompted her to seek treatment. Her hearing was normal. Caloric testing revealed reduced sensitivity in the left ear. Previous history was unremarkable, with the exception of an upper respiratory tract infection a number of weeks earlier. What is the most likely diagnosis for this patient?

A. Labyrinthitis

B. Vestibular neuronitis

C. Ménière's disease

D. Benign positional paroxysmal vertigo (BPPV)

E. Migraine

11. A 56-year-old man presents with slurring of speech and left gaze palsy. During neurological testing, the angle of his mouth deviated toward the right on attempted smiling, and he was unable to forcefully close his left eye against resistance. Which of the following is a likely location for his lesion?

A. Midbrain tegmentum

B. Midbrain base

C. Pontine tegmentum

D. Pontine base

E. Internal capsule

12. A family makes an appointment with their primary care physician as they are concerned about the behavior of their 5-month-old infant. Of particular concern was a noted difficulty in swallowing during breast feeding, concurrent with the skin taking on a bluish color and the nailbeds taking on a purplish color. Upon neurological examination, it is determined that the infant has an upper extremity weakness and downbeat nystagmus. Diagnostic radiology is performed with the following results:

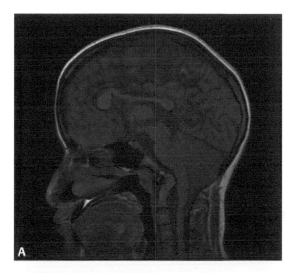

A

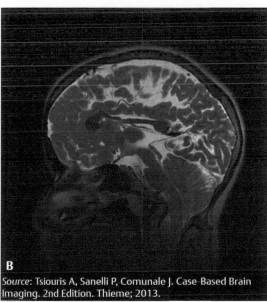

B

Source: Tsiouris A, Sanelli P, Comunale J. Case-Based Brain Imaging. 2nd Edition. Thieme; 2013.

Which of the following is the most likely diagnosis for the infant?

A. Chiari I malformation

B. Chiari II malformation

C. Chiari III malformation

D. Dandy–Walker malformation

E. Posterior fossa subarachnoid cyst

13. A 62-year-old male has worked in a paper mill for the previous 43 years. During that time, he has been exposed to noxious odors on a frequent basis and has lost the ability to distinguish between certain smells. Upon retirement, his exposure to the fumes ends but his ability to distinguish odors remains impaired. When visiting his neurologist, it is explained that all those years of exposure have altered the neural basis of olfactory discrimination in his brain. Which of the following neural properties has been disrupted?

A. Activity within groups of olfactory glomeruli

B. Activity within groups of cells within the amygdala

C. Activity within groups of cells within the lateral olfactory stria

D. Activity within groups of cells within the medial olfactory stria

E. Activity within groups of cells within the anterior olfactory nucleus

14. A 72-year-old male has the following Weber and Rinne test results:

Test	Left ear result	Right ear result
Weber	No lateralization	Lateralization
Rinne	AC > BC	BC > AC

Abbreviations: AC, air conduction; BC, bone conduction

Which of the following conditions is most consistent with these test results?

A. Otosclerosis involving the left ear

B. Otosclerosis involving the right ear

C. Sensorineural loss involving the right ear

D. Sensorineural loss involving the left ear

E. A normal examination

15. A severely malnourished 68-year-old male, who eats out of garbage dumpsters, was brought to the ER unconscious. Upon regaining consciousness, he presents as ataxic and apathetic. On interrogation, he fails to provide the correct address of where he lives. He also narrates that he had played several memorable matches for his team in the NFL, and suffered an injury during one of his matches, which is the primary cause for his current physical symptoms. He, however, fails to name his team and provide any documents to support his statement. Which of the following structures might be found involved in a CT scan of the brain for him?

A. Ventromedial hypothalamic nucleus

B. Dorsomedial hypothalamic nucleus

C. VPL thalamic nucleus

D. Dorsomedial thalamic nucleus

E. Lateral geniculate bodies

F. Medial geniculate bodies

Consider the following case for questions 16 to 19:

A 60-year-old man presents with medication-refractory essential tremor and parkinsonism. Deep brain stimulation targeting the VLo nucleus of thalamus is being considered as the potential next line of intervention.

16. Which of the following structures sends direct input to the VLo nucleus?

A. Globus pallidus, external segment

B. Globus pallidus, internal segment

C. Substantia nigra, pars compacta

D. Substantia nigra, pars reticulata

E. Putamen

F. Dentate nucleus, posterior cerebellar lobe

17. Which of the following areas of the cerebral cortex receives primary inputs from the VLo nucleus?

A. Anterior paracentral cortex

B. Posterior paracentral cortex

C. Cingulate cortex

D. Primary auditory cortex

E. Primary visual cortex

18. Which of the following pathways is utilized by fibers from the VLo nucleus to reach the cerebral cortex?

A. Anterior limb of internal capsule

B. Genu of internal capsule

C. Posterior limb of internal capsule

D. Sublentiform limb of internal capsule

E. Retrolentiform limb of internal capsule

19. Which of the following is the primary supply for the VLo nucleus?

A. Thalamoperforating branch of posterior cerebral artery (P1)

B. Thalamogeniculate branch of the posterior cerebral artery (P2)

C. Medial posterior choroidal branch of the posterior cerebral artery (P2)

D. Lenticulostriate branch of middle cerebral artery

E. Medial striate branch of the anterior cerebral artery

20. A 60-year-old woman presents with ataxic gait, left hand incoordination, and tremor affecting her left hand, associated with intentional movement. Which of the following might be the site of a lesion for her?

A. Left putamen

B. Left primary motor cortex

C. Left premotor cortex

D. Left thalamus

E. Left dentate nucleus

21. A 38-year-old right-handed male presented to the emergency department with a complaint of acute headache. Neurological testing revealed right-sided facial weakness and left-sided weakness in the body. Ophthalmologic exam revealed right gaze palsy. Which of the following is the most likely diagnosis?

A. Ataxic-hemiparesis syndrome

B. Ventral pontine (Millard–Gubler) syndrome

C. Ventromedial pontine (Raymond's) syndrome

D. Pontine locked-in syndrome

E. Dorsal pontine (Foville's) syndrome

Consider the following case for questions 22 and 23:

A first-year resident in radiology expresses concern over a mass lying within a ventricle, which displayed greater signal intensity than deep cerebral grey matter in a T2-weighted spin echo. He is convinced that it is a tumor, which is filling up the ventricle and is encroaching on its lateral walls. To his surprise, he finds that the patient has no neurological symptoms that can be correlated to such a tumor. The attending, from his experience and location of the structure, explains that it could be the glomus of the choroid plexus.

22. Which of the following locations for the structure would confirm its diagnosis as the glomus?

A. Anterior horn of lateral ventricle

B. Body of lateral ventricle

C. Atrium of lateral ventricle

D. Temporal horn of lateral ventricle

E. Roof of third ventricle

23. Which of the following is the primary supply of the glomus?

A. Anterior choroidal artery

B. Medial posterior choroidal artery

C. Lateral posterior choroidal artery

D. Anterior inferior cerebellar artery

E. Posterior inferior cerebellar artery

24. A 28-year-old woman presents with gaze symptoms consistent with demyelination of the left medial longitudinal fasciculus due to multiple sclerosis. What type of gaze deficits are most likely to be observed with this patient?

Left gaze   Right gaze

A.

B.

C.

D.   Nystagmus

E.   Nystagmus

25. A 77-year-old woman presents to her primary care physician concerned about general loss of olfaction. It is determined that she has suffered damage of an unknown etiology to the olfactory glomerulus. In the following image, which area best corresponds to the location of this damage?

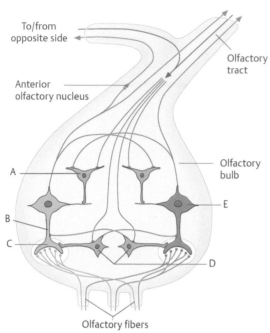

Source: Schünke M, Schulte E, Schumacher U et al. THIEME Atlas of Anatomy: Head, Neck, and Neuroanatomy. 2nd Edition. Thieme; 2016. Illustration by Karl Wesker/Markus Voll.

A. Area A

B. Area B

C. Area C

D. Area D

E. Area E

26. A 22-year-old woman is brought to the ER following carbon monoxide exposure from a faulty stove. Neuroimaging consult revealed lesion confined to the cortical areas of the left occipital pole, which represent the macula. What pattern of visual field deficit would you expect?

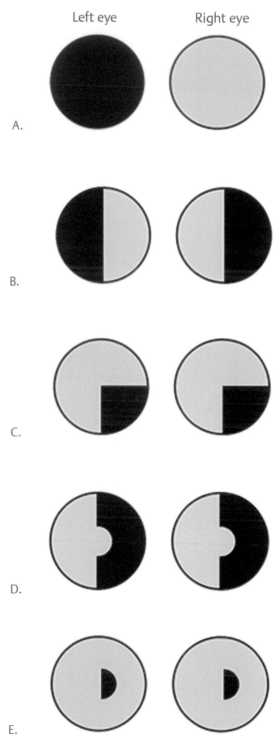

Source: Schünke M, Schulte E, Schumacher U et al. THIEME Atlas of Anatomy: Head, Neck, and Neuroanatomy. 2nd Edition. Thieme; 2016. Illustration by Karl Wesker/Markus Voll.

Consider the following case for questions 27 and 28:

A 35-year-old left-handed male self-presented to the emergency department fearing he had experienced a stroke. Upon neurological examination, he had paralysis of conjugate upward gaze, abnormalities in pupil response (dissociated near-light response), convergence (a retraction nystagmus on upward gaze), and signs of lid lag.

27. Which is the most likely diagnosis?

A. Weber's syndrome

B. Claude's syndrome

C. Benedikt's syndrome

D. Parinaud's syndrome

E. Nothnagel's syndrome

28. Neurodiagnostic imaging revealed the presence of a tumor within the pineal region. Which structure was most likely compressed by this tumor, resulting in the upward gaze paralysis reported?

A. Inferior colliculi

B. Superior colliculi

C. Oculomotor nucleus

D. Optic nerves

E. Trochlear nucleus

29. A 71-year-old woman experiences a stroke that results in a left-sided cortical lesion to her primary auditory cortex. Which symptoms would this patient most likely display?

A. Hearing loss in the ear ipsilateral to the site of the lesion, along with other listening, learning, communication, and related difficulties

B. Hearing loss in the ear contralateral to the site of lesion, along with other listening, learning, communication, and related difficulties

C. Hearing loss in both ears, along with other listening, learning, communication, and related difficulties

D. No hearing loss, but complex listening, learning, communication, and related difficulties

E. All of the above are possible

30. A 36-year-old male patient presented to the emergency department following a collapse at his workplace. Upon admission, he had a Glasgow Coma Scale score of 9. Preoperative CT scanning revealed a large idiopathic subdural hematoma resulting in a transtentorial herniation that disrupted function of the left CN III. Which of the following symptoms would be expected in this patient?

A. Diplopia

B. Cycloplegia

C. Miosis

D. A + B

E. B + C

F. A + C

31. A 51-year-old woman is taken to the emergency department displaying apparent signs of loss of regulation of blood pressure and heart rate. It is determined that a lesion is affecting the function of the hypothalamus. Which of the following structures, through its connections with the hypothalamus, is involved in maintaining homeostasis?

A. Ventral horns of the spinal cord

B. Lateral dorsal nucleus of the thalamus

C. Dorsal motor nucleus of the vagus nerve

D. Solitary nucleus

E. Nucleus accumbens

32. A 37-year-old male undergoes surgery to remove a large tumor within his left parietal lobe. As part of this surgery, an inadvertent injury to the optic tract occurs. Which of the following types of visual defect would be expected in him?

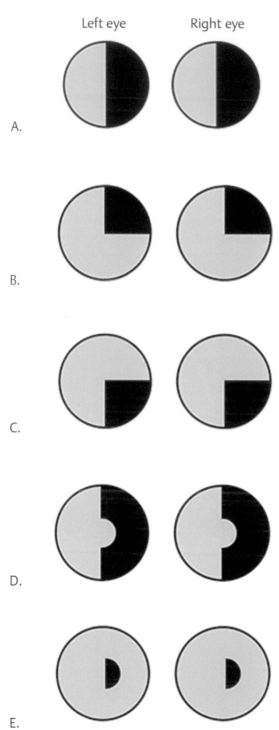

Left eye   Right eye

A.

B.

C.

D.

E.

Source: Schünke M, Schulte E, Schumacher U et al. THIEME Atlas of Anatomy: Head, Neck, and Neuroanatomy. 2nd Edition. Thieme; 2016. Illustration by Karl Wesker/Markus Voll.

33. A 22-year-old male presents with memory impairment following surgical removal of colloid cysts from his third ventricle. MRI scan determined there was complete bilateral destruction of the fiber pathway connecting the hippocampus to the mammillary bodies. Which of the following structures was affected?

A. Fornix
B. Cingulum
C. Internal capsule
D. Corpus callosum
E. Entorhinal cortex

34. A physician-scientist has developed an antibody that can target excitatory neurons in the central nervous system. Which of the following neurons within the cerebellar cortex can be studied, utilizing the antibody?

A. Granule cell
B. Golgi cell
C. Stellate cells
D. Basket cells
E. Purkinje cells

35. A 40-year-old male is brought into the ER following a traumatic brain injury of unknown origin. When assessed, he received a Glasgow Coma Scale of 3. To test brainstem function, a caloric test was performed in which the patient's head was elevated to 30 degrees from the horizontal and cold water was injected into the right external auditory meatus. If his brainstem was intact, which of the following ocular reflexes would be expected?

A. Horizontal nystagmus to the left
B. Deviation of the eyes to the left
C. Horizontal nystagmus to the right
D. Deviation of the eyes to the right
E. Vertical lower nystagmus

36. A 56-year-old female presents to the emergency department following a visual sensation that she described as the "curtain coming down" in her field of vision. There is no associated pain. For approximately 2 weeks prior to this, she had been noticing flashing lights and "floaters" in her visual field. Which areas on the presented image are most related to these clinical findings?

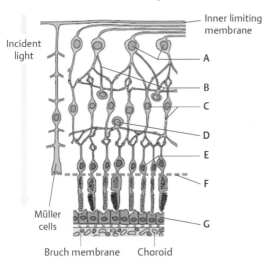

Source: Schünke M, Schulte E, Schumacher U et al. THIEME Atlas of Anatomy: Head, Neck, and Neuroanatomy. 2nd Edition. Thieme; 2016. Illustration by Karl Wesker/Markus Voll.

A. Areas A and C
B. Areas C and D
C. Areas D and E
D. Areas E and G
E. Areas G and choroid

37. A 51-year-old right-handed male visits a neurologist after he continually experiences an odor that he cannot define, and that others are unable to verify. An MRI scan determines a tumor is found, which, as narrated to the patient, is responsible for the olfactory hallucinations he is experiencing. Seizure activity in which of the following regions, due to the tumor, may be responsible for the patient's symptoms?

A. Orbitofrontal cortex
B. Posterior parietal cortex
C. Fusiform gyrus
D. Anterior temporal lobe
E. Basal ganglia

38. A 56-year-old man presents with an infarction of the anterior inferior cerebellar artery that involves his middle cerebellar peduncles. Which of the following fibers would specifically be damaged in him?

A. Ventral spinocerebellar fibers
B. Dorsal spinocerebellar fibers
C. Vestibulocerebellar fibers
D. Pontocerebellar fibers
E. Dentatorubrothalamic fibers

39. A man in his early 20s is brought to the emergency department after being found unconscious in an alleyway behind a bar. Shortly after being admitted to the local hospital, he regains consciousness and shows signs of oculomotor nerve palsy. Which of the following extraocular muscles would be spared following the injury (see accompanying image)?

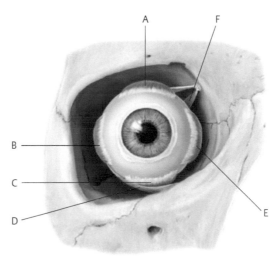

Source: Schünke M, Schulte E, Schumacher U et al. THIEME Atlas of Anatomy: Head, Neck, and Neuroanatomy. 2nd Edition. Thieme; 2016. Illustration by Karl Wesker/Markus Voll.

A. A and B
B. A and E
C. B and E
D. B and F
E. E and F

40. A 66-year-old woman presents with a visual scotoma as seen in the following image:

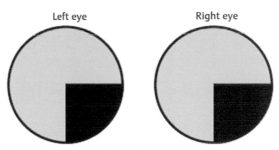

Source: Schünke M, Schulte E, Schumacher U et al. THIEME Atlas of Anatomy: Head, Neck, and Neuroanatomy. 2nd Edition. Thieme; 2016. Illustration by Karl Wesker/Markus Voll.

Based on this information, what is the most likely location of the corticovisual pathway damage in her?

A. Left optic nerve lesion
B. Optic chiasm lesion
C. Left optic tract lesion
D. Lesion of optic radiation in left anterior temporal lobe
E. Lesion of optic radiation in left parietal lobe

24.2 Answers and Explanations

Easy	Medium	Hard

1. Correct: Middle third of the right crus cerebri in the midbrain (E)

The tongue deviates to the side of the weakness (by pushing of the strong contralateral genioglossus muscle), on attempted protrusion. The angle of the mouth deviates to the strong side (by the pull of intact facial muscles), on attempted smiling. Therefore, this patient is suffering from left-sided tongue and left lower facial weakness. Multiple cranial nerve involvement and affection of the lower face hint toward a UMN lesion (e.g., crus cerebri, internal capsule). Corticobulbar fibers contained within the crus cerebri control the contralateral, not ipsilateral (F), side of tongue and face.

Ventromedial medullary paralysis (A and B) might cause hypoglossal nucleus palsy (LMN type), but will not cause facial paralysis.

Damage to the caudal pontine tegmentum (C and D) might involve the facial nerve nucleus. The paralysis will be of LMN type and will involve the whole face. Also, it will cause ipsilateral face and contralateral tongue palsies—the same side of face and tongue will not be affected.

2. Correct: Erection mediated by parasympathetic fibers of the S2–S4 spinal cord; ejaculation mediated by sympathetic fibers of the L2–L4 spinal cord (B)

Male sexual function is controlled by both the sympathetic and parasympathetic autonomic nervous system. Erection is mediated by parasympathetic motor fibers from the S2–S4 spinal cord via the pelvic splanchnic nerves (nervi erigentes). Ejaculation is mediated by sympathetic motor fibers from the intermediolateral cell column of the L2–L4 spinal cord via the hypogastric nerves.

3. Correct: Normal physiological variant (B)

The diagnosis of anisocoria is made when there is a difference of 0.4 mm or more between the sizes of the pupils of the eyes. While it could be the result of a number of etiologies, the difference of less than 1 mm and normal reaction to light make the diagnosis of normal physiological variant most appropriate.

Horner's syndrome (A) is a combination of symptoms that arises following damage to the sympathetic nervous system, of which anisocoria would be expected. However, other prominent symptoms consistent with the diagnosis (ptosis, anhidrosis, and enophthalmos) were not present.

Mechanical anisocoria (C) can be caused by previous trauma, surgery, or inflammation of the eye. Lack of such history makes the diagnosis less probable.

Adie (tonic) pupil (D) is caused by a degeneration of the ciliary ganglia and the postganglionic parasympathetic fibers that normally constrict the pupil and affect accommodation. It most often presents in young women and can result in anisocoria. The reactions to light and near focus are present but are extremely sluggish, and have a prolonged latent period prior to onset of constriction.

Lastly, while many pharmacological agents (E) may cause anisocoria, most of these present with a much larger pupil deviation.

4. Correct: Deficits in orienting responses to stimuli (E)

The tectospinal tract arises from the superior colliculus in the roof (tectum) of the midbrain and then courses in the contralateral ventral white column to provide synaptic input to ventral gray interneurons. It receives input from the retina and visual cortex and has reciprocal connections with the vestibular nuclei, and causes head turning in response to sudden visual or auditory stimuli.

Ataxia and postural instability (A) can be caused by a wide range of conditions including focal lesions to the cerebellum or dorsal columns, exogenous substances such as alcohol, and cerebellar degeneration such as an autoimmune disorder, but are not likely to occur from damage to the tectospinal tract.

Similarly, diplopia (B) can be caused by various etiologies (paralysis of extraocular muscles, for example), but not due to tectospinal tract involvement.

An intention tremor (C), also known as a cerebellar tremor, is most common in multiple sclerosis, with a variety of other causes possible such as cerebellar damage or damage to the superior cerebellar peduncle, brainstem, or thalamus.

A disruption of the maintenance of gaze reflex (D) is most often observed following damage to the medial longitudinal fasciculus, such as is most often seen in relatively early stages of multiple sclerosis.

5. Correct: Dysmetria (C)

The patient is suffering from dysmetria, which is a form of appendicular ataxia characterized by abnormal movement trajectories, such as difficulty in accurately pointing to a moving object.

Asterixis (A), or flapping tremor, is a form of brief rapid movement that is often seen in metabolic encephalopathies, particularly in hepatic failure.

Ataxic movements with abnormal timing are referred to as dysrhythmia (B).

Dysdiadochokinesia (D) is a form of appendicular ataxia characterized by abnormalities of rapid alternating movements.

Titubation (E) is a peculiar tremor of the head or the trunk that occurs with midline cerebellar lesions.

6. Correct: Dentate nucleus (A)

Output from the neocerebellar cortex is mainly to the dentate nucleus, which in turn projects to the red nucleus (parvocellular part) and from there to the VLC of the thalamus (known as the dentatorubrothalamic tract). From the thalamus, information projects back to motor (primary and association) areas of the cortex. This circuit is involved in planning the motor program for the extremities. Lesion to the involved structures causes different forms of appendicular ataxia including dysmetria.

The flocculonodular lobe (C), via its bidirectional connections with the vestibular nuclei, influences the medial longitudinal fasciculus and plays an important role in maintaining balance and vestibulo-ocular reflexes. Lesion of this part of the cerebellum leads to truncal ataxia, vertigo, and nystagmus.

Afferents from the vestibular nuclei also project to the vermis (D). The midline vermis projects to fastigial nuclei (B) and is important in the control of proximal limb and trunk muscles. Lesions of these structures will primarily cause truncal ataxia.

Ventral spinocerebellar tract (E) originates from leg interneurons within the spinal cord and projects to the intermediate or paravermal area within the cerebellum. Lesion of this structure is unlikely to cause upper limb ataxia.

7. Correct: Vertical diplopia affecting right eye (D)

A lesion affecting the paramedian area of the caudal midbrain will affect the left trochlear nucleus. This will, in turn, lead to a paralysis of the superior oblique muscle of the right eye, which will result in deviation of the right, but not the left (C), eyeball upward and slightly inward. This causes vertical diplopia which is at a maximum on downward gaze.

Mydriasis (A and B) might result from oculomotor nerve and/or nuclear palsy. These will be involved in rostral, but not caudal, midbrain lesions.

Loss of pain sensation from arms (E and F) could result from lesions of the anterolateral system (spinothalamic tracts), which would be involved in lateral, but not paramedian, midbrain lesions.

8. Correct: VPL nucleus, left thalamus (B)

The input to VPL is from the ipsilateral posterior column—medial lemniscus and spinothalamic tracts, which carry all modalities of sensation from the contralateral upper and lower limbs, and trunk.

A lesion to the right VPL nucleus (A) would involve the left upper limb.

The input to VPM (C and D) is from the anterior and posterior trigeminothalamic tracts carrying all modalities of sensation from the face. Therefore, lesion of this nucleus would most likely cause numbness of the contralateral face.

Paracentral lobules (E and F) represent cortical areas responsible primarily for lower, and not upper, limbs.

9. Correct: Thalamogeniculate branch of left posterior cerebral artery (P2) (C)

The thalamogeniculate branch of the left, and not right (D), posterior cerebral artery supplies the posterior region of the left thalamus, including the VPL nucleus.

Supply of anterior cerebral arteries (A and B) includes motor and sensory cortical areas that control the lower limbs.

Supply of thalamoperforating branch of posterior cerebral artery (E and F) includes the anterior part of the thalamus, including the anterior, VA, and VL nucleus.

10. Correct: Vestibular neuronitis (B)

In this case, the patient is presenting with symptoms most consistent with vestibular neuronitis. The proposed etiologies for it include viral infection, vascular occlusion, and immunologic mechanisms. Symptoms typically consist of continuous vertigo and reduced sensitivity of the affected ear during caloric irrigation.

Labyrinthitis (A) and Ménière's disease (C) could be ruled out as the patient has no hearing loss.

BPPV (D) is one of the most common types of peripheral vertigo, arising commonly as a result of debris in the posterior semicircular canal. Patients complain of sudden onset of vertigo that lasts 10 to 20 seconds with certain head positions. The triggering positions include rolling over in bed into a lateral position, getting out of bed, etc.

Migraine (E) could present with vertigo, but the caloric stimulation test would be normal.

11. Correct: Pontine tegmentum (C)

The patient is suffering from left complete facial palsy (LMN type) and left abducens nucleus palsy. This leads to the diagnosis of pontine tegmental lesion, affecting both facial and abducens nucleus.

The midbrain tegmentum (A) is not associated with UMN or LMN involved with facial or abducens nerves.

A lesion to the base of the brainstem (B and D) would involve the corticospinal tract and the patient would present with contralateral hemiplegia.

Technically, lesion of the pontine base (D) could involve the emerging facial and abducens nerve fibers. However, abducens nerve involvement, in contrast to abducens nuclear lesion, will produce inability to abduct his left eye, but not left gaze palsy.

Midbrain base (B) and internal capsule (E) lesions can be ruled out as these would produce UMN type of lesions for the facial nerve and his upper face would be spared.

12. Correct: Chiari II malformation (B)

The presented images in question demonstrate a small posterior fossa, protrusion of the inferior cerebellar tonsils, enlarged massa intermedia, stenogyria, tectal beaking, dysplastic corpus callosum, and enlarged anterior portions of the third and fourth ventricle due to aqueductal stenosis. These are consistent with Chiari type II malformation. Clinical features of the infant are also consistent with the diagnosis, since stretching of the lower brainstem frequently causes apnea, cyanosis, bradycardia, dysphagia, nystagmus, upper limb weakness, etc.

Type I Chiari malformation (**A**) may present with similar symptomology including upper extremity weakness and nystagmus, but the onset is usually in young adulthood and imaging would indicate herniation of the cerebellar tonsils, with an elongated appearance rather than the herniation of the cerebellar vermis observed here. Also, herniation of lower medulla would be absent.

Chiari type III malformation (**C**) typically presents with an occipital encephalocele containing a variety of abnormal neuroectodermal tissues, a much rarer condition.

Dandy–Walker malformation (**D**) and posterior fossa arachnoid cyst (**E**) may appear similar on neuroradiology scans, but both with enlarged, rather than small, posterior fossa.

Components of Dandy–Walker syndrome (**D**) include enlarged posterior fossa, elevated tentorial attachment, agenesis of cerebellar vermis, and cystic dilation of the fourth ventricle. Symptoms typically include mental retardation, ataxia, and seizures.

A posterior fossa arachnoid (**E**) cyst typically causes mass effect and the clinical and imaging features will not be consistent with the findings for the infant.

13. Correct: Activity within groups of olfactory glomeruli (A)

Different olfactory glomeruli respond to different kinds of olfactory stimuli, and therefore activities within these structures are involved in the ability to distinguish olfactory stimuli. No such organization has been found within other listed (**B–E**) components of the olfactory system.

Cells within the amygdala (**B**) are activated by olfactory stimuli, and may relate to the role of amygdala in olfactory memory. Both the lateral (**C**) and medial (**D**) olfactory striae have axons of the olfactory tract and make connections with different regions. Lastly, dendrites of the anterior olfactory nucleus (**E**) synapse with fibers of the olfactory tract, while their axons project to the olfactory nucleus and bulb of the opposite side. These form a feedback circuit that modulates the sensitivity of olfactory sensation.

14. Correct: Otosclerosis involving the right ear (B)

Based on these results, the patient seems to have otosclerosis of the right ear (conduction deafness). Such patients hear the vibration more loudly in the affected ear (Weber test), and bone conduction is greater than air conduction for the affected ear (Rinne test).

Otosclerosis involving the left ear (**A**) would have an opposite pattern of results to those reported (lateralization and bone conduction > air conduction for left ear).

With sensorineural hearing loss (**C** and **D**), the patient would hear the vibration louder in the normal ear (Weber test), and air conduction would be greater than bone conduction for the normal ear (Rinne test).

A normal examination (**E**) would not include lateralization (Weber test), and air conduction would be greater than bone conduction for both ears (Rinne test).

15. Correct: Dorsomedial thalamic nucleus (D)

The patient is suffering from Korsakoff's psychosis, with classical features of amnesia and confabulation consequent to thiamine deficiency (commonly results from chronic malnutrition). This almost always follows Wernicke's encephalopathy (results in ataxia, nystagmus, etc.), which causes lesions localized to periventricular structures at the level of third and fourth ventricles. The dorsomedial and anterior nuclei of thalamus, and the mammillary bodies are severely atrophied in Wernicke's encephalopathy.

None of the other listed structures (**A, B, C, E,** and **F**) are as significantly involved.

16. Correct: Globus pallidus, internal segment (B)

The VL nucleus of thalamus has been subdivided into two main parts: VLo and VLc. The internal segment of the globus pallidus projects to VLo, while the deep cerebellar nuclei (**F**) project to part VLc.

The magnocellular part of the ventral anterior nucleus (VAmc) receives afferents from the substantia nigra pars reticulata (**D**), while its principal or parvocellular part (VApc) receives afferents from internal segment of the globus pallidus.

Other listed structures (**A, C,** and **E**) have no direct inputs to thalamus.

17. Correct: Anterior paracentral cortex (A)

The VL nucleus projects to the primary and premotor cortices. Anterior paracentral cortex controls motor activities of the lower limbs and will, therefore, be fed by the nucleus.

Posterior paracentral (**B**, sensory areas for lower limb), cingulate (**C**, limbic functions), primary auditory (**D**), or primary visual (**E**) areas are not motor in function and will not receive projections from VL nucleus.

18. Correct: Posterior limb of internal capsule (C)

The posterior limb of the internal capsule carries corticopontine, thalamocortical (from VPL, VPM, VA, and VL), and corticospinal (pyramidal) fibers.

The anterior limb (**A**) carries frontopontine and thalamocortical (anterior thalamic radiation from DM and ANT nuclei) fibers.

The genu (**B**) conveys corticobulbar/corticonuclear fibers.

The sublentiform (**D**) part conveys the auditory (inferior thalamic) radiation.

The retrolentiform (**E**) part of the internal capsule conveys the optic (posterior thalamic) radiation.

19. Correct: Thalamoperforating branch of posterior cerebral artery (P1) (A)

The thalamoperforating branch of posterior cerebral artery supplies the anterior part of the thalamus, including the anterior, VA, and VL nucleus.

The thalamogeniculate branch of the posterior cerebral artery (**B**) supplies the posterior thalamus, including the LGB, MGB, pulvinar, VPL, and VPM nuclei.

The DM nucleus of the thalamus is supplied by the medial posterior choroidal branch of the posterior cerebral artery (**C**).

The genu and posterior limb of the internal capsule are supplied by the lenticulostriate branch of middle cerebral artery (**D**), but it has no supply for thalamus.

Lastly, the medial striate branch of the anterior cerebral artery (**E**) supplies the head of caudate nucleus, anterior part of the lenticular nucleus, and the anterior limb of the internal capsule among other structures, but has no supply for thalamic nuclei.

20. Correct: Left dentate nucleus (E)

The dentate nucleus is a deep cerebellar nucleus, and cerebellar disorders involve the same side of the body. Ataxia, incoordination, and intention tremor are classical signs of cerebellar disorder as well.

While lesions of putamen (**A**), primary motor (**B**) and premotor (**C**) cortices, or thalamus (**D**) could mimic some of the motor symptoms, these would affect contralateral limbs.

21. Correct: Dorsal pontine (Foville's) syndrome (E)

Foville's syndrome, a consequence of dorsal pontine injury, includes ipsilateral gaze palsy (lesion of abducens nucleus), ipsilateral facial palsy (lesion of facial nucleus), and contralateral hemiparesis (lesion of corticospinal fibers).

Ataxic-hemiparesis syndrome (**A**) presents with contralateral ataxia (transverse pontine fibers) and hemiparesis (corticospinal fibers). Ataxia primarily involves the upper limbs, while hemiparesis primarily involves the lower limbs.

Millard–Gubler syndrome (**B**), from ventral pontine injury, is similar to Foville's syndrome except for the eye findings. There is lateral rectus weakness only, instead of gaze palsy, because the abducens fascicle is injured rather than the nucleus.

Raymond's syndrome (**C**) presents similar to Millard–Gubler syndrome, but may also involve ipsilateral ataxia (middle cerebellar peduncle) and ipsilateral facial hemisensory loss (CN V root).

Pontine locked-in syndrome (**D**), a lesion of bilateral ventral pons, typically includes weakness in all extremities (lesion of bilateral corticospinal fibers), aphonia (lesion of bilateral corticobulbar fibers), and bilateral loss of horizontal eye movements (lesion of bilateral CN VI fibers).

22. Correct: Atrium of lateral ventricle (C)

Glomus of the choroid is an enlargement of the choroid plexus located within the atrium of the lateral ventricles. Its primary function is to produce CSF. It can produce variable signals in T2-weighted sequences on MRI and often can be confused as a tumor to the inexperienced eye.

Other listed structures (**A, B, D,** and **E**) are not common locations for glomus choroideum.

23. Correct: Lateral posterior choroidal artery (C)

The lateral posterior choroidal artery is the primary supply of the glomus within the atrium of the lateral ventricles.

Anterior choroidal artery (**A**) supplies choroid plexus within the temporal horn of lateral ventricle. Medial posterior choroidal artery (**B**) supplies choroid plexus within roof of the third ventricle. Anterior inferior cerebellar artery (**D**) supplies choroid plexus sticking out of foramen of Luschka. Posterior inferior cerebellar artery (**E**) supplies choroid plexus within fourth ventricle.

24. Correct: (D)

Due to the role of the medial longitudinal fasciculus in programming eye movements, a left-sided lesion would produce a left internuclear ophthalmoplegia, consisting of an impaired adduction of the left eye (paralysis of medial rectus) and a nystagmus in the right eye, on right gaze. The nystagmus in this case is a result of increased drive to the extraocular muscles thought to be due to an attempt by the oculomotor system to drive the nonfunctioning eye.

Deficits in both leftward and rightward gaze bilaterally (**A**) would result from damage to both abducens nuclei.

Impaired abduction of the right eye but intact movement of the left eye, on right gaze (**B**), would result from a right-sided abducens nerve lesion. Left gaze is intact.

Impaired abduction of the right eye and adduction of the left eye, on right gaze, (**C**) would be associated with a right abducens nucleus lesion. Left gaze is intact.

Lastly, the patient in option **E** has left internuclear ophthalmoplegia (similar to patient in option **D**) plus left-gaze palsy. This can happen if both the left abducens nucleus and left medial longitudinal fasciculus is damaged.

25.   Correct: Area C (C)

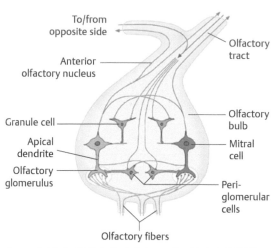

Source: Schünke M, Schulte E, Schumacher U et al. THIEME Atlas of Anatomy: Head, Neck, and Neuroanatomy. 2nd Edition. Thieme; 2016. Illustration by Karl Wesker/Markus Voll.

The olfactory glomeruli are made up of dendrite plus the synapses from the axons of primary sensory cells. Within each glomerulus, the axons of the receptor organ contact the apical dendrites of mitral cells, which ultimately make up the principal projection neurons within the olfactory bulb.

As evident from the image, area A represents the granule cells, area B represents apical dendrite of the mitral cells, and area E represents the mitral cells. Last, area D in the image represents the periglomerular cells, which, in combination with the granule cells, are involved in lateral inhibition within the olfactory system.

26.   Correct: (E)

Unilateral lesion confined to the cortical areas of the left occipital pole that represent the macula will lead to right homonymous hemianopic central scotoma.

Complete blindness of left eye (**A**) can result from lesion of the left optic nerve.

Bitemporal hemianopia (**B**) results from lesion of the optic chiasm.

Right lower quadrantanopia (**C**) might result from lesion in the medial part of the optic radiation in the left parietal lobe.

Right homonymous hemianopia, with macular sparing (**D**), is observed in some left occipital lobe lesions.

27.   Correct: Parinaud's syndrome (D)

Parinaud's syndrome, also known as dorsal midbrain syndrome, is caused by compression of the rostral midbrain and pretectum. Features include paralysis of upward gaze, a convergence-retraction nystagmus on upward gaze, lid lag, and dissociated near-light pupillary response.

Infarction of the ventromedial midbrain results in distinct symptoms of Weber's syndrome (**A**). This is characterized predominantly by an ipsilateral CN III palsy and contralateral hemiplegia (damage to the corticospinal tract).

Claude's syndrome (**B**), a result of dorsal tegmentum infarction, is described as ipsilateral oculomotor nerve palsy with contralateral ataxia (involvement of red nucleus, brachium conjunctivum, or fibers of the superior cerebellar peduncle).

Benedikt's syndrome (**C**), also a result of dorsal tegmentum infarction, includes incoordination (involvement of the superior cerebellar peduncle and/or red nucleus) and oculomotor nerve palsy. In addition, damage to the corticospinal tract resulting in contralateral hemiparesis is a distinct finding.

Nothnagel's syndrome (**E**), a lesion within the midbrain tectum involving the quadrigeminal plate, presents as unilateral or bilateral CN III palsy and ipsilateral ataxia (involvement of SCP).

28.   Correct: Superior colliculi (B)

The most common cause of Parinaud's syndrome is compression of the rostral midbrain and pretectum near the level of the superior colliculus, usually due to mass effect from an adjacent pineal tumor. Limited upward gaze is the distinguishing symptom, as the vertical gaze center lies in close vicinity to the superior colliculus.

Compression of the inferior colliculi (**A**) would result in auditory deficits, as the major ascending auditory pathways (the lateral lemnisci) converge within the inferior colliculi.

Damage to the oculomotor nuclei (**C**) would result in CN III palsy, usually consisting of a down and out position of the eye. Lesion of the trochlear nucleus (**E**) might cause vertical diplopia, with the eye turned upward and slightly inward. Neither of these, however, will cause upward gaze palsy.

Damage to the optic nerves (**D**) would result in significant loss of vision (blindness).

29.   Correct: No hearing loss, but complex listening, learning, communication, and related difficulties (D)

Due to the complex nature of sound processing within primary auditory cortex, in addition to the extensive crosstalk between the primary auditory cortices of both hemispheres, unilateral lesions of primary auditory cortex do not usually result in hearing loss, but rather result in complex listening, learning, communication, and related difficulties in auditory comprehension. Hearing loss (**A, B, C,** and **E**), as a result of cortical lesions, is only observed with bilateral primary auditory cortex damage, such as seen with bilateral embolic stroke to the area of Heschl's gyrus.

30. Correct: A + B (D)

Oculomotor paralysis is frequently observed following transtentorial herniation as a result of either subdural or epidural hematoma. Oculomotor paralysis often results in diplopia (**A**) due to extraocular muscle paresis, cycloplegia (paralysis of accommodation, **B**) due to paralysis of ciliary muscles, and mydriasis (pupillary dilation due to paralysis of constrictor pupillae muscle).

Miosis (**C, E,** and **F**) is caused by paralysis of the sympathetic system, as occurs in Horner's syndrome.

31. Correct: Solitary nucleus (D)

The caudal part of the solitary nucleus of the medulla (also known as the cardiorespiratory nucleus) plays a role in the control of autonomic functions receiving input from the hypothalamus, periaqueductal gray, amygdala, and visceral afferents of the glossopharyngeal and vagus nerves.

The ventral horns of the spinal cord (**A**) contain motor neurons that affect skeletal muscles.

The lateral dorsal nucleus of the thalamus (**B**) primarily receives information from the entorhinal cortex and projects to the cingulate and parietal cortex.

The dorsal motor nucleus of the vagal nerve (**C**) serves parasympathetic functions, primarily for the thoracoabdominal organs.

The nucleus accumbens (**E**) is one of the primary constituents of the reward system, playing an important role in processing rewarding stimuli and the reinforcement of behavior, but has no direct role in control of blood pressure and heart rate.

32. Correct: (A)

Lesion to the left optic tract would produce right homonymous hemianopia, since it interrupts fibers from temporal and nasal parts of the left and the right retina, respectively. This results in loss of vision from the nasal and temporal fields of vision for the left and the right eyes, respectively.

Right upper quadrantanopia (**B**) might result from lesion of the optic radiation in the left temporal lobe (Meyer's loop).

Right lower quadrantanopia (**C**) might result from lesion in the medial part of the optic radiation in the left parietal lobe.

Right homonymous hemianopia, with macular sparing (**D**), is observed in some left occipital lobe lesions.

Unilateral lesion confined to the cortical areas of the left occipital pole that represent the macula will lead to right homonymous hemianopic central scotoma (**E**).

33. Correct: Fornix (A)

The fiber pathway connecting the hippocampus to the mammillary bodies is the fornix.

The cingulum (**B**) is a collection of white matter fibers projecting from the cingulate gyrus to the entorhinal cortex (**E**).

The internal capsule (**C**) is projection fiber carrying both ascending and descending information to and from the cerebral cortex.

The corpus callosum (**D**) is the commissural pathway joining identical areas of two cerebral hemispheres.

34. Correct: Granule cell (A)

Refer to the following image:

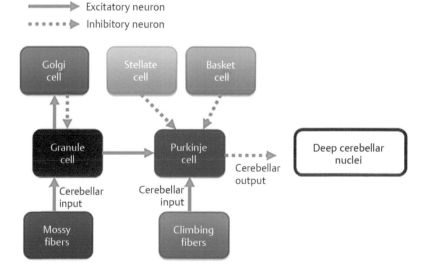

As seen in the image, granule cells are the only excitatory neurons, among those listed, within the cerebellar cytoarchitecture. These, therefore, would be the targets for the developed antibody.

35. Correct: Deviation of the eyes to the right (D)

This patient has scored the minimum possible on the Glasgow Coma Scale, indicating he is nonresponsive to any stimuli. Caloric testing with cold water in the comatose patient with an intact brainstem will result in a horizontal deviation of the eyes toward the side of the irrigated ear (the right side in this case).

Nystagmus (**A, C,** and **E**) is not observed in the comatose patient.

The use of warm, but not cold, water in the comatose patient results in deviation of eyes away from the irrigated ear (**B**).

36. Correct: Areas E and G (D)

Refer to the following image:

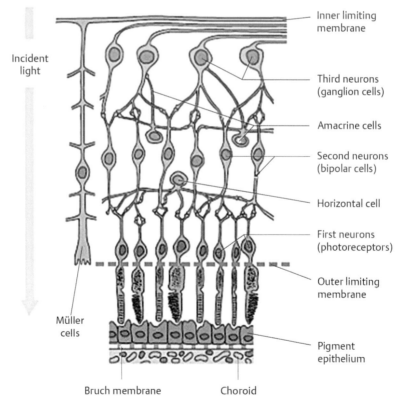

Source: Schünke M, Schulte E, Schumacher U et al. THIEME Atlas of Anatomy: Head, Neck, and Neuroanatomy. 2nd Edition. Thieme; 2016. Illustration by Karl Wesker/Markus Voll.

Detachment of the retina is actually separation of the neurosensory layer (i.e., the photoreceptors [area E] and inner retinal layers) from the retinal pigment epithelium (area G). Subretinal fluid accumulates under the neurosensory layer. The patient complains of painless decrease in vision and may give a history of flashes of lights or sparks. Loss of vision, as in this case, may be described as a curtain in front of the eye.

No other combinations of retinal structures (**A, B, C,** and **E**) are related to retinal detachment.

37. Correct: Anterior temporal lobe (D)

Uncinate fits, often involving olfactory hallucinations of foul smelling odors, are most often associated with seizure activity within the anterior aspect of the temporal lobes. Specifically, seizure activity often includes the uncus (hence the name of the condition), parahippocampal gyrus, and the pyriform cortex.

Orbitofrontal cortex (**A**) seizures are associated with alimentary automatisms, alterations of awareness, and vigorous motor automatisms.

Posterior parietal cortex (**B**) seizures would be associated with visuospatial perception and/or spatial awareness deficits.

Fusiform gyrus seizures (**C**) may result with problems in face and body processing, word recognition, within-category identification, and possibly color hallucinations.

Basal ganglia seizures (**E**) are associated with dyskinesia.

38. Correct: Pontocerebellar fibers (D)

The middle cerebellar peduncle (or brachium pontis) only carries afferent fibers of the pontocerebellar tract.

The superior cerebellar peduncle (or brachium conjunctivum) carries afferent fibers of ventral spinocerebellar tract (**A**) and efferent fibers to the red nucleus and thalamus (**E**).

The inferior cerebellar peduncle (or restiform body) carries afferent fibers through the dorsal spinocerebellar (**B**), vestibulocerebellar (**C**, via juxtarestiform body), and olivocerebellar (major constituent) tracts; efferent fibers through cerebellovestibular (via juxtarestiform body) and cerebello-olivary tracts.

39. Correct: B and F (D)

Refer to the following image:

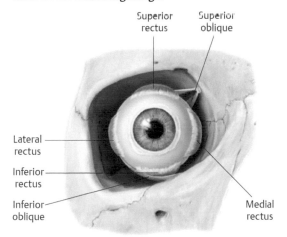

Source: Schünke M, Schulte E, Schumacher U et al. THIEME Atlas of Anatomy: Head, Neck, and Neuroanatomy. 2nd Edition. Thieme; 2016. Illustration by Karl Wesker/Markus Voll.

The oculomotor nerve supplies most of muscles controlling eye movement, and in particular the superior rectus, inferior rectus, inferior oblique, and the medial rectus.

The lateral rectus muscle is innervated by the abducens nerve, whereas the superior oblique muscle is innervated by the trochlear nerve.

40. Correct: Lesion of optic radiation in left parietal lobe (E)

The visual field defect illustrated would result from lesion of the optic radiation in left parietal lobe. This results in right lower quadrantanopia, and occurs since the affected fibers for the lower quadrant course superior to those for the upper quadrant in the Meyer's loop in the anterior temporal lobe.

A left optic nerve lesion (**A**) would produce complete blindness in the left eye.

A lesion of the optic chiasm (**B**) would produce bitemporal hemianopia, as it disrupts fibers from the nasal portion of each retina (that would typically cross over to contralateral primary visual cortex).

A lesion of the left optic tract (**C**) would cause right homonymous hemianopia.

Lastly, a lesion of optic radiation in left anterior temporal lobe (**D**) would result in right upper quadrantanopia, as the affected fibers for the upper quadrant wind around the inferior horn in the temporal lobe and are separated from those for the lower quadrant.

Index